P9-AOV-234

GARY GREENBERG is a practicing psychotherapist and author of *Manufacturing Depression* and *The Noble Lie*. He has written about the intersection of science, politics, and ethics for many publications, including the *New Yorker*, *Wired*, *Discover*, and *Rolling Stone*. He is a contributor at *Mother Jones*, and a contributing editor at *Harper's*. Dr. Greenberg lives with his family in Connecticut.

Praise for *The Book of Woe*

"[I]ndustrious and perfervid . . . Mr. Greenberg [argues] that the [DSM] and its authors, the American Psychiatric Association, wield their power arbitrarily and often unwisely, encouraging the diagnosis of too many bogus mental illnesses in patients (binge eating disorder, for example) and too much medication to treat them. . . . Mr. Greenberg argues that psychiatry needs to become more humble, not more certain and aggressive. . . . Greenberg is a fresher, funnier writer. He paces the psychiatric stage as if he were part George Carlin, part Gregory House."   —*The New York Times*

"Greenberg's documentation of the *DSM-5* revision process is an essential read for practicing and in-training psychotherapists and psychiatrists and is an important contribution to the history of psychiatry."
                                                              —*Library Journal*

"The rewriting of the bible of psychiatry shakes the field to its foundations in this savvy, searching exposé. Deploying wised-up, droll reportage from the trenches of psychiatric policy-making and caustic profiles of the discipline's luminaries, Greenberg subjects the practices of the mental health industry— his own included—to a withering critique. The result is a compelling insider's challenge to psychiatry's scientific pretensions—and a plea to return it to its humanistic roots."   —*Publishers Weekly* (starred review)

"Greenberg is an entertaining guide through the treacheries and valuable instances of the *DSM*, interviewing members on both sides of the divide and keeping the proceedings conversational even when discussing the manual's pretensions toward epistemic iteration. He also brings his own practice into [*The Book of Woe*], with examples of the *DSM* falling woefully short in capturing the complexity of personality. Bright, humorous, and seriously thoroughgoing, Greenberg takes all the *DSM*s for a spin as revealing as the emperor's new clothes."   —*Kirkus Reviews*

"[A] brilliant look at the making of *DSM-5* . . . entertaining, biting, and essential . . . Greenberg builds a splendid and horrifying read. . . . [He] shows us vividly that psychiatry's biggest problem may be a stubborn reluctance to admit its immaturity."
—David Dobbs, Nature.com

"[Greenberg's] fascinating history of the *Diagnostic and Statistical Manual of Mental Disorders* (the *DSM*) . . . show[s] just how muddled the boundaries of mental health truly are."
—Chloë Schama, *Smithsonian*

"Greenberg argues persuasively that the current *DSM* encourages psychiatrists to reach beyond their competence. . . . I'm impressed by Greenberg's reporting, his subtlety of thought, his dedication to honesty, and his literacy . . . a very good book."
—Benjamin Nugent, Slate.com

"The process of assembling [*DSM-5*] has been anything but smooth, as *The Book of Woe* relates. . . . Greenberg argues—persuasively—that this fifth edition of the *DSM* arises not out of any new scientific understanding but from one of the periodic crises of psychiatry . . . invaluable."
—Laura Miller, Salon.com

"In *The Book of Woe*, Greenberg takes the lay reader through a history of the *DSM*, which is really a history of psychiatry. . . . [A] fascinating and well-researched account."
—*The Boston Globe*

"[E]ngaging, radical, and generally delectable . . . Greenberg is a practicing psychotherapist who writes with the insight of a professional and the panache of a literary journalist . . . [A] brilliant take-down of the psychiatric profession . . . *The Book of Woe* offers a lucid and useful history."
—*The Chicago Tribune*

"This is a landmark book about a landmark book. . . . Greenberg paints a picture so compelling and bleak that it could easily send the vulnerable reader into therapy. . . . [He] takes the reader deep inside the secretive world of the panels and personalities that have spent years arguing about which disorders and symptoms they would keep and which they would discard in the new *DSM*."
—Robert Epstein, *Scientific American*

"Gary Greenberg is a thoughtful comedian and a cranky philosopher and a humble pest of a reporter, equal parts Woody Allen, Kierkegaard, and Columbo. *The Book of Woe* is a profound, and profoundly entertaining, riff on malady, power, and truth. This book is for those of us (i.e., all of us) who've ever wondered what it means, and what's at stake, when we try to distinguish the suffering of the ill from the suffering of the human."
—Gideon Lewis-Kraus, author of *A Sense of Direction*

"This could be titled *The Book of . . . Whoa!* An eye-popping look at the unnerving, often tawdry politics of psychiatry."
— Gene Weingarten, two-time Pulitzer Prize–winning author
of *The Fiddler in the Subway*

"Bringing the full force of his wit, warmth, and tenacity to this accessible inside account of the latest revision of psychiatry's diagnostic bible, Gary Greenberg has written a book to rival the importance of its subject. Keenly researched and vividly reported, *The Book of Woe* is frank, impassioned, on fire for the truth—and best of all, vigorously, beautifully alive to its story's human stakes."
— Michelle Orange, author of *This Is Running for Your Life*

"Gary Greenberg has become the Dante of our psychiatric age, and the *DSM-5* is his *Inferno*. He guides us through the not-so-divine comedy that results when psychiatrists attempt to reduce our hopelessly complex inner worlds to an arbitrary taxonomy that provides a disorder for everybody. Greenberg leads us into depths that Dante never dreamed of. *The Book of Woe* is a mad chronicle of so-called madness."
— Errol Morris, Academy Award–winning director,
and author of *A Wilderness of Error*

"In this gripping, devastating account of psychiatric hubris, Gary Greenberg shows that the process of revising the *DSM* remains as haphazard and chaotic as ever. His meticulous research into the many failures of *DSM-5* will spark concern, even alarm, but in doing so will rule out complacency. *The Book of Woe* deserves a very wide readership."
— Christopher Lane, author of *Shyness:
How Normal Behavior Became a Sickness*

"Gary Greenberg's *The Book of Woe* is about the *DSM* in the way that *Moby-Dick* is about a whale—big-time, but only in part. An engaging history of a profession's virtual bible, *The Book of Woe* is also a probing consideration of those psychic depths we cannot know and those social realities we pretend not to know, memorably rendered by a seasoned journalist who parses the complexities with a pickpocket's eye and a mensch's heart. If I wanted a therapist, and especially if I wanted to clear my mind of cant, I'd make an appointment with Dr. Greenberg as soon as he could fit me in."
— Garret Keizer, author of *Privacy* and *The Unwanted Sound of
Everything We Want*

"*The Book of Woe* is a brilliant, ballsy excursion into the minefield of modern psychiatry. Greenberg has wit, energy, and a wonderfully skeptical mind. If you want to understand how we think of mental suffering today—and why, and to what effect—read this book."
— Daniel Smith, author of *Monkey Mind*

Also by Gary Greenberg

Manufacturing Depression:
The Secret History of a Modern Disease

The Noble Lie: When Scientists Give the Right Answers
for the Wrong Reasons

THE
BOOK
OF WOE

The DSM and the Unmaking
of Psychiatry

Gary Greenberg

A PLUME BOOK

PLUME
Published by the Penguin Group
Penguin Group (USA) LLC
375 Hudson Street
New York, New York 10014

USA | Canada | UK | Ireland | Australia | New Zealand | India | South Africa | China
penguin.com
A Penguin Random House Company

First published in the United States of America by Blue Rider Press,
a member of Penguin Group (USA) Inc., 2013
First Plume Printing 2014

ℙ REGISTERED TRADEMARK—MARCA REGISTRADA

THE LIBRARY OF CONGRESS HAS CATALOGED THE BLUE RIDER PRESS EDITION AS FOLLOWS:
Greenberg, Gary.
The book of woe : the DSM and the unmaking of psychiatry /
Gary Greenberg.
p.   cm.
Includes bibliographical references and index.
ISBN 978-0-399-15853-7 (hc.)
ISBN 978-0-14-218092-1 (pbk.)
1. Mental illness—Classification.   2. Psychiatry—Philosophy.   3. Diagnostic and statistical manual of mental disorders.   I. Title.
RC455.2.C4G74   2013   2013002239
618.89—dc23

Printed in the United States of America
10 9 8 7 6 5 4 3 2

Original hardcover design by Gretchen Achilles

The names, identifying characteristics, and details of the case histories (including session dialogues) of patients have been changed to protect their privacy.

THE
BOOK
OF WOE

Chapter 1

Shortly after New Orleans physician Samuel Cartwright discovered a new disease in 1850, he realized that like all medical pioneers he faced a special burden. "In noticing a disease not heretofore classed among the long list of maladies that man is subject to," he told a gathering of the Medical Association of Louisiana, "it was necessary to have a new term to express it." Cartwright could have followed the example of many of his peers and named the malady for himself, but he decided instead to exercise the ancient Greek he'd learned while being educated in Philadelphia. He took two words—*drapetes*, meaning "runaway slave," and the more familiar *mania*—and fashioned *drapetomania*, "the disease causing Negroes to run away."

The new disease, Cartwright reported in *The New Orleans Medical and Surgical Journal*, had one diagnostic symptom—"absconding from service"—and a few secondary ones, including a sulkiness and dissatisfaction that appeared just prior to the slaves' flight. Through careful observations made when he practiced in Maryland, he developed a crude epidemiology and concluded that environmental factors could play a role in the onset of drapetomania.

Two classes of persons were apt to lose their Negroes: those who made themselves too familiar with them, treating them as equals; and on the other hand those who treated them cruelly, denied them the common necessaries of life, neglected to protect them, or frightened them by a blustering manner of approach.

But the most evenhanded treatment would not prevent all cases, and for those whose illness was "without cause," Cartwright had a prescription: "whipping the devil out of them."

Lest anyone doubt that drapetomania was a real disease—and, evidently, some Northern doctors did—Cartwright offered proof. First of all, he said, we know that Negroes are descended from the people of Canaan, a name that means "submissive knee-bender," so it's clear what God had in mind for the race. And in case a reader subscribed to the notion, taught in the "northern hornbooks in Medicine," that "the Negro is only a lampblacked white man . . . requiring nothing but liberty and equality—social and political—to wash him white," Cartwright called as witnesses the prominent European doctors who had "demonstrated, by dissection, so great a difference between the Negro and the white man as to induce the majority of naturalists to refer him to a different species." Africans' blood was darker, he said, and "the membranes, tendons, and aponeuroses, so brilliantly white in the Caucasian race, have a livid cloudiness in the African." This historical and biological evidence, Cartwright concluded, proved that running away is neither willfulness nor the normal human striving for freedom, but illness plain and simple.

Drapetomania was never considered for the *Diagnostic and Statistical Manual of Mental Disorders*, the American Psychiatric Association's compendium of mental illnesses, but that may be only because there was no such book in 1850. (Indeed, the Association of Superintendents of American Institutions for the Insane, the organization that eventually became the APA, was only six years old at the time, and the word *psychiatry* had just come into use.) Certainly it met many of the criteria for inclusion. It was a condition that caused distress for a certain group of people. It had a known and predictable onset, course, and outcome.

Its diagnostic criteria could be listed in clear language that a doctor could use, for instance, to distinguish normal stubbornness from pathological dissatisfaction, or to determine whether a slave was running away because he was sick or just evil. Many people besides Cartwright had observed it. Its discovery was announced in a respected professional journal. Its definition was precise enough to allow other doctors to develop tests that distinguished normal (or, as the DSM puts it, *expectable*) from disordered dissatisfaction, and to conduct research that confirmed (or didn't) that most runaway slaves had been sulky prior to absconding, or that slaves treated too familiarly or too cruelly were more likely to contract drapetomania, or that whipping prevented the disease from running its full course. Still other doctors might have recommended potions that would relieve its symptoms. As the years wore on, some doctors might have objected that the disease pathologized a normal response to atrocious conditions, while others might have fought bitterly and publicly over smaller issues: whether or not *defiance* also belonged on the list of criteria; whether to add Dr. Cartwright's other discovery, *dyaesthesia aethiopica*, the malady causing slaves to "slight their work," to the diagnostic manual; which gene predisposed slaves to drapetomania and dyaesthesia; where the thirst for freedom could be found in the brain; and, perhaps, whether or not these were real illnesses or only constructs useful to understanding what Dr. Cartwright called the "diseases and physical peculiarities of the Negro race."

Dr. Cartwright's disease, in short, and the promise it held out—that a widely observed form of suffering with significant impact on individuals and society could be brought under the light of science, named and identified, understood and controlled, and certain thorny moral questions about the nature of slavery sidestepped in the bargain—might have spawned an entire industry. A small one, perhaps, but one that would have no doubt been profitable to slave owners, to doctors, maybe even to slaves grateful for their emancipation from their unnatural lust for freedom—and, above all, to the corporation that owned the right to name and define our psychological troubles, and to sell the book to anyone with the money to buy it and the power to wield its names.

Even if you're one of the many people who are suspicious of psychiatry and skeptical of its claims to have identified the varieties of our suffering and collected them in a single volume, you might be thinking that I'm not being entirely fair here, that even if the Civil War hadn't come along ten years later and rendered Cartwright's outrageous invention moot, doctors would have quickly consigned drapetomania to the dustbin of medical history. You might point out that even at the time sensible people objected—Frederick Law Olmsted, for instance, whose *Journeys and Explorations in the Cotton Kingdom* includes a mordant account of "the learned Dr. Cartwright" and his diseases, and the unnamed doctor who satirized Cartwright in the *Buffalo Medical Journal* by suggesting that drapetomania occurs when "the nervous erythism of the human body is thrown into relations with the magnetic pole ... thus directing [the slave's] footsteps northward." You might say that in introducing a book about the DSM with an anecdote about a diagnosis that is so obviously specious, and in implying that this is somehow emblematic of the diagnostic enterprise, I am taking a cheap shot.

And you may be right.

On the other hand, especially if you are a gay person, you might not be so quick to think that drapetomania is merely a low-hanging cherry that I've picked to flavor my tale. Because you might be old enough to remember back forty or fifty years, to a time when homosexuality was still listed in the DSM. Which meant that doctors could get paid to treat it, scientists could search for its causes and cures, employers could shun its victims, and families could urge them to seek help, even as gay people conducted their intimacies in furtive encounters, lived in fear and shame, lost jobs, forwent careers, and chained themselves to marriages they didn't want. They underwent countless therapies—shocks to the brain and years on the couch, behavior modification and surrogate sex, porn sessions that switched from homo to hetero at the crucial moment—in desperate attempts to become who they could not be and to love whom they could not love, to get free of their own deepest desires, all in the name of getting well. And all this, at least in part, because a society's revulsion had found expression in the official diagnostic manual of a medical profession, where it gained the imprimatur not of a church or a state, but of science. When doctors said homosexuality was a disease, that was not an opinion, let alone bigotry. It was a fact. When they wrote that fact down in the DSM, it was not a denunciation. It was a diagnosis.

Or maybe you're among the 11 percent of the U.S. adult population whose daily regimen includes taking a dose or two of Lexapro or Paxil or some other antidepressant, and you've been doing that for years, ever since a doctor told you that you had Major Depressive Disorder (or maybe she just said you had clinical depression), meaning that your sulkiness and dissatisfaction were symptoms of a mental disorder, and that this was a chemical imbalance that those drugs would fix. And maybe they did, because at least for a little while you felt better; but then you got tired of feeling numb, of gaining weight, of not wanting sex and not being able to have an orgasm even if you did; and then you tried to get off the drugs only to find that your brain off drugs is an unruly thing, that your old difficulties returned or new ones arose when you stopped taking them. Which might mean, you told yourself, that you indeed have that disease, but every once in a while—when you read about the placebo effect, or you hear that this chemical imbalance does not, as far as doctors know, really exist, or when you look at the DSM and realize that there are more than seventy combinations of symptoms that can result in this one diagnosis and that any two people with the diagnosis may have only one symptom in common—you wonder whether what your doctor told you is true and whether you have now changed your brain chemistry, perhaps irreversibly, to cure a disease that doesn't exist.

Or maybe you're a parent of a child who drove you to despair with his tantrums and defiance, whom you took to doctor after doctor until finally you found the one who told you that he had Bipolar Disorder, but that this was really good news, because that disease could be cured with a daily dose of Depakote or Risperdal. And sure enough, your kid calmed down, but now he weighs twice what he should and there's sugar in his urine and dark circles under his eyes, and you're beginning to think—especially since you heard about how drug industry money influenced doctors to make that diagnosis and how pharmaceutical companies still haven't fully tested these drugs on children and how doctors massaged those diagnostic criteria to fit your kid—that maybe your psychiatrist was wrong when he said that Bipolar Disorder is the same kind of disease as diabetes, a chemical problem that you leave untreated only if you are a bad parent.

Or maybe you're like me—a mental health professional who has been faithfully filling out insurance forms for thirty years, jotting down those five-digit codes from the DSM that open the money taps, rendering diagnoses even though you are pretty sure you're not treating medical conditions, and for just a moment you hesitate, contemplating the bad faith of pouring a lie into the foundation of a relationship whose main and perhaps only value is that it provides an opportunity to look someone in the eye and, without fear of judgment or the necessity to manipulate, speak the truth. And, having contemplated it, you tell yourself whatever story you have to and you sign the paper, and the best you can do is to curse the DSM in a kind of incantation against your own bad faith.

Or maybe you've never had truck with the mental health industry, but the other day you were talking with a friend and explaining to her that you had to wash your dishes before you could leave your house, and you found yourself saying, "I'm just so OCD, you know?" Or you've heard your friends do the same thing with their own or others' quirks. "He's pretty ADHD," they might say. Or, "She's clinically depressed." Or, "Sorry, that's just my PTSD." And maybe you've been brought up short by the way the DSM's lingo has infiltrated our self-understanding or wondered what it says about us that we describe the habits of our hearts in a pastiche of medical clichés.

If you are one of those people, which is to say if you have had occasion to take the DSM seriously (and even the book's most ardent defenders will tell you this was your first mistake), then you may be sympathetic to my rhetorical move. You may understand that Dr. Cartwright did what he did because he could, because the power to give names to our pain is a mighty thing and easy to abuse. Cartwright seems to have intended to serve the interests of slave owners and white supremacists and their economic system by providing "another [of] the ten thousand evidences of the fallacy of the dogma abolition is built on," but surely the doctors who insisted that homosexuality was a disease were not all bigots or prudes. Nor are the doctors who today diagnose with Hoarding Disorder people who fill their homes with newspapers and empty pickle jars, but leave undiagnosed those who amass billions of dollars while other people starve, merely toadying to the wealthy. They don't mean to turn the suffering inflicted by our own peculiar institutions, the depression and anxiety spawned by the displacements of late capitalism and postmodernity, into markets for a criminally avaricious pharmaceutical industry.

The prejudices and fallacies behind psychiatric diagnoses, and even the interests they serve, are as invisible to all of us, doctors and patients alike, as they were to Dr. Cartwright's New Orleanian colleagues or to all those doctors who "treated" homosexuals. The desire to relieve suffering can pull a veil over our eyes. And sometimes it takes an incendiary example or two to rip that veil away.

———

So I apologize for my cheap shot. I apologize to the epidemiologists and sociologists alarmed by ever-rising rates of mental illness and disability; and to the patients who have benefited from a diagnosis; and to the interested civilians who have the intuition that there is such a thing as mental illness, that it belongs under the purview of medicine and that as such it ought to be cataloged, whatever the difficulties; and to the doctors who can argue cogently that the advantages of doing so far outweigh the costs. I apologize to the reasonable folks who think, reasonably, that the DSM is the culmination of a lot of honest hard work by smart and well-intentioned people doing their best at an impossible task, and that it should be given the benefit of the doubt. I apologize to the people who acknowledge that even if the DSM is not the Bible it's cracked up to be, it still, as the backbone of a medical specialty that has done yeoman service, deserves its authority over our inner lives.

But that doesn't mean I'm sorry. By *apologize*, I mean what the ancient Greeks meant. I mean to explain. Because I think drapetomania is not a historical novelty or an anomaly or an accident. It is not the exceptional error that proves the rule that science is self-correcting and will ultimately punish arrogance and incompetence. The story of drapetomania is a cautionary tale, just as the ones about homosexuality and childhood Bipolar Disorder are, and just as the story about a disorder that sits quietly today in the DSM-5 (my vote is for Internet Use Disorder) will be in some tomorrow. All these stories tell us why our inner lives are too important to leave in the hands of doctors: because they don't know as much about us as they claim, because a full account of human nature is beyond their ken.

While I'm explaining myself, let me tell you a story.

In 2012, I got a voice-mail message from a former patient; I'll call him Sandy. I last saw him about ten years ago. I'd worked with him from the time he was in his junior year in high school until he finished his graduate studies. He'd been plagued by anxiety so severe that he was unable to attend school and, eventually, to leave his house at all. Early on in therapy, he'd told me that he was sure he was gay, and that this was what had led him to hole up in his room contemplating suicide as the preferable alternative to what his parents and pastor, who hadn't deleted homosexuality from their book of sins, called "the gay lifestyle." We talked about this, and more generally about what therapists and patients talk about: parents, friends, regrets, confusion, and fear. I can't tell you why, but therapy worked, at least enough to get him to overcome his self-loathing and his parents' disapproval and to come out, in all senses of that phrase. Last I knew, he had a job and a life in a faraway city. He could work, love, and stay alive, which, by my lights, is about all we can ask for. He kept in touch sporadically via e-mail or phone to tell me what he was up to or to let me know he'd seen something I'd written in a magazine.

The message went like this:

"I know I shouldn't call you, and I promise I won't call you again. But you've got to help me. They've sucked all the bones out of my body. I'm here in this hotel room and my bones are gone. My mother and my father and James. They've done this to me. And I don't want to die. Please don't let them kill me. Don't let them. You're the only one who can help. You know I love you, and I love Ellen Goldstein, too. Good-bye. Good-bye." (I made up those names.)

He didn't leave a number, but according to caller ID, he was calling from a Holiday Inn a thousand miles from where, as far as I knew, he had last been living. Sandy had checked out by the time I tried to return the call. I don't know where he went next. But I am pretty sure about one thing: his parents and James, whoever he was, did not suck the bones out of his body, and they probably weren't about to cook Sandy up in a stew, or whatever he was sure they were going to do. I would guess they didn't even know where he was. I'm not even sure Sandy knew where he was. As I write this, I still don't know what became of him.

Now, if you're like me and most everyone I know, the first thing that you think when you hear a story like this is that Sandy is mentally ill. But what do we mean when we say this?

The first answer is that he is crazy. That is, he is behaving in a way that is abnormal, bizarre, out of touch with reality. The technical term here is *psychotic* or *delusional*. I think this is self-evident, and even if I didn't care about Sandy, I wouldn't think it is benign, a sane response to an insane world, say, or some salutary plunge into the collective unconscious. He was in trouble; he was, as the current jargon goes, *dysfunctional*; his inner life had gone haywire; he needed help.

But what kind of trouble? And what kind of help?

This brings us to the second answer: that his craziness is best understood as the manifestation of a disease that is medical in nature, that is in some essential way no different from all the other diseases that afflict us, and that is best left to doctors to understand and treat.

We have become accustomed to thinking of *disease* in a very specific way: as a pathology of the body, something gone wrong in our tissues or our cells or our molecules. You secrete too much of this or don't produce enough of that, or the rate of the other thing is too high or low, and that is why you can't walk up stairs without losing breath, or why you are in pain or are losing weight, and why, if you don't do what the doctor says to do, if you don't take his pill or let him plunge his scalpel into your skin or drip poison into your veins, you will continue to suffer, or your suffering will get worse, or you will die.

But before you will submit to the cure, you have to believe that the doctor knows something about your pain that you do not, that she can identify that disease, that she is on familiar terms with it, that she knows it by name. She must, in other words, give you a diagnosis.

Diagnosis, not unlike *drapetomania*, comes from two Greek words, meaning "to learn" and "apart." It is a knowledge that sorts one thing from another. The Greeks understood how hard it is to parse the world, especially when it comes to complex experiences. "Love is a madness,"

Socrates tells Phaedrus, and to understand that madness, to untangle it from other experiences, he says that two principles must be upheld. "First, the comprehension of scattered particulars in one idea" that is clearly and consistently described. But, Socrates continues, we can't gather the particulars together under just any idea. No matter how vividly described or comprehensive the categories, and no matter how well they seem to cohere, they must also be fashioned "according to the natural formation, where the joint is, not breaking any part as a bad carver might." A good diagnosis must be more than the fancy of the diagnostician, more than merely deft. It must also be accurate. It must carve nature at its joints.

What is true for the madness that is love is true for any madness at all—or, for that matter, any suffering that doctors purport to understand. The diagnostician's job is to find the disease that unites the scattered symptoms and makes them manifest in precisely the way they do, to say with certainty that this distress is the result of that illness and no other. The diagnostic enterprise hinges on an optimistic notion: that disease is part of a natural world that only awaits our understanding. But even if this is true, nature gives up its secrets grudgingly, and our finite senses are in some ways ill suited to extracting them. More important, our prejudices lead us to tear nature where we want it to break. Science, especially modern medicine, is founded on this equally optimistic idea: that experts can purge their inquiry of prejudice and desire, and map the landscape of suffering along its natural boundaries.

Greek doctors, as it turned out, were not so good at this. They had some ideas about what those natural formations were, largely having to do with four bodily humors—blood, bile, phlegm, and melancholy—that, if thrown out of balance, could cause illness. But humoral theory was more metaphysics and wishful thinking than truth. Even Hippocrates and his disciples seemed to know this, as they traded mostly in *empiricism*—the painstaking observation of the way symptoms appeared to the doctor's senses, the courses they took, the outcomes they reached, and the interventions that affected them.

In the nineteenth century, most doctors still believed that humoral imbalances caused disease. Before John Snow could persuade the local government to close the infected well that caused the 1854 cholera outbreak in London, he had to overcome the common idea that the disease was carried by a *miasma*, bad air that could upset humoral balance. Louis Pasteur and Robert Koch had to work hard to convince their colleagues that germs caused diseases like rabies and anthrax, and that they (the germs, not the colleagues) could be targeted and killed. As the microscope and the chemical assay provided incontrovertible evidence of germs and their destruction, doctors were won over to the germ theory, and soon it seemed that they had begun to fulfill Socrates' dictum to find the natural joints that separated our ills from one another.

By the turn of the twentieth century, doctors were stalking disease like Sherlock Holmes stalked criminals. Under the magnification of their microscopes, syphilis, diabetes, and streptococcus, to name just a few, soon yielded their secrets and their terrifying hold on us. With their newfound ability to parse suffering, to track it down to the bodily processes causing it, and then to dispatch it with a potion or a surgery, doctors gained prestige—and with it, money and power. They were rewarded as much for their prowess in relieving suffering as for the promise they now embodied: that they could use science to give a name to someone's suffering and then, having named it, to relieve it.

This revolution in medicine accounts in part for the immense appeal of considering craziness to be just another disease. If scientific understanding and cure were possible for the suffering of the body, then why not for the suffering of the mind? If Sandy's conviction that his bones have been sucked out of his body is some kind of metaphor, if the content of his delusion brims with meaning—an expression of impotence, a lack of backbone, an inability to hold himself up—then it is out of the reach of the microscope and the X-ray. It requires what the ancient doctors offered: interpretation and the invocation of metaphysics, of something beyond the symptom. But if the delusion is only another symptom, if it is not, in principle, different from the malaise and relentless thirst of an untreated diabetic, or the narrowing of vision of a glaucoma patient, or the fever of someone with malaria, then it can be brought under the physician's purview. It doesn't need to be understood in itself any more than fever or thirst does. It can be explained, it can be treated, and it can be cured.

If you've gotten sick or injured and a doctor has restored you to health or if you've seen this happen to someone else—and who hasn't?—then you know the lure of this promise. If you've watched your child descend into psychosis or your husband spin out into mania or yourself struggle to get off the bed onto which depression has laid you, then you know it even better.

On the other hand, if you've been involved with the mental health industry, then you probably also know that the promise is not always fulfilled. Even if doctors can settle on a name for Sandy's illness—and this is not a sure thing; they are likely to be torn between Schizophrenia and Bipolar Disorder—they will not be able to scratch out a prescription, tell him to take two and call in the morning. He may end up taking a drug indicated for a different diagnosis, or a cocktail of pills—one to quell his hallucinations, one to temper his agitation, one to relieve his depression, and one to help him sleep—and the combination may change monthly or even weekly, or it may work for a while and then stop. No one will be able to explain why that happened, any more than they will be able to explain why the drugs worked in the first place. No honest psychiatrist will claim that she cured Sandy's, or anyone's, mental illness; and while she is being honest, she may acknowledge that, for the most part, her treatments are targeted at symptoms, not diseases, and that she selects them as much by intuition and experience as by scientific evidence.

But psychiatry's appeal is not just about the possibility of cure, which is why the profession continues to flourish even when it cures nothing and relieves symptoms only haphazardly. It's in the naming itself. What Wallace Stevens called the "blessed rage to order" is so deep in us that it is in our origin story: the first thing the Bible's authors have Adam and Eve do to establish their dominion over Eden is to name its flora and fauna. That story doesn't have a happy ending, and neither does the one I'm about to tell you (although in the latter case, there is good reason for that). But the rage itself is surely blessed, or at least as blessed as we humans can be, and as noble. Give a name to suffering, perhaps the most immediate reminder of our insignificance and powerlessness, and suddenly it bears the trace of the human. It becomes part of our story. It is redeemed.

But what kind of story? And what kind of names?

The DSM-IV, the most recent edition of the manual,* sorts psychiatric problems into chapters like "Mood Disorders" and "Feeding and Eating Disorders" and from there into individual illnesses like Major Depressive Disorder (MDD) or Bulimia Nervosa, each of which might have its own specifiers, so that a complete diagnosis might read Major Depressive Disorder, Recurrent, Severe, with Melancholic Features. For each disorder, criteria are listed. There are, for instance, nine criteria for a Major Depressive Episode; if you meet five of them, then you have fulfilled the necessary condition for that diagnosis; and if you meet four others in addition, then you have sufficient symptoms to earn the MDD label. In addition to the criteria, the DSM supplies *text*, a not-quite-narrative account of the prevalence, family and gender patterns, and other associated features of the disorder, and instructs doctors how to differentiate among disorders that resemble one another. Depending on

*Since the first DSM, published in 1952, there have been three major revisions: DSM-II (1968), DSM-III (1980), and DSM-IV (1994). There have also been two interim revisions, more limited in scope: DSM-III-R (1987) and DSM-IV-TR (2000). The DSM-IV-TR is the edition in effect until DSM-5 is released. For brevity, I will refer to this current edition as DSM-IV.

how you count—whether or not you consider each subtype its own disorder, for instance—the DSM-IV lists around three hundred disorders in its nearly one thousand pages.

You could think of the DSM as a handbook designed to help doctors recognize the varieties of psychological travail, not unlike the way Audubon's field guides help ornithologists recognize birds. You could think of it, as some people (especially its critics) do, as the Bible of psychiatry, providing a scriptural basis for the profession. You could think of it—and this is what the APA would like you to do with the DSM-5*—as a living document, akin to the U.S. Constitution, a set of generalizations about the present, flexible and yet lasting enough to see an institution into the future. Or you could think of the DSM as a collection of short stories about our psychological distress, an anthology of suffering. You could think of it as the book of our woes.

All of these work; I favor the last one, but then again, I'm hardly unprejudiced, and even I have to admit that the DSM barely qualifies as literature. It's lacking in plot, and it bears all the traces of having been written by committee; it is, as Henry James said of the nineteenth-century novel, a "loose, baggy monster." But then again, unlike the works of Tolstoy and Thackeray, the DSM belongs to a genre that is forgiving of poor writing, that ends up inviting and rewarding it. The book avoids the Latinate jargon that physicians tend to favor, but it is written by doctors and designed to be used in medical offices and hospitals around the world; it is a medical text. Which, nowadays anyway, means it is a scientific text, one that casts its subjects into dry, data-driven stories, freed from the vagaries of hope and desire, of prejudice and ignorance and fear, and anchored instead in the laws of nature.

---

*After the DSM-5 revision got under way, the American Psychiatric Association decided to abandon Roman numerals in favor of Arabic. I will be using the Arabic throughout, but some quoted material from early in the process will use Roman.

I'm not sure that this is the right genre for understanding us, and I'm not alone in my doubts. Psychiatry didn't always have dominion over the landscape of mental suffering, at least not the kind that shows up in everyday life. Psychiatrists, once known as "alienists," originally presided over asylums housing people too crazy to function outside them. The treatments the doctors doled out, if they doled out any at all, varied from hospital to hospital and took place largely out of the view of polite society. Psychiatrists did not appear on television to give relationship advice. They did not suggest ways to beat the winter blues. They did not prescribe cocktails of psychoactive drugs to accountants and schoolteachers while telling them what they suffered from.

Not that there weren't doctors doing those things or their equivalents. But most of them were neurologists like George Beard, who suggested, toward the end of the nineteenth century, that symptoms ranging from "insomnia, flushing, drowsiness, bad dreams" through "ticklishness, vague pains and flying neuralgias" to "exhaustion after defecation" added up to a disease that, in his bestselling *American Nervousness*, he christened *neurasthenia*. Or Silas Weir Mitchell, author of the bestselling *Fat and Blood*, his account of how to treat neurasthenia and hysteria (the details of which I won't go into; just use your imagination on the title and you'll get the idea), who was the inspiration for "The Yellow Wallpaper," Charlotte Perkins Gilman's famous fictionalized account of the rest cure she took at his hands. Or John Harvey Kellogg, who teamed up with his industrialist brother, Will, to introduce America's fatigued brain workers to the wonders of flaked cereals, electric light baths, and pelvic massage. Or Sigmund Freud, whose ideas about intrapsychic conflict as the source of psychological turmoil, which he called neurosis, landed on American soil (along with Freud himself) in 1909.

Whatever the merits of their particular theories, these doctors had one thing in common. People flocked to them, to the spas where nurses swaddled them for their naps, to the offices where they were shocked or steamed or vibrated, and to the analysts' couches where they disburdened themselves of their family secrets and lurid fantasies. The everyday psychopathology of the masses was a burgeoning and protean market, especially among the swelling ranks of the affluent; and doctors, armed with the authority of the microscope and the pharmacy, had seized it.

The enormous opportunity created by the democratizing of mental illness, and exploited by neurologists, was not lost on psychiatrists. In the first third of the twentieth century, they began to escape the asylum, setting out mostly for private offices, where they, too, began to minister to the walking wounded, mostly by practicing psychoanalysis. Their colleagues/competitors included neurologists, but they also included anthropologists and art historians and social workers—nonmedical people who had been trained in psychoanalysis and had hung out their shingles. Given the ascendant power of medicine, these lay analysts might well have failed to capture much of the market from doctors, but the New York Psychoanalytic Society, dominated by psychiatrists, was not content to wait for the invisible hand to lift them to dominance. In 1926, for reasons it didn't spell out explicitly, it declared that only physicians could practice psychoanalysis.

Back in Vienna, Freud, who had long loathed America as a land of the shallow and unsophisticated, was livid. "As long as I live," he thundered, "I shall balk at having psychoanalysis swallowed by medicine." He spelled out the reasons for his objections in *The Question of Lay Analysis*. Medical education, he wrote, was exactly the wrong training for the therapist's job. "It burdens [a doctor] with too much . . . of which he can never make use, and there is a danger of its diverting his interest and his whole mode of thought from the understanding of psychical phenomena." Instead of learning from "the mental sciences, from psychology, the history of civilization and sociology," Freud wrote, would-be physician analysts would learn only "anatomy, biology and the study of evolution." They would thus be subject to "the temptation to flirt with endocrinology and the autonomous nervous system," and to turn psychoanalysis into just another "specialized branch of medicine, like radiology."

Steeped in the wrong genre, Freud worried, doctors would not provide the densely layered readings of their patients' suffering that he had offered in his essays on subjects like melancholia and narcissism, in case studies about delusional characters like the Wolf Man and the Rat Man, and in books declaring the significance of the seemingly insignificant, of dreams and jokes and slips of the tongue. They would not try, as analysts surely would, to understand the reason Sandy thought someone had sucked out his bones, as opposed to the infinity of other delusions he could have had. Instead, they would offer the kind of cure suggested in their medical texts, the kind that doesn't care what, if anything, the delusion itself might actually mean.

Freud might not have minded that first DSM, which was issued in 1952, thirteen years after his death. He might have recognized his legacy in the names of the sections—"Disorders of Psychogenic Origin" and "Psychoneurotic Disorders"—and of diagnoses such as anxiety reaction and sexual deviation. He might have been pleased by the literary descriptions, steeped in psychoanalysis, which turned up, for instance, in the definition of *depressive reaction* as the result of "the patient's ambivalent feeling toward his loss." Buoyed by the continued presence in the book's 132 pages of his notion that the mind was a host of inchoate and often contradictory feelings, Freud might have been willing to acknowledge that his forecast of a hostile takeover of psychoanalysis by medicine had been wrong. He might even have admired his descendants for their cleverness in avoiding that fate and yet still claiming the perquisites of the doctor, for having figured out how to have it both ways.

But Freud might also have predicted that it was only a matter of time before the strain between the reductive impulse of medicine and the expansive nature of psychoanalysis raised internal havoc. The problems began in 1949, before the first DSM was published, when a psychologist showed that psychiatrists presented with the same information about the same patient agreed on a diagnosis only about 20 percent of the time. By 1962, despite various attempts to solve this problem, clinicians still were agreeing less often than they disagreed, at least according to a major study. In 1968, at just around the time the second edition of the DSM came out, research showed that for any given psychotic patient, doctors in Great Britain were more likely to render a diagnosis of manic depression than schizophrenia, while doctors in the United States tended to do the opposite—a difference that was obviously more about the doctors than the patients.

In the meantime, one of psychiatry's own had turned against it. Thomas Szasz, an upstate New York doctor with a libertarian bent, argued in *The Myth of Mental Illness* (1961) that psychiatrists had mistaken "problems of living"—the age-old complaints that characterize our inner lives—for medical illnesses, and the result was a loss of personal responsibility (and a sweetening of the pot for doctors). Also in the early 1960s, Erving Goffman and Michel Foucault, among other academics, chimed in with their view that mental illness was more sociological than medical, and that psychiatrists were pathologizing deviancy rather than turning up genuine illness—which they (along with Szasz) believed existed only in cases where physiological pathology could be identified as the source of the trouble.

The arguments about diagnostic agreement and the nature of mental illness might have remained arcane academic topics had it not been for a Stanford sociologist, David Rosenhan, who, in 1972, sent a cadre of healthy graduate students to various emergency rooms with the same vague complaint: that they were hearing a voice in their heads that said "Thud." All the students were admitted with a diagnosis of schizophrenia, and although they acted normally once they were hospitalized (or normally for graduate students; they spent much of their time making notes, behavior that was duly jotted down in their charts as indicative of their illness), the diagnosis was never recanted. Some were released by doctors, and others had to be rescued from the hospital by their colleagues, but all were discharged with a diagnosis of Schizophrenia, in Remission.

Rosenhan's recounting of his exploit, "On Being Sane in Insane Places," appeared in the January 1973 edition of *Science*. Later that year, gay activists, including some psychiatrists, after years of increasingly public and contentious debate, finally persuaded the APA to remove homosexuality from the DSM—a good move, no doubt, but one that, especially after what had happened to the graduate students, couldn't help but reveal that even when psychiatrists did agree on a diagnosis, they might have been diagnosing something that wasn't an illness. Or, to put it another way, psychiatrists didn't seem to know the difference between sickness and health.

Forty years, two full rewrites, and two interim revisions of the DSM later, they still don't. Psychiatrists have gotten better at agreeing on which scattered particulars they will gather under a single disease label, but they haven't gotten any closer to determining whether those labels carve nature at its joints, or even how to answer that question. They have yet to figure out just exactly what a mental illness is, or how to decide if a particular kind of suffering qualifies. The DSM instructs users to determine not only that a patient has the symptoms listed in the book (or, as psychiatrists like to put it, that they *meet the criteria*), but that the symptoms are "clinically significant." But the book doesn't define that term, and most psychiatrists have decided to stop fighting about it in favor of an I-know-it-when-I-see-it definition (or saying that the mere fact that someone makes an appointment is evidence of clinical significance). Instead, they argue over which mental illnesses should be admitted to the DSM and which symptoms define them, as if reconfiguring the map will somehow answer the question of whether the territory is theirs to carve up.

This kind of argument leads to all sorts of interesting drama, much of which you will soon be reading about, but none of it can answer the question I posed about Sandy: Is *disease* really the best way to understand his craziness? How much of our suffering should we turn over to our doctors—especially our psychiatrists?

I don't know the answer to that question. But neither do psychiatrists. Even in a case as florid as Sandy's, they cannot say exactly how they know he has a mental illness, let alone what disorder he has or what treatment it warrants or why the treatment works (if it does), which means that they cannot say why his problem belongs to them. That's no secret. Any psychiatrist worth his or her salt will freely acknowledge (and frequently bemoan) the absence of blood tests or brain scans or any other technology that can anchor diagnosis in a reality beyond the symptoms. What they are more circumspect about is the disquieting implication of this ignorance: that if a physician wants to claim that drapetomania and homosexuality and, as the DSM-5 has proposed, at one time or another, Hypersexuality and Internet Use Disorder and Binge Eating Disorder are medical illnesses, there is nothing to stop him from doing so and if he is shrewd and lucky and smart enough to persuade his colleagues to follow him, the insurers, the drug companies, the regulators, the lawyers, the judges, and, eventually, the rest of us will have no choice but to go along.

So while the psychiatrists who author the DSM and I share an ignorance about how much of our inner travail should be considered illness, only the psychiatrists have the power to decide, and only the American Psychiatric Association claims those decisions as intellectual property that is theirs to profit from. That's why I think you should be more disturbed by their ignorance than mine. After all, if the people who write the DSM don't know which forms of suffering belong in it, and can't say why, then on what grounds can the next instance in which prejudice and oppression are cloaked in the doctor's white coat be recognized? Or, to put it more simply, why should we trust them with all the authority they've been granted?

———

That's a question that psychiatrist Allen Frances has been asking recently. Frances knows a great deal about power and psychiatry. Indeed, *The New York Times* once called him "perhaps the most powerful psychiatrist in America." That was in 1994, when Frances, who then headed the psychiatry department at Duke University School of Medicine, was chair of the DSM-IV task force, the APA committee responsible for that revision. He's retired now, and not as powerful, but he's a lot more famous, mostly because he has spent the last four years waging a scorched-earth campaign against his successors, largely on the grounds that they are abusing their power. He's warned anyone who will listen that the DSM-5 will turn even more of our suffering into mental illness and, in turn, into grist for the pharmaceutical mill.

Frances is seventy years old, a big, swarthy man with a prominent brow set off by a shock of white hair. I once heard a bartender tell him he looked like a cross between Cary Grant and Spencer Tracy. The bartender may have been flirting or fishing for a bigger tip, but he had one thing right: Frances, like those stars, exudes charm and authority in equal measure. He's soft-spoken, his voice high and reedy, and his patter is compulsively self-effacing, but like certain dangerous animals, he's unpredictable, and always ready to spring.

I hadn't known Frances for very long before he said something to me that he came to regret. It was just before dawn on a morning in August 2010. He'd finished his workout and cracked open his first Diet Coke of the day in the kitchen of the California home he shares with his psychiatrist wife, Donna Manning. The jihad Frances had launched against his former colleagues had made him appealing to magazines like *Wired*, which had sent me to get the skinny on this loyalist denouncing the new regime. Since I'd arrived the day before, he'd been giving it to me, volubly and forcefully; and now we returned to one of the recurring themes of yesterday's conversation: the way the DSM seemed to grant psychiatrists dominion over the entire landscape of mental suffering, a perch from which they could proclaim as a mental disorder any aberration they could describe systematically. I asked him whether he thought a good definition of mental disorder would establish the bright boundary that would sort the sick from the unusual, and thus keep psychiatry in its proper place.

"Here's the problem," Frances said. "There is no definition of a mental disorder."

I mentioned that that hadn't stopped him from putting one into the DSM-IV, or the people who were then making the DSM-5 from fiddling with it.

"And it's bullshit," he said. "I mean you can't define it."

This was the comment that Frances would come to regret—or at least, when it appeared in the lead of the *Wired* article, to regret having said to me. He soon found himself explaining it—to other writers, to his mildly titillated grandchildren, to attorneys who used it to discredit his testimony as a forensic expert, and, worst of all from his point of view, to Scientologists and other opponents of psychiatry who used it to draft Frances into their cause. Frances never quite blamed me for having turned his words into aid and comfort to the enemy. But even so, he was pretty sore about it, especially, he said, because my use of his words might encourage mentally ill people to go off their medications. I had turned him into my Charlie McCarthy, he complained—not by putting words in his mouth, but by throwing my tone into his voice.

I'm sure Frances would have used a different phrase if he'd thought about it. He didn't intend to dismiss the diagnostic enterprise, let alone all of psychiatry, but rather to say only that it is impossible to find that bright line and probably not worth the bother, that a good clinician can be trusted to determine significance and then, with the help of a decent diagnostic manual, figure out which disorder to diagnose and get on with the treatment. He was shooting from the hip, and even though I don't regret reporting his comment, I can see why he wishes I hadn't.

On the other hand, metaphors often have significance beyond their author's intent, although, as Freud pointed out, sometimes analysis is required to ferret it out. Fortunately for us, there is a philosopher of bullshit. His name is Harry Frankfurt, and he's taught at Yale and Princeton, and in 2005 he published a tiny gem of a book called *On Bullshit*. "Bullshit is unavoidable whenever circumstances require someone to talk without knowing what he is talking about," writes Frankfurt. "Thus the production of bullshit is stimulated whenever a person's obligations or opportunities to speak about some topic exceed his knowledge of the facts relevant to that topic." Filling in the gap between opportunity and knowledge requires the bullshitter to stand "neither on the side of the true nor on the side of the false," he adds. "His eye is not on the facts at all, as the eyes of the honest man and of the liar are, except insofar as they may be pertinent to his interest in getting away with what he says."

For the last fifteen years, some of the smartest psychiatrists in the world, people who have studied diagnosis for their entire careers, people motivated, at least in part, by the desire to relieve suffering, have worked longer and harder, and taken more fire, than they ever expected as they revised the DSM-IV. But if you ask any one of them (and I have asked many) about the DSM's diagnoses and criteria—new and old— he or she will tell you they are only "fictive placeholders" or "useful constructs," the best the profession can do with the knowledge and tools at hand. They are fully aware, in other words, that their opportunity (although they may call it an obligation) to name and describe our psychological suffering far exceeds their knowledge. They have intentionally, if unhappily, stood on the side of neither the true nor the false, and for the sixty years since the first DSM was published, they have gotten away with it.

I don't mean to say that the DSM is nothing more than bullshit, or that the APA is merely trying to hoodwink us in order to maintain its franchise or make a buck (or a hundred million of them, which is what the DSM-IV has earned it). That would be as glib as tarring the entire diagnostic enterprise with Dr. Cartwright's brush. And as uninteresting: finding bullshit in a professional guild's attempt to strengthen its market position would be no more remarkable than discovering gambling in Casablanca. But what are neither glib nor uninteresting are the circumstances that make it necessary and possible for the 150 men and women on the DSM-5 task force and work groups to have it both ways, to manufacture fiction and yet act as if it were fact. If the story of the DSM-5 has any redeeming value, if it is more than a story about parochial disputes and internecine warfare, it is that it can reveal the conditions that motivate the publication of the DSM and the interests that another revision serves.

Some of those circumstances are straightforward enough, and depressingly banal. If fully 10 percent of your guild's revenue, and an uncountable amount of your authority, depend on a single book, a book that once saved your profession from oblivion and since then has brought it fabulous riches, you don't give it up easily. But other circumstances are less obvious and more dangerous, and the idea that gives psychiatry the power to name our pain in the first place—that the mind can be treated like the body, that it is no more or less than what the brain does, that it can be carved at its joints like a diseased liver—is perhaps the most important of all. It reflects what is best about us: our desire to understand ourselves and one another, to use knowledge to relieve suffering, even if it results in a kind of reductionism that insults our sense of ourselves as unfathomably complex and even transcendent creatures. It also reflects what is worst—the desire to control, to manipulate, to turn others' vulnerabilities to our advantage. The first impulse demands a search for truth at all costs. The second makes it imperative to get away with whatever you can in order to exploit a market opportunity. When those impulses collide, commerce—and often bullshit—will prevail.

Chapter 2

Allen Frances is not the first psychiatrist to draw a bead on his profession's inability to distinguish between illness and health. Neither is he the first to worry about the effects of this uncertainty on public confidence in his profession. The two concerns have gone hand in hand since at least 1917, when Thomas Salmon gave a talk in Buffalo, New York, to the American Medico-Psychological Association (the new name for the Association of Superintendents, which would later be renamed the American Psychiatric Association).

"The present classification of mental diseases is chaotic," Salmon told his colleagues. "This condition of affairs discredits the science of psychiatry and reflects unfavorably upon our association." He proposed a solution: a classification of twenty different mental diseases "that would meet the scientific demands of the day."

Although his organization was already seventy years old, Salmon's list was one of the first proposals for a psychiatric *nosology*, or classification of diseases. Earlier psychiatrists had kept track of their patients, but their concerns ran much more to the statistical than to the diagnostic. In part, this was because they were making their count at the behest of the Census Bureau, which, starting in 1840, had wanted to know just how many people were "insane," but not which forms of insanity they had. When those numbers increased dramatically throughout the mid–nineteenth century—especially in neighborhoods where new asylums had been built—their explanations were more sociological than physiological or psychological. "It cannot be supposed that so many people were suddenly attacked with insanity when these establishments were opened or enlarged," said Massachusetts doctor Edward Jarvis, head of his state's Commission on Lunacy. Rather, he explained, "the more the means of healing are provided and made known to the people, the more they are moved to intrust [sic] their mentally disordered friends to their care." Supply, at least when it came to mental hospitals, could create demand.

But what had driven these recently discovered patients insane in the first place? "Within the last fifty years, there has unquestionably been a very great real increase of the malady [insanity] in the progress of the world from the savage to the civilized state." Not that "these two great facts, the development of mental disorder and the growth of human culture, stand as cause and effect," he added quickly. But then again, Jarvis was more than just saying. There were two types of causes of insanity—physical (as in "palsy, epilepsy, fever, and blows on the head") and moral, "those which first affect the mind and the emotions." This second type of cause was surely on the increase, a by-product of all that progress and the brave new world it had ushered in.

In an uneducated community, or where men are born in castes and die without stepping beyond their native condition; where the child is content with the pursuit and the fortune of his father, and has no hope or expectations of any other, these undue mental excitements and struggles do not happen, and men's brains are not confused with new plans nor exhausted with the struggle for a higher life, nor overthrown with the disappointment in failure. In such a state of society, these causes of insanity cannot operate.

Upward mobility carried risks with it, and so did modern education. Indeed, the "professional insane"—doctors, lawyers, teachers, and the like—were uniquely subject to the demands that "arise from excessive culture and overburden the mental powers." Which is why, he thought, 3.75 percent of them were on the rolls in Massachusetts.

"From all this survey," Jarvis concluded in 1872, "we are irresistibly drawn to the conclusion that insanity is a part of the price we are paying for the imperfection of our civilization."

Jarvis's conclusion made the particulars of his patients' afflictions less important than their demographics and geography and economics, and their relief more a matter of social than medical remedy. This may well have reflected some idealism on his part and a sense that psychiatry's job was to help perfect civilization rather than to cure individuals. But there is a less noble reason for Jarvis's and his colleagues' nosological inattention: they simply couldn't compete with their microscope-armed brethren. As the magnificently named psychiatrist Pliny Earle complained in 1886:

In the present state of our knowledge, no classification of insanity can be erected upon a pathological basis, for the simple reason that, with slight exceptions, the pathology of the disease is unknown. Hence, for the best understood foundation for a nosological scheme for insanity, we are forced to fall back upon the symptomatology of the disease—*the apparent mental condition*, as judged from the outward manifestations.

All the statistical analysis in the world, and all the recommendations for the perfection of society, would not make psychiatrists real doctors; real medicine was practiced upon individual patients, upon their errant physiologies and the bugs that had made them go haywire. As if this weren't trouble enough, the democratization of mental illness had so favored neurologists that by the time World War I broke out, psychiatry, according to historian Edward Shorter, "had become marginal to the mainstream of medicine." So when Thomas Salmon presented his classification of diseases to his colleagues in Buffalo, it was clear that they risked professional demise if they could not fill in the gap between opportunity and knowledge by meeting those scientific demands.

Salmon's solution took inspiration from an earlier attempt to solve the same problem. In the late nineteenth century, a German doctor named Emil Kraepelin had noted the nosological chaos in which psychiatrists claimed with certainty that their patients suffered from "masturbatory insanity" or "wedding night psychosis" or "dementia praecox," but couldn't say how they knew what these conditions were, or where one started up and another left off, or, most important, whether or not they existed.

Kraepelin would have liked to ground his nosology as his colleagues in other specialties did. "Pathological anatomy," he wrote, offered "the safest foundation for a classification," but the brain, where that pathology would most likely be found, was way beyond the reach of the instruments of the time. So he settled for what Pliny Earle had lamented as second best. He proposed that the landscape of mental suffering could be effectively mapped if a doctor observed it carefully and systematically enough, if, that is, he stuck faithfully to the phenomenon as it presented itself in the clinic. Discern how symptoms grouped together in patients, how, for example, delusions of grandeur went together with mania, or how hallucinations dogged the same patients who were paranoid, and then chart the course and outcome of those cases, and you have the basis for an accurate taxonomy of insanity, one that, or so Kraepelin promised, would line up with the pathological anatomy that doctors were sure to discover in the future.

Kraepelin's method required patience and discipline and, above all else, a steely determination not to indulge in "poetic interpretation of the patient's mental process, [which] we call empathy."

"Trying to understand another human being's emotional life," he once told his students, "is fraught with potential error . . . It can lead to gross self-deception in research."

Early in his career, Kraepelin got a job in an Estonian asylum. He didn't speak the local language, so it was a perfect opportunity to hone his method for discerning the nature of his patients' illnesses undistracted by empathy. He observed their behaviors, noted them on cards, sorted them according to which ones appeared together, and chronicled what happened to the patients who had those groups of symptoms. In 1893 he published the first in a series of textbooks in which he gave names to the illnesses he claimed to have discerned and provided descriptions of how they could be recognized.

Kraepelin's taxonomy had to compete with Freud's rich and riveting accounts, and it languished, especially in the United States. But when Salmon introduced his nosology, he didn't write about Oedipal complexes or reaction formations. Instead he took a Kraepelinian approach, laying out neat categories of mental illness, many of which, including dementia praecox and manic-depressive insanity and involutional melancholia, were cribbed directly from his German forebear.

Salmon shared something else with Kraepelin: ignorance about the biochemical origins of mental illness, coupled with the assumption that when they were finally discovered, as they inevitably would be, they would prove that the diseases existed in the way we expect diseases to exist, and that psychiatrists had known all along what they were talking about.

Salmon had renewed the promissory note issued by Kraepelin, and the market was quick to take on the debt. A year after his talk, the association issued the *Statistical Manual for the Use of Institutions for the Insane*, based largely on Salmon's nomenclature. The book pleased the Census Bureau enough that it adopted the categories for its own ongoing attempt to include the mentally ill in its count of Americans. The *Statistical Manual* was revised ten times between 1918 and 1942, but it remained, as the title implied, primarily a guide to data collection, focused mostly on institutionalized patients whose ills were presumably biological in origin. It also remained brief: its last edition ran to seventy-one pages covering, besides Salmon's original handful of diagnoses, eight "psychoneuroses" added in response to the ascendancy of psychoanalysis.

By 1940, the American Psychiatric Association (the name Salmon's organization had adopted in 1921) had a membership of only 2,295 doctors. But World War II, with its influx of soldiers suffering war neuroses (later to be known as Posttraumatic Stress Disorder), had induced the army to increase the ranks of its psychiatrists, and by the end of the war, thanks to some quick on-the-job training, there were 2,400 psychiatrists serving in the army alone. It wasn't long before the swelling ranks of psychiatrists sought to extend their success to the civilian walking wounded. "Our experiences with therapy in war neuroses have left us with an optimistic attitude," wrote two prominent psychiatrists in 1944. "The lessons we have learned in the combat zone can be well applied . . . at home."

But neither psychoanalysis, the dominant mode of therapy, nor the *Statistical Manual* was entirely well suited to these new psychiatrists. Psychoanalysis, with its focus on early childhood as the fount of all pathology, couldn't really explain why so many soldiers, presumably normal before the war, became mentally ill after exposure to its horrors. Neither could the *Statistical Manual*, with its focus on constitutional and presumably incurable illnesses, account for what seemed to be transient and dramatic reactions to the environment.

Psychoanalysis proved easy enough to adapt, especially now that Freud was dead and couldn't object. Freud's insistence that only early childhood trauma caused neurosis could be modified without losing the basic idea that intrapsychic conflict was the culprit. Trauma later in life, such as a war, could also disrupt intrapsychic functioning and leave people unable to adapt to new and difficult circumstances. This failure could be understood as a *psychoneurotic reaction*, and analysts, armed with this notion, recast psychoanalysis as a theory of adaptation to life circumstances, and their practices as a ministry to the walking wounded.

But the *Statistical Manual* presented a different kind of problem. Its basic terms didn't even come close to describing what psychiatrists were seeing in the clinic. Indeed, they complained, only 10 percent of their cases fit into the classification system. So they began to improvise, stretching diagnostic categories to fit their patients, inventing labels when that didn't work, and borrowing disease names from other medical specialties whenever they could. The armed forces developed their own nosology, as did the Veterans Administration, and these began to compete for primacy with the edition of the *Statistical Manual* that had been issued in 1942. In 1948, George Raines, chair of the APA's committee on nomenclature, summed up the situation he faced:

> At least three nomenclatures were in general use, and none of them fell into line with the International Statistical Classification . . . One agency found itself in the uncomfortable position of using one nomenclature for clinical use, a different one for disability rating, and the International for statistical work. In addition, practically every teaching center had made modifications of [the *Statistical Manual*] for its own use and assorted modifications of the Armed Forces nomenclature had been introduced into many clinics and hospitals by psychiatrists.

Psychiatry, or at least the APA, was once again mired in the chaos that Salmon had lamented three decades earlier as a threat to the viability of his profession.

Raines decided to put off a revision of the *Statistical Manual* scheduled for 1948 in favor of a total revamping. Drawing on the armed forces' classification, input from psychiatric teaching hospitals, polls of the APA's membership, and reviews of the scientific literature, he and his committee assembled a revised manual, which they submitted to the membership in 1950. The proposed book still provided labels and descriptions for conditions presumed to be unresponsive to the environment as either cause or cure. But it also contained definitions of *reactions*, disorders resulting from traumatic life circumstances and accounted for by the updated, adjustment-focused version of psychoanalysis that had emerged since the war.

Raines's revision offered something for private practice and hospital psychiatrists alike. It also had a different focus from the earlier manual—largely, Raines explained, because the recent establishment of the National Institute of Mental Health meant that statistical analysis, once the "stepchild of [the] Federal Government," would now be handled by public officials. Freed from that drudgery, psychiatrists could pay closer attention to diagnosis, and the new revision stood ready to aid them with eighty-seven diagnoses to choose from, each with a paragraph describing a prototypical patient. If, for instance, a patient was complaining of "diffuse" anxiety, "not restricted to situations or objects . . . not controlled by any specific psychological defense mechanism . . . characterized by anxious expectation and . . . associated with somatic symptomatology," then the doctor could diagnose Anxiety Reaction. On the other hand, if "the anxiety . . . is allayed, and hence partially relieved, by depression and self-depreciation . . . precipitated by a current situation . . . associated with a feeling of guilt for past failures or deeds . . . [and] dependent on the intensity of the patient's ambivalent feeling toward his loss," then the patient had Depressive Reaction. Because of this new focus, the manual had a new name: *The Diagnostic and Statistical Manual: Mental Disorders*.

When it was released in 1952, the DSM's nomenclature imposed some order on the professional landscape. As insurance payments came to play an increasing role in the medical marketplace, those new diagnoses proved useful, especially to private-practice doctors. But these successes came at a cost: by delineating a realm of "disorders of psychogenic origin or without clearly defined physical cause or structural change in the brain," the DSM represented a partial abandonment of Kraepelin's promise that mental disorder could be understood like physical disease, and eventually would be explained as the manifestation of brain pathologies. And by incorporating Freudian concepts like *defense mechanism* and *ambivalence toward loss*, the DSM glossed over a question that had been looming since the New York Psychoanalytic Society claimed psychoanalysis for medicine. Were those psychogenic disorders really medical problems? Should psychiatrists continue to try to carve up the landscape of mental suffering in the way that the rest of medicine was carving up the afflictions of the body?

By 1963, leading psychiatrists such as Karl Menninger were beginning to think the answer was no. "Instead of putting so much emphasis on different kinds . . . of illness," he wrote, "we propose to think of all forms of mental illness as being essentially the same in quality and differing quantitatively." Menninger didn't think the search for "what was behind the symptom" should be abandoned. Rather, he believed, like Edward Jarvis, that psychiatrists should focus their attention not on hypothetical brain disturbances or quasi-medical psychogenic diseases, but on "Man in transaction with his universe"—the economic, political, and social world in which psychological life was lived.

Many of his colleagues shared Menninger's dour view of diagnosis, and, glad as they were to use the book to get insurance payments, they otherwise ignored not only the DSM, but nosology in general. By the late 1960s, it had become a professional backwater; discussions of disease classification were relegated to the last session of the last day of professional conferences. But even if the DSM had managed to put Kraepelin's promissory note into abeyance, if not to abandon it entirely in favor of Menninger's transactional view, still a market based on confidence cannot tolerate outstanding debt forever. After the repeated blows to psychiatry's credibility in the late 1960s and early 1970s—the reliability fiascos, the Rosenhan caper, the homosexuality debacle— the note was finally called in. In 1975, a Blue Cross executive told the *Psychiatric News*, the APA's house organ, that his industry was reducing mental health treatment benefits because "compared to other types of services, there is less clarity and uniformity of terminology concerning mental diagnoses." And in 1978, a presidential commission, convened, among other reasons, to set priorities for federal funding, concluded that "documenting the total number of people who have mental health problems . . . is difficult not only because opinions vary on how mental health and mental illness should be defined, but also because the available data are often inadequate or misleading."

Whatever their patients were suffering from, the doctors' problem was obvious. The DSM did a lousy job of helping them figure out and agree on which disease belonged to which patient, and even in the cases where it succeeded (after all, how hard is it to diagnose homosexuality?), the DSM didn't help doctors prove that patients were suffering from medical diseases rather than the human condition. Turning away from Kraepelin and toward Freud had been a boon, but it had now become an embarrassment. Unless something was done, it was going to be increasingly difficult for psychiatrists to make a living.

The war over the homosexuality diagnosis finally came to an end in 1973, when a Columbia psychiatrist, Robert Spitzer, sat down with both sides and hammered out a compromise. The DSM would no longer list homosexuality as a disease, but it would still provide a diagnosis for people who were gay and didn't want to be: Ego-Dystonic Homosexuality, a condition, clinicians were advised, that was the result, at least in part, of "negative social attitudes [that] have been internalized." It was a win-win: gay people would no longer be subject to bizarre and pointless therapies (or to psychiatrist-assisted discrimination), the APA would stop getting humiliated by protests, and therapists everywhere would continue to get insurance dollars to treat gay patients.

Like most compromises, this one left some bad feelings. "If groups of people march and raise hell, they can change anything in time. Will schizophrenia be next?" one psychiatrist fulminated. "Referenda on matters of science [make] no sense," said another. But the compromise at least kept the profession from splitting at its seams even as it began to regain its dignity and the confidence of its patrons in government and industry. And it showed that Spitzer had a great command of both the political and the scientific issues at stake.

When I met with him, Spitzer, nearing eighty and hobbled by Parkinson's disease, was barely able to walk from the easy chair in his sunny living room to the kitchen table, where sandwiches whipped up by his full-time aide awaited, but his mind seemed undiminished. He certainly remembered what his profession was up against after the homosexuality crisis, and he was not mincing words about it.

"Psychiatry was regarded as bogus," he said. "I knew it would be better off if it was accepted as a medical discipline."

Like Salmon before him, he believed that a nosology that met the scientific demands of the day was the key to restoring credibility to his profession. He also knew that if he managed to fashion that solution, "my colleagues would think I had done something very worthwhile." So he volunteered for the job of revising the DSM, and, given his successful nosological diplomacy on the homosexuality front, the APA was delighted to have him.

Spitzer also knew that even if his job was to carve nature at its joints with the scalpel of scientific knowledge, he was stuck with the same dull instruments that Salmon and Kraepelin used—which were not all that different from what ancient doctors like Hippocrates had at their disposal: their senses, and the empirical world they could apprehend. And while ancient doctors could taste a patient's urine or smell his sweat or peer into body cavities for information the patient couldn't provide directly, psychiatrists were limited to the symptoms a patient could describe and the signs embedded in his behavior and comportment.

Still, as Kraepelin had demonstrated, it was possible to make observations carefully and group them systematically. Spitzer's attraction to this method wasn't so much a matter of conviction as predilection. "Ever since I was a child, I liked to sort things," he said, recalling that at summer camp he graphed his attractions to different female campers. Of course, to sort out the girls successfully, you have to know which categories to put them in, and what makes them belong in one or the other. You have to believe that beauty and intellect and sense of humor are real properties, and that your way of discerning them is accurate and consistent. Like Kraepelin, Spitzer was certain that if he was careful enough in observing them, the outward manifestations would reveal the underlying mental condition.

To Spitzer, it wasn't the unfulfilled promise of Kraepelin and Salmon, but rather psychoanalysis—with its claims that psychopathology was the human condition, that same-sex love was the result of damage inflicted in childhood by absent fathers and overbearing mothers, and that, in general, mental suffering was the result of the eternal war among ego, id, and superego—that had led psychiatry to near shipwreck. It was psychoanalysis that had led psychiatrists like Menninger to abandon the idea of sorting suffering into medical categories. It was psychoanalysis that had persuaded doctors to sort mental disorders according to the inner turmoil that had allegedly caused them—the Oedipal conflict, say, or a fixation on the anal stage of infantile sexual development. And it was psychoanalysis that claimed that when it came to our psychological lives, the line between illness and health could be drawn by determining if the problem was the result of intrapsychic conflict, of the lies we tell ourselves about ourselves, of the truths we dance around or repress and transmute into symptoms.

Spitzer hadn't much liked the psychoanalytic training that had been required of him and most psychiatrists of his era, and he really didn't like being an analyst. "I was uncomfortable with not knowing what to do with their [patients'] messiness," he said. "I just didn't know what the hell to do." And it was obvious to him that Freud's theory of mind was a poor substitute for pathological anatomy, and the complexes and resistances and defense mechanisms—the psychoanalyst's stock-in-trade—were far too ungrounded in any kind of empirical reality to be useful. Proving the existence of ego, id, and superego was like proving the existence of the Holy Trinity. These notions were more metaphysics than physics, psychoanalysis more religion than science, and the crises of the 1960s and 1970s were the result.

Of course, this was exactly the problem: psychoanalysis had thrived in the theoretical vacuum left by the continued ignorance of how the brain works. So it wasn't like there was a theory waiting in the wings to replace it. But, Spitzer reasoned, if his only options were a theory that couldn't be proved (and that was leading his profession to disaster after disaster) or no theory at all, then the correct choice was obvious. It was time to abandon Freud's pretense to understanding the origin and nature of mental illness, and to return to the one thing Kraepelin said psychiatrists could safely claim to know: what they could observe.

Spitzer was already working with a group of researchers at Washington University in St. Louis to resurrect Kraepelin. By 1972, the group had described fourteen different diagnostic groupings, established the criteria by which patients could be placed into one or another of them, and conducted research showing that the diagnoses were reliable. Six years later, the Washington University group issued the Research Diagnostic Criteria (RDC), twenty-one categories with checklists of the criteria by which each one could be known.

The RDC bore virtually no resemblance to the DSM, then in its second edition. Where the DSM-II listed illnesses like Depressive Neurosis, defined as a "disorder manifested by an excessive reaction of depression due to an internal conflict," the RDC created Major Depressive Disorder, defined not in a paragraph full of Freudian jargon, but as a list of symptoms:

A. One or more distinct periods with dysphoric mood or pervasive loss of interest or pleasure. The disturbance is characterized by symptoms such as the following: depressed, sad, blue, hopeless, low, down in the dumps, "don't care anymore," or irritable . . .

B. At least five of the following symptoms are required to have appeared as part of the episode for definite and four for probable (for past episodes, because of memory difficulty, one less symptom is required).

   1. Poor appetite or weight loss or increased appetite or weight gain (change of 0.5 kg a week over several weeks or 4.5 kg a year when dieting)
   2. Sleep difficulty or sleeping too much
   3. Loss of energy, fatigability [sic], or tiredness
   4. Psychomotor agitation or retardation (but not mere subjective feeling of restlessness or being slowed down)
   5. Loss of interest or pleasure in usual activities, including social contact or sex (do not include if limited to a period when delusional or hallucinating) (The loss may or may not be pervasive.)
   6. Feeling of self-reproach or excessive or inappropriate guilt (either may be delusional)
   7. Complaints or evidence of diminished ability to think or concentrate, such as slowed thinking, or indecisiveness (do not include if associated with marked formal thought disorder)
   8. Recurrent thoughts of death or suicide, or any suicidal behavior

C. Duration of dysphoric features at least one week, beginning with the first noticeable change in the subject's usual condition (definite if lasted [sic] more than two weeks, probable if one to two weeks).

Purged of shaggy concepts and imprecise language, the RDC could tell clinicians exactly what to look for and what they had found if they saw it—a method that would leave much less room for disagreement.

The RDC may have renewed Kraepelin's promissory note, but, so Spitzer claimed, it also provided the means for paying it off. Of course, Socrates' observation still held: to gather together scattered particulars into groups was not to carve nature at its joints. But, Spitzer contended, all those observations, made by many researchers using the same language, would add up to a body of knowledge for each disorder, and the nosology would inexorably gain substance. Two different teams researching depression, for example, would be able to claim that they were looking at the same phenomenon, and as findings converged and solidified, so would the case for the existence of depression as a disease. And if that convergence couldn't or didn't occur, then that would be an indication that there was something wrong with the category, that it had been ill conceived or poorly defined, or that it just plain didn't exist. *Reliability*—the extent to which diagnostic criteria would yield agreement among clinicians—was not the same as *validity*, or the extent to which the diagnosis described an actual disease. But beefed-up reliability could at least make the profession seem less bogus.

"The use of operational criteria for psychiatric diagnosis is an idea whose time has come!" Spitzer wrote in 1978. Of course, he knew that twenty-one diagnoses wouldn't be nearly enough to cover the entire terrain over which psychiatrists claimed dominion, or to ensure that all their patients would qualify for a diagnosis and thus insurance reimbursement. He invited his colleagues to name the disorders they thought they were treating, and he found many of them eager to get in on the ground floor of the new scheme. He and his committees winnowed the suggestions, developed the criteria by which the survivors would be known, and assembled them into a diagnostic manual the likes of which had never been seen. A 500-page hardbound tome, the DSM-III made the spiral-bound, 134-page DSM-II look like a mere pamphlet. And by nearly doubling the number of mental disorders, it also vastly expanded the manual's scope, turning it into an entirely new psychopathology of everyday life.

Even so, the DSM-III was not universally popular among psychiatrists. Some thought its symptom lists, its plain language, and its workaday disorder names degraded the profession. "Clerks rather than experts can make this kind of classification," one grumbled.

This, of course, was exactly the point. Imagination was what had led psychiatry to founder; a Kraepelinian nosology was the best way to prevent psychiatrists from steering their profession back onto the shoals of unreliability. Spitzer had fashioned a dictionary of disorder that allowed psychiatrists to identify our foibles without recourse to the troublesome Freudian mumbo jumbo or, for that matter, any other mumbo jumbo.

And the result was sensational. The DSM-III not only restored both internal and external confidence in psychiatry; it was also an international bestseller. "It made an unbelievable amount of money for the APA," Spitzer said. "That was a huge surprise." And looking back on it, Spitzer has no question where the book's popularity came from. "DSM-III looks very scientific," he told me. "If you open it up, it looks like they must know something."

The psychiatrists who wrote and used the DSM-III indeed knew something. They knew that certain symptoms tended to group together and that psychiatrists could reliably identify the people who belonged in those groups. But Spitzer acknowledges that the book did not solve the validity problem. He doesn't even think it was supposed to. Indeed, he told me, the APA hired him to achieve only the smallest of bureaucratic goals—to bring the DSM into harmony with the World Health Organization's International Classification of Diseases, known as the ICD. When I pressed him, he allowed that, of course, increasing reliability was also on his—and the APA's—mind. But validity? "No, no," he said, "not at all." That's not what they wanted, and that's not what he meant to do.

Even now, in fact, the man who crafted the deal to delete homosexuality isn't sure that homosexuality is not a valid disorder. "It has a distinct course, there's no doubt about that," he said, adding that there are gender differences in prevalence and evidence that it is a familial trait. But, he cautioned, "to decide whether it's a disorder or a normal variant, you'd have to decide whether homosexuality represents a dysfunction. People who think it is a disorder would argue from an evolutionary viewpoint that we are hardwired for heterosexual attraction."

Some of those people would also argue that a lack of heterosexual attraction is a disease to be cured, and in 2003, after interviewing two hundred people who claimed to have been "cured" of their sexual orientation by "reparative therapy," Spitzer determined that "highly motivated" patients could indeed change their preference, a conclusion he published in the *Archives of Sexual Behavior*. The journal accompanied the article with fiercely critical commentary, and in the popular press gay activists pilloried the man who had freed them from psychiatry. Spitzer defended his work then, but more recently, he told me, he had come to regret the paper and was considering "writing something in which I would say the critiques are largely or in many ways true."

In May 2012, Spitzer did exactly that. His assumption that "participants' reports of change were credible and not self-deception or outright lying" had been incorrect, he wrote in a letter to the *Archives*. His subjects had *told* him they were no longer attracted to people of the same sex, but "there was no way to determine if [their] accounts of change were valid." Spitzer apologized to the "gay community" for making "unproven claims of the efficacy of reparative therapy" and to "any gay person who wasted time and energy undergoing [it]."

Spitzer's recantation, and his ongoing uncertainty about homosexuality, reflect his questing and curious mind, which seeks empirical answers to difficult questions and is always open to new evidence. It also reflects his honesty about the limitations of his paradigm, which can elicit detailed accounts of what people are experiencing, but can't say exactly what, if anything, to make of those accounts. Descriptive psychiatry can't determine whether or not a person's story about his sexual orientation is a true one. More important, it can't tell us whether the list of symptoms, no matter how reliable, constitutes a disease. It can gather scattered particulars into a category called *gay*, but it can't say whether those amount to the natural formation known as *disease*. It can't carve nature at its joints.

Spitzer is also honest about the fact that the decisions he made to admit or exclude a diagnosis from the DSM-III were not entirely scientific. "The categories that were added were concepts that clinicians in those days thought were important," he said, and their criteria consisted of what "clinicians said was a good way of defining them." Spitzer was the nosological diplomat among clinicians squaring off over pet concepts. He was perfectly suited to this role because, in addition to his predilection for sorting, he said, "I love controversy. I love it!"

Spitzer no doubt had in mind the controversy he had presided over as his committees fought about diagnoses and criteria—but it was only a matter of time before a different kind of controversy set in. It was exactly the kind of controversy that Thomas Salmon had worried about, and the culprit was none other than Bob Spitzer's DSM.

Chapter 3

Allen Frances often sings praise as a prelude to criticism, and sometimes in exact proportion. So when he tells me how brilliant Bob Spitzer is, how valuable he has been to psychiatry, and then adds, "I don't want anything in your book that would hurt him the slightest bit," which he does repeatedly, it is pretty clear that he's winding up to plunk him. Not that he doesn't deeply respect Spitzer—that's obvious as soon as you see the two of them together—or doesn't mean the praise. But he definitely has a beef with the man he replaced at the DSM's helm.

The problem isn't the DSM-III. The move to descriptive diagnosis was, Frances believes, necessary and beneficial for psychiatrists and patients alike. But almost immediately after that book came out in 1980, the APA decided to revise it. The new book would be called DSM-III-R, to reflect the fact that it was not a new edition, but a minor revision to correct textual errors and tweak criteria that were proving unwieldy. Spitzer was hired to direct the effort, but, according to Frances, "Bob couldn't resist playing with it. He couldn't resist the committee meetings, all the new diagnoses, all the excitement" as experts, once again given the opportunity to enshrine their pet ideas, advocated for new labels or criteria.

"In the morning, everyone would be screaming ideas," Frances recalled. "Bob [Spitzer] and Janet [Williams, Spitzer's wife and a member of the revision committees] would be on a blackboard, trying to put it into some kind of order. Then we'd have lunch, usually a big lunch." While the others ate, Spitzer and Williams would refine the morning's arguing into diagnostic criteria. When the group reconvened, Frances said, "we'd be sleepy and much more subdued," making it that much easier "for the most powerful person in the room to rule." The wrangling continued after the sessions, as doctors collared Spitzer and lobbied for their proposals.

The backroom dealing was bad enough, Frances thought, but even worse, the fighting was in many ways pointless. "The things that looked so different to the people involved never amounted to a hill of beans," Frances said. "Should the threshold for a diagnosis be four or five symptoms, should the criterion be this item or that? The answers are almost always arbitrary." So in 1987, when Harold Pincus, then the APA's director of research, offered him the job of running the DSM-IV revision, Frances told him he'd accept only if the process was entirely different. "The last thing I wanted was to be in rooms full of people pontificating without evidence about things that didn't matter," he said. As much as he might have coveted the job, "I never wanted to be in one of those meetings again."

Frances didn't always feel this way. In fact, at one time he was among the pontificators. "I knew the instinct," he said—the one that leads a doctor to think that he's seeing a cluster of symptoms that no one has put together before, and thus has discovered a new disorder. "You think you're smarter than everyone else, and that what you're seeing in this patient should be in the DSM."

Frances himself had once followed the instinct, nominating Masochistic Personality Disorder for DSM-III, aimed at people who "employ self-sacrificing and self-defeating behavior in service of maintaining relationships or self-esteem." His proposal came under withering attack from feminists who considered it a way of blaming abusive relationships on women's psychopathology. It also, Frances said, turned out to be a "dumb idea, because all the behaviors in a diagnostic manual of mental disorders are by definition self-defeating. The concept really adds nothing." By 1980, he had abandoned the proposal, having learned an important lesson about diagnostic manuals. "Realizing in retrospect how dumb my own off-the-cuff suggestion was made me more alive to the fallibility of the many other off-the-cuff suggestions DSMs necessarily attract."

As much as he wished to steer clear of the dumb arguing, however, Frances was even more intent on avoiding the pitfall that had snared Spitzer when he ran the DSM-III-R effort. "It's much better to have a common language than a Babel of different languages," he said, and the DSM-III had achieved that. But whatever stability and respectability this success had brought to the field was threatened by DSM-III-R. When that book came out in 1987, a year late, over budget, and even longer than the original, clinicians once again had to master new diagnoses, researchers had to piece together the new disorders with the old literature, and psychiatry, which had just barely settled down, was once again in turmoil.

The DSM-III had systematized the description of mental disorders, put labels on clusters of symptoms, but, as the DSM-III-R process had proved, those clusters could be arranged and rearranged indefinitely. Descriptive psychiatry was no small achievement, but the categories, the boundaries between them, and the criteria within them—these were not discoveries of nature at work, at least not in the same way that the identification of streptococcus and influenza, their characteristics, and the boundaries between them were. They were approximations, and even if they were based on careful observations, they were forever in debt to expert opinion.

The expert who led the move to delete homosexuality from the DSM might come to believe that homosexuality is a disease, and then once again decide that it is not. With each change of opinion comes the potential for instability and discord; and to Frances, this meant that the DSM-III's achievement was a fragile one. "The fact that we had a descriptive system only revealed our limitations," he said. "If you believe that labels are only labels, you don't want to keep changing the language arbitrarily. It just confuses everybody." If the DSM is not the map of an actual world against whose contours any changes can be validated, then opening up old arguments, or inviting new ones, might only sow dissension and reap chaos—and annoy Frances in the bargain. If he was going to revise the DSM, Frances told Pincus, then his goal would be stabilizing the system rather than trying to perfect it—or, as he put it to me, "loving the pet, even if it is a mutt."

Frances thought there was a way to protect the system from both instability and pontificating: meta-analysis, a statistical method that, thanks to advances in computer technology and statistical modeling, had recently allowed statisticians to compile results from large numbers of studies by combining disparate data into common terms. The result was a statistical synthesis by which many different research projects could be treated as one large study. "We needed something that would leave it up to the tables rather than the people," he told me, and meta-analysis was perfect for the job. "The idea was you would have to present evidence in tabular form that would be so convincing it would jump up and grab people by the throats."

"We put a lot of faith in meta-analysis," Frances told me.

Not that he expected to use meta-analysis to sort out the arguments, at least not very often. "You need lots of data from lots of sources for a meta-analysis," he said. "And I knew that the literature didn't have the data. I knew we couldn't do a real meta-analysis of most of what would come up." If someone brought up one of those off-the-cuff ideas in a meeting, or collared him with a pet proposal at dinner, Frances would just tell him to bring him the data, which he was pretty sure didn't exist. Meta-analysis would protect the DSM-IV (not to mention Frances) from the pontificators, the profession from confusion, the common language from its own tenuousness. With statistics guarding the gate, the revision would be modest. It might also be boring, but, Frances says, "dull is better than arbitrary." Seven years after he met with Pincus, when the DSM-IV was released, it was nearly four hundred pages longer than the DSM-III-R, but most of the expansion was in the explanatory sections. Only a few new diagnoses had crossed Frances's threshold, and the book remained fundamentally the same kind of manual. Just as he had promised, Frances had deferred to the tradition originated by Spitzer.

Not every psychiatrist loved the mutt. Among its more prominent detractors was Steven Hyman, who in 1996 became the head of the National Institute of Mental Health. A neurogeneticist by training, Hyman hadn't thought much about nosology before taking over at NIMH. It "seemed a bit like stamp collecting," he once wrote, "an absorbing activity perhaps, but not a vibrant area of inquiry." But then he realized that the DSM was "a critical platform for research." Its categories and criteria were the basis of decisions made by journal editors, grant reviewers, regulators, and the Food and Drug Administration, which meant that scientists were bound to frame their proposals in the DSM's language. "DSM-IV diagnoses controlled the research questions they could ask, and perhaps, even imagine."

"The tendency [is] always strong," John Stuart Mill wrote in 1869, "to believe that whatever receives a name must be an entity or being, having an independent existence of its own." To Hyman, who quoted Mill approvingly, this tendency had led all the stakeholders in nosology—scientists, regulators, editors, doctors, drug companies, and, of course, patients—to take the labels as more than labels, as the names of actual diseases. They had, at least according to Hyman, *reified* what were intended only as concepts. And this was no mere abstract concern.

It became a source of real worry to me, that as Institute director, I might be signing off on the expenditure of large sums of taxpayers' money for ... projects that almost never questioned the existing diagnostic categories despite their lack of validation.

The DSM, Hyman concluded, had "created an unintended epistemic prison," and anyone with a stake in the mental health treatment system was trapped inside.

While he was at NIMH, Hyman had occasion to confide his reservations to at least one colleague: Steven Mirin, then medical director of the APA. Both men had been affiliated with Harvard and lived in the Boston area, but they'd become friends only after they had both arrived in Washington and their kids started attending the same schools. On a weekend afternoon in the summer of 1998, they were eating lunch by the side of Mirin's suburban swimming pool when Mirin asked Hyman if NIMH would give the APA money to get the next revision of the DSM up and running.

Mirin's request for taxpayer money to kick-start a project from which a private organization would reap huge profits was not as untoward as it might seem. After all, the DSM is indispensable to public health, and NIMH had helped fund the DSM-IV. Nonetheless, and despite their friendship, Hyman said no. He told Mirin that a revision was premature, not only because the ink was barely dry on the DSM-IV, but more important, because psychiatrists had yet to come up with a better way to carve up the landscape of mental illness. All they could do, Hyman thought, was continue to create and refine concepts that would then be mistaken for real disease entities, and further trap psychiatry in its epistemic prison. Until someone figured out how to fashion a key, Hyman didn't think there was much point to another revision, and he wasn't going to provide any public money for one. After all, you don't remodel a house when the foundation is infested with termites.

Mirin didn't fight back—mostly, he says, because he didn't disagree. "The DSM was a system based on descriptive criteria influenced by experts in the field," Mirin told me. "They had lots of opinions, but these couldn't necessarily be validated." The uncertainty out of which the diagnoses were fashioned could not help but show up in the clinic.

"It's one thing to guess and another to biopsy a tumor or to measure an enzyme," Mirin said. And both he and Hyman knew which method the DSM had saddled them with. Spitzer may have freed them from Freudian metaphysics, but still, as Mirin put it, "we were stuck with making diagnoses based on scripture."

Even so, America's leading psychiatrists weren't about to renounce the only scriptures they had—mostly because, as much as they knew the DSM was flawed, they didn't have anything with which to replace it. "I realized that it got me nowhere to criticize the DSM because that did not offer a constructive alternative," Hyman told me. "In fact, given the way the DSM had controlled the imagination of scientists, there was little information with which to see beyond it."

Hyman may have been anguishing about psychiatry's predicament, but Mirin wasn't losing any sleep over the fact that his profession was stuck guessing about categories that didn't really exist. "I don't recall feeling particularly tortured about it. The DSM was essential to being paid for treatment. Without its methodology, payors would see mental illnesses as figments of a provider's imagination." It was also essential to the APA's finances. After all, Mirin told me, "coming down the mountain with the Ten Commandments sure sells a lot of books."

Of all his accomplishments during his tenure in Washington, Steve Mirin seems proudest of the time he persuaded *The Washington Post* to support legislation requiring insurers to pay for mental health care at the same level as other medical services. So far, *parity*, as this mandate was called, had only been implemented in a few states, and often only for mental disorders considered by insurers to be biological in origin. In

2002, there was a bill pending in Congress that would make it binding everywhere and for the entire range of DSM-IV diagnoses. President George W. Bush had endorsed it, but the bill seemed likely to sink into the mud of the legislative process, in part, Mirin thought, because the *Post*—"the hometown paper of every member of Congress," as he put it—had twice come out against parity. So he arranged to meet on September 3 with an editorial page editor to see if he could sway the paper's opinion.

Mirin arrived expecting an hour with a single editor, so he was surprised and pleased when six editors and a reporter filed into the conference room and talked with him for nearly ninety minutes. He may not have been losing sleep over it, but the editors did their best to torment him with the discrepancy between the DSM's authority and the actual science behind it. They "asked questions such as 'How do you diagnose mental illness?' and 'How do you tell if it's real?' and 'Do you have a science base like the rest of medicine does?'" Mirin told the *Psychiatric News*.

Mirin was prepared for this inquisition. His press office had briefed him about the ways of reporters, and his staff had subjected him to a mock grilling. Nor did he have to face it alone. He'd brought with him an expert on diagnostic questions: Darrel Regier, whom he had recently hired to head up the APA's research arm, the American Psychiatric Institute for Research and Education. Mirin had recruited Regier from the National Institute of Mental Health, where he had risen to the rank of vice admiral in the Public Health Service. Regier was attractive to Mirin in part because of his familiarity with the ways of government bureaucracies, but at least as important was the fact that Regier, an epidemiologist as well as a psychiatrist, had been measuring the levels of mental illness in the population since the earliest days of DSM-III.

What Regier had seen didn't inspire confidence. As the head of the NIMH's Epidemiological Catchment Area (ECA) team, he had overseen a group of researchers who, starting in 1980, fanned out across five U.S. cities armed with a questionnaire keyed to the diagnostic criteria in DSM-III. They'd asked twenty thousand people, selected to reflect the general population, about their worries and their sadness, about whether they heard voices, about how they slept and ate. They tabulated the results and, in 1984, began to release them in a series of journal articles.

The ECA's findings were stunning. In any given year, more than 20 percent of Americans qualified for a DSM-III diagnosis. Nearly one-third of us—eighty million people, according to the 1990 census—would have a mental illness in our lifetimes. And the sick among us were really sick. Sixty percent of those diagnosed with a mental illness had a *comorbid disorder*, meaning they qualified for at least two diagnoses. Ninety-one percent of people with schizophrenia had at least one other diagnosis, as did 75 percent of people with a depressive disorder. Fifteen percent had three or more diseases. More than half of the people with a drug-related diagnosis, such as Cannabis Abuse, also had a second (or third) diagnosis. Even more alarming, only 19 percent of the afflicted had sought help for their troubles, a number that dropped to 13 percent in the cases where only one diagnosis was warranted. It seemed that America had an enormous but unacknowledged and untreated public health problem whose effects on productivity, on family life, and on the body politic were unfathomable.

This potential fivefold increase in the size of the market for psychiatry wasn't so much an embarrassment of riches as a plain embarrassment. Even accounting for the fact that epidemiological studies, in which researchers go out looking for trouble, almost always yield bigger numbers than studies that rely on numbers gleaned from doctors' offices and hospitals, the results beggared imagination. They also cast doubt on the DSM. The questions at least had to be asked: Was the problem in the minds of the people or in the methods of the doctors? Did the DSM-III make it too easy to turn people's everyday troubles into disease? Was the book that saved the profession going to lead it to another downfall?

Two decades later, Regier thinks the answers are all too clear. I interviewed him in 2010, in his spacious office on a high floor of APA headquarters in Arlington, Virginia. At sixty-seven, he has a smooth, unlined face. His tie is tightly knotted, his shirt as crisp and neat as his office. He gives off a quiet confidence, the certainty of a man who has crunched the numbers and seen the results, and concluded that "we just don't have good thresholds for identifying what we would consider mental disorders." Having eliminated any account of the origin or nature of mental illness in favor of pure observation, the DSM-III had also eliminated the thresholds, vague as they might be, provided by Freud's insistence that mental illness was distinguished by its origins in intrapsychic conflict. The resulting symptom-based diagnosis is binary; if you have five of the nine symptoms of depression, you have the same disorder as a person with all nine, just as if you have a small stage 1 tumor in your lung, you have the same disease as someone with the same kind of tumor who is about to die. With those five symptoms, as with the first appearance of the tumor, you have crossed the line from health to illness, and the rest is only a question of severity.

But, as those prevalence numbers made clear, doctors using DSM checklists were all too likely to find disease everywhere. There was no governor, no way to say this person was sick and that one was simply unhappy, nothing like the CT scan that confirms that the patient with the persistent cough and fatigue has a tumor in his lung. A doctor who diagnosed strep entirely on the basis of symptoms was practicing bad medicine, while a doctor who diagnosed depression only on the basis of symptoms was practicing standard psychiatry. It seemed that in his attempt to make psychiatry look more like the rest of medicine, Spitzer had actually fashioned a book that only highlighted the differences.

The comorbidity rates—the frequency with which people qualified for more than one diagnosis—were another embarrassment. Here again, Regier said, the ECA studies pointed not so much to a sick population as to a flawed manual. Spitzer had anticipated the possibility of multiple diagnoses, and in the introduction to DSM-III he suggested that there was a hierarchy of mental illness, that some disorders only had a narrow range of symptoms while others contained multitudes. Schizophrenia, for instance, was far more encompassing than major depression, so clinicians confronted with a patient presenting symptoms of both were advised to render only a schizophrenia diagnosis on the assumption that the low mood was part of the more comprehensive disorder. Regier pointed out that this amounts to a claim that the depression itself is "just noise," of no inherent interest or value in understanding the patient or their disorders. But the ECA team found that people with symptoms of both schizophrenia and depression were different from people with only schizophrenia in many ways. Ignoring their depression meant failing to get a complete diagnostic picture and losing "an enormous amount of data" about mental health. "The ECA blew the hierarchy out of the water," Regier said proudly. "It just didn't make any sense when we started looking at the data."

Concerns like this led the APA to abandon the hierarchy in the DSM-III-R, but the real problem, Regier told me, was not the approach but something much more basic: the idea that DSM disorders are discrete diseases that exist in nature in the same way as cancer and diabetes. This, to Regier, is the fundamental flaw of the DSM, the one that accounts for the high rates of both prevalence and comorbidity. "It makes it seem like an anxiety disorder doesn't have any mood symptoms and a mood disorder doesn't have any anxiety symptoms. But it isn't that simple. It's just not the way people present."

But it is the way the DSM presents mental illness; indeed, that neat separation is the signal innovation of the DSM-III. Fortunately for Mirin and Regier, by the time of their fateful meeting with the *Post* editors, they'd turned their skepticism into a strategy. "We walked them through how we understood mental illness, and what our thoughts were about diagnosis and the DSM," Mirin recalled. Not, of course, their thoughts about the book's failure to correspond to clinical reality or about the way the categorical approach trapped diagnosticians in a tautological loop (which, after all, were highly technical matters, known and understood only by experts), but rather their thoughts about the troubles reported in the daily paper that might make the average editor skeptical: the shifting sands of psychiatric diagnosis, the prevalence rates, the frequent and repeated revisions of the nosology, the disorders that came and went with dismaying regularity. These they readily acknowledged, but then they turned them to advantage. The problem wasn't that psychiatry was inexact when compared with the rest of medicine, but rather that the rest of medicine was nowhere near as certain as it was cracked up to be. The glucose levels that constitute diabetes, the cholesterol counts that call for treatment, the blood pressure that qualifies as hypertension—these numbers had all changed over time, and after no small amount of wrangling. To hold psychiatry to a more stringent standard was unfair and would make victims of doctor and patient alike.

This approach was exactly the right one for his audience. "They were smart people," Mirin said. "They were sophisticated enough to understand that what their doctor told them about hypertension was not carved in stone, either." If the *Post*'s editors noticed the intellectual sleight-of-hand at work here, the way that these leading psychiatrists were distancing themselves from the same claims to certainty that had allowed the DSM to rescue psychiatry from the pseudoscience precipice (or, for that matter, if they wondered whether or not they should keep taking their diuretics), they didn't say, at least not in print. Perhaps they were afraid they'd seem unsophisticated or just plain dumb. Either way, six days after the meeting, the paper came out in favor of parity, Congress passed a limited version of the bill, and mental health professionals everywhere rejoiced. Six years and many editorials later, parity became the law of the land. Mirin and Regier's strategy succeeded. They had spun the dross of diagnostic uncertainty into gold.

Maybe you're not smart or sophisticated enough to understand this argument, either. Maybe you think Mirin and Regier were just trying to have it both ways. You might then suggest that those prevalence numbers were still a little fishy. You might wonder out loud what would happen if 25 or 30 percent of the population exceeded the standard glucose or blood pressure thresholds, but only 19 percent of that group—about 5 percent of the population—ever got sick enough to even show up at their doctor's office. You might then ask what exactly those numbers added up to, whether they measured disease at all, and if the whole idea of hypertension or type 2 diabetes had been created by an industry too interested in selling treatments to people who were actually healthy. You might point out that regardless of whether or not they are diseases in themselves or only risk factors, blood pressure and glucose levels can at least be measured with a high degree of certainty. And you might raise the question of whether or not it's really fair to compare conditions such as high glucose and blood pressure to mental illnesses, whether or not telling a patient he has hypertension for which he should take diuretics is really the same kind of intervention as telling him he has a chemical imbalance that antidepressants will correct.

Darrel Regier would have an answer for some of those questions. You think those numbers are high? Well, he would tell you, or at least he told me, you should see the Midtown Manhattan Study. Regier started his training with the people who ran that project, which began in 1952, took ten years to complete, and was conducted exactly where you think it was. Researchers canvassed 1,911 Manhattanites and concluded, according to Regier, that 85 percent of the population had a mental illness.

When Regier graduated from Indiana University's medical school in 1970, the Midtown Manhattan Study still constituted the standard epidemiology of mental illness. "I was just coming out of a residency where I was seeing really sick patients," he said, "and I'm saying to myself, 'What are they talking about over here with all of these people who have an occasional symptom but are never going to go into treatment? What is normality if 85 percent have a mental illness?'"

The Midtown Manhattan Study is a talking point for most defenders of the DSM. They cite that 85 percent number as evidence that even if the DSM is an imperfect document, and even if it catches an improbable number of people in its diagnostic net, at least it's better than what we had in the old days. We in the mental health business call this a *downward comparison*, and we sometimes recommend one to our patients to help them put their problems in perspective. "Yes, it's true your wife left you for your next-door neighbor," you might say, "but at least your kids won't have to commute as far as most children of divorce." It's usually a pretty lame intervention, as that example indicates, and to the extent that it's successful, it's often because you're actually bolstering the patient's self-esteem by pointing out that he's better off than the next guy. Schadenfreudian therapy, you might call it.

You can't exactly blame psychiatrists for grasping at this straw. But some straws are flimsier than others. Take that 85 percent number, for instance. The Midtown Manhattan Study team, which was headed by sociologist Leo Srole, never said that 85 percent of its subjects were mentally ill. In fact, Srole and his colleagues hadn't set out to diagnose New Yorkers at all. Indeed, they wrote, they didn't want to use the DSM or any other diagnostic system because they were "designed for classifying full-blown pathology"—and didn't do such a good job of defining it in the first place. So rather than ask about symptoms of mental illnesses, they asked about childhood fears of thunder and strangers, and current attitudes toward drinking and gambling. They solicited subjects' worries about the atom bomb and old age. They asked whether they thought people talked behind their backs or if they wondered whether "anything is worthwhile" or if they believed that "most people think a lot about sex." They paid attention to whether the interviewees were sloppy or neat, nervous or relaxed, if they were facetious, dull, or rambling. They attempted, in other words, to capture the everyday experience of the average citizen and to determine how much psychological suffering it entailed.

To make their assay, Srole's team devised a six-point classification of *symptom formation*. People at the "healthy extreme" got a zero. At the next two stages were people who had "emotional disturbance without apparent constriction or disability," and the last three ratings "span[ned] the morbidity range of the mental health spectrum." These were the people whose symptoms had "crippling effects on the performance of . . . daily life roles"—as close to a working definition of mental illness as Srole's team ventured.

Like Karl Menninger and most mainstream psychiatrists and sociologists at the time, Srole and his colleagues subscribed to the Freudian notion that between the dynamics of our psyches and the demands of civilization, virtually everyone was bound to be troubled and that, as they wrote, "mental illness and mental health [differed] in degree rather than in kind." So when it turned out that something like 85 percent of the subjects (the actual number is 81.5 percent) scored more than a zero, the researchers could have been no more surprised than the audience at a Woody Allen movie would be to discover that most Manhattanites are at least a little neurotic. But Srole and his team weren't making the ridiculous claim that 85 percent of us are mentally ill. Rather, they were reporting the unremarkable finding that if you sit down with people and ask them about their emotional lives, you will find that most of them will confess to some difficulty.

The abnormal people in this study, as in most studies, were those at the ends of the spectrum—the 15 percent who claimed to be free of psychic turmoil, and the 23.4 percent who scored in the morbid range.

This latter finding, Srole noted, was a bit of a surprise. It was mo
double the rate of mental illness found in an earlier study of Balti
eans. But it was fully one-third *less* than the number of people wh
would, twenty-five years later, turn up as mentally ill in Regier's ECA
study, and surely nowhere near 85 percent.

Regier knows that Srole's study didn't really conclude that 85 percent of its subjects were mentally ill. Indeed, he cited the 23 percent figure accurately in a 1978 report to a presidential commission on mental health. He also knows about the Baltimore study, and about a National Institutes of Health study conducted by his mentor, psychiatrist Michael Shepherd, which found a prevalence rate of around 15 percent. That, in fact, was the figure he used in his report to the president: on any given day, he wrote, about 15 percent of Americans were mentally ill.

Regier thinks Shepherd's study is "a classic," and the 15 percent figure "wonderful." It's easy to see why he didn't lead his presentation to the *Post* editors with his conviction, based on a quarter century of studying the subject, that prevalence rates had been inflated by the DSM—published, remember, by the organization he was working for—or, for that matter, that the categorical approach to diagnosis didn't reflect the reality of mental illness. He and Mirin had a guild to represent, and telling the editors that parity laws would force insurers to pay for the treatment of people who didn't necessarily have illnesses that didn't really exist would probably not have been the best way to do that.

Besides, by the time they took on the *Post*, Mirin and Regier were already beginning to plan for the DSM-5. The book they had in mind was no mere sequel. If it worked out the way they wanted it to, it would be a DSM to end all DSMs.

Chapter 4

Steve Mirin took Steve Hyman's refusal to give the APA money for a new DSM as a challenge. "Steve was putting pressure on the field to start to consider a different approach to diagnosis," he told me. Mirin shared both Hyman's wish to put psychiatry on a new footing and an idea about what that foundation should be. "Steve and I had an agenda," Mirin told me. "To introduce neuroscience into diagnosis."

The 1990s had been, by presidential decree, the Decade of the Brain. Billions of dollars had been spent trying to get the brain to give up its secrets. Much of that money had gone to brain scanning devices, especially the functional magnetic resonance imager (fMRI), a miracle machine that allowed scientists to glimpse the brain at work. No university research lab worth its salt lacked one, and scientists, flush with grant money, slid their subjects inside to perform innumerable tasks. They solved math problems and played video games, remembered sad times and anticipated pleasures, considered moral dilemmas, took drugs, looked at porn, and even (in France, of course) had sex. All the while, the machines whirred and clanked, recording a comprehensive account of the brain at work.

Actually, all the machines were tracking was the movement of oxygen carried by blood through the brain, a record reassembled by computers into images colorized for greater effect. Like kids in the pee-wee league chasing a soccer ball, your blood races around your brain to sites that are becoming active, and scientists inferred from observing this movement that those areas were the parts of the brain responsible for the behavior or experience under study. And so there was an unceasing flow of news reports, accompanied by those increasingly familiar full-color fMRI images, about what the brain did when it thought no one was looking, about which area of the brain gave rise to this faculty or that thought, about the latest secret of consciousness uncovered by science.

The enthusiasm was contagious. By the time the Decade of the Brain had ended, Nobel laureate Eric Kandel was proclaiming that "the mind is a set of operations carried out by the brain, much as walking is a set of operations carried out by the legs." The fact that the pictures that seemed to prove this were only prettied-up shots of the blood rocketing around in the brain and that they left unobserved the networks that connect these lit-up areas, not to mention that they ignored the enormous philosophical questions begged by these claims—Was the brain *causing* the experience, or simply *responding* to the mind's demand? Could mind be reduced to body? Was the whole of consciousness no more than the sum of its parts?—had disappeared in the enthusiasm of conquering what had only recently seemed to be an impenetrable terrain.

Kandel, a psychiatrist, believed that scientists now knew enough to say something else with confidence about the mind: that "all mental disorders involve disorders of brain function." He never specified what *involve* meant, but Thomas Insel, Hyman's successor at NIMH, didn't hesitate to turn this idea into something less equivocal—and less tautological. "We can think of mental disorders not just as brain disorders but as disorders of brain circuits," he told psychiatrists at a conference. This equivalence meant that psychiatry would one day be transformed into "clinical neuroscience." Psychiatrists could finally move beyond the observation of symptoms and signs, and uncover the world behind the world of mental illness, so they could finally say with authority which mental disorders exist and who has them. They would be able to leave behind the approach that was at once its salvation and its scourge: a classification of diseases based on description and observation but with no account of what caused them. And then they would be able to meet the scientific demands of the day.

Neuroscience was not new to psychiatrists. In the 1930s and 1940s, even as Freudian theory was coming to dominate American psychiatry, powerful biological treatments—electroshock therapy, insulin comas, and lobotomies—were convincing many doctors that the brain could be treated like any other organ in the body. Its workings were immensely complex, the biological psychiatrists allowed, but the difficulty of unraveling them was only a formidable technical challenge. There was no reason that the mysteries of consciousness could not be solved by understanding the brain. Long before the first subject slid into the first fMRI machine, at least some doctors thought it was only a matter of time before mental illness was vanquished by the same weapons that had undone pneumonia.

Other psychiatrists were less sanguine. As early as 1917, Adolf Meyer, director of the psychiatry department at Johns Hopkins and the unofficial dean of American psychiatry, worried that biological psychiatry was a collection of "neurologizing tautologies." Sure, the brain was involved in consciousness and its troubles, Meyer said, but to single it out as the *cause* of suffering was to go beyond the existing evidence, and perhaps beyond any possible evidence. Post hoc, as the logicians say, does not mean propter hoc. That a depressed patient emerged from a shock treatment undepressed does not prove that the cause of depression was in the brain's electrical activity. Indeed, some shock therapists in the 1930s wondered if they weren't merely "driving the Devil out of our patients with Beelzebub."

The doctors' assertion that they had found the source of mental illness was based on deduction; they had to assume that the brain was the causal agent in order to conclude that mental illness was an effect. They also had to assume that the neurological dysfunction, whatever it was,

was both the necessary and the sufficient condition for the psychological problem. Brain-based psychiatry was in this respect no less tautological than symptom-based psychiatry, the brain's role as a causal agent more myth than science. Scientists and laypeople alike, Meyer warned, should approach these findings with caution.

But it was hard to argue with the biological psychiatrists when their schizophrenic patients awoke from insulin-induced comas coherent and rational (if only temporarily) or when their shock machines roused depressed people from their torpor. It was even harder to argue with the doctors who in the early 1950s experimented on themselves and lab animals with LSD, discovered that the drug was closely related to a recently discovered brain chemical—serotonin—and, based on the profound alterations of consciousness the drug induced, concluded that the brain conducted its business in an electrochemical currency. Most persuasive of all, however, was the serendipitous discovery of drugs that seemed to target specific mental illnesses, presumably by targeting those chemicals—Thorazine for schizophrenia, for instance, and imipramine for depression. These developments were all accidental, and scientists could not fully explain any of them, but even so, they could not help but reinforce the idea that mental illnesses existed in nature, specifically in the brain, and that they were not unlike infectious diseases—the result of a biochemical process that could be found and turned into a target for one of medicine's magic bullets.

By the mid-1960s, biological psychiatrists thought they were zeroing in on the process in question: deficiencies or surpluses in the chemicals known as neurotransmitters. In 1965, Joseph Schildkraut, a National Institutes of Health scientist, claimed to have reverse-engineered antidepressants and found that they worked by increasing levels of dopamine and adrenaline in the brain; depression, he announced, must be the result of deficiencies in those two neurotransmitters. Within a decade, however, scientists had determined that Schildkraut was wrong, and they settled on another possibility, their old friend serotonin. What seemed never to be in doubt as the doctors rushed from theory to theory was the idea that one brain chemical or another was the cause of mental suffering, just as one bacterium or another must be the cause of infection.

By the early 1990s, millions were taking Prozac for their serotonin deficiencies. Biological psychiatry had established a foothold deep in the popular and professional culture. Our everyday understanding of ourselves now included the idea that we are neurotransmitter-powered thinking and feeling machines. All that was left was to figure out the particulars.

But these details were especially devilish. By the time Mirin and Hyman began dreaming of a DSM-5, near the end of the Decade of the Brain, there was still not one biological test for a DSM disorder. The idea that a lack of serotonin caused depression had been abandoned for lack of evidence (and for contradictory findings) almost as quickly as it arose, except in doctors' offices, where it proved immensely useful to physicians trying to persuade reluctant patients to take their drugs. The attempt to find the genetic underpinnings of mental disorders had also been frustrated.

In part, of course, the failure to find the pathological anatomy of psychological suffering could be blamed on the complexity of our neurochemistry and genetic architecture, especially when it came to the brain. But Hyman thought there was an additional problem. "The gold standard was the DSM criteria," he told me. "It struck me as a fool's errand to try to develop a biomarker for a fictive category." The lack of molecular evidence only reinforced what doctors like Mirin and Hyman already knew—that the DSM-III's nosology only *looked* scientific, that the empire of psychiatry was still built on air.

In 2002, the APA officially announced that Spitzer's mutt had had its day. In *A Research Agenda for DSM-V*, a book that kicked off the official revision effort, the APA acknowledged that the reification of the DSM-IV's categories, "to the point that they are considered to be the equivalent of diseases," had most likely "hindered research." Nor was "research exclusively focused on refining the DSM-defined syndromes [likely to] be successful in uncovering their underlying etiologies." Searching for the causes of the illnesses listed in the DSM was proving to be not unlike a drunk looking for his car keys under a streetlight even if that's not where he dropped them. Scientists were unlikely to find the causes of Generalized Anxiety Disorder or Major Depressive Disorder or any of the other DSM categories—as descriptive psychiatrists had been promising to do since Kraepelin—because it increasingly seemed unlikely that they really were the equivalent of diseases.

So the APA did what organizations everywhere do when they find themselves flummoxed. They convened a committee. To be exact, they convened thirteen committees that, beginning in 2004, held a series of "planning conferences" at APA headquarters. Because the conferences were explicitly devoted to finding that new paradigm—which, according to the *Research Agenda*, was "yet unknown"—the NIMH helped pay for them.

Among the people Regier appointed to organize the conferences was a Columbia University psychiatrist named Michael First. First had been the text editor for the DSM-IV and the editor of the DSM-IV-TR. Since 1990, part of his salary at Columbia had been paid by the APA, for which he consulted on all matters related to the DSM. He'd already worked on DSM-5, editing the *Research Agenda* and writing its foreword.

When he's not traveling around the world, lecturing on diagnostic issues or consulting to the Centers for Disease Control or the World Health Organization or teaching clinicians how to use the DSM, First can be found in a basement office at the New York State Psychiatric Institute, part of Columbia Presbyterian hospital on the northern tip of Manhattan. He's bent over in his office chair when I arrive, searching for something amid the piles of papers that have spilled over from his desk and tables and onto the floor. Bearded and rumpled, he looks like a psychiatrist in a *New Yorker* cartoon. When he talks, thoughts tumble out like the papers in his office, one on top of another, but somehow usually making sense. So you'd be mistaken to think that he's absentminded. If I hadn't interrupted him, he would surely have reached into the mess and found just what he was looking for, just as he seems to be able to rummage around in his memory and retrieve the slightest detail of the DSM's history.

"In a way, I was born to do the DSM," First told me. But he didn't always think so. "When I first saw DSM-III"—at the University of Pittsburgh's medical school in 1978—"I thought it was preposterous. I saw the Chinese-menu approach and thought, 'This is how they do diagnosis in psychiatry?' It seemed overly mechanical and didn't fit my idea of what the study of the mind and psychiatry should be."

First had a second love: computer science, which he had pursued as an undergraduate at Princeton. He'd almost chucked pre-med for computers, and during medical school, he continued his interest, working with a team using artificial intelligence for diagnosis in internal medicine. He took a year off to earn a master's degree in computer science, working on a program to diagnose neurological problems. When he returned to medical school, he settled on psychiatry as his specialty, and his interest in using computers to aid diagnosticians made that Chinese menu approach seem not quite so preposterous. "I thought, 'Well, psychiatry is actually relatively straightforward. It's got a book with rules in it already—an obvious good fortune if I was going to try to get a computer to be able to do this." Which he was, and which is why he decided to go to the New York State Psychiatric Institute, the professional home of Bob Spitzer, where he planned to exploit his good fortune.

Spitzer had already flirted with computer-assisted diagnosis in the 1970s, when he was first developing the criteria-based approach. He'd abandoned the attempt, however, and soured on the idea. First managed to negotiate a bargain: he could work on his program so long as he helped out with one of Spitzer's—an old-fashioned paper-and-pencil test Spitzer was developing called Structured Clinical Interview for DSM Disorders, or SCID. The SCID, which is still in use, is straightforward to use. If you answer yes when the doctor asks you if you've been sad for two weeks or more, then he is directed to ask you about the next criterion for depression—whether or not you have lost interest in your usual activities. If you answer no, then he moves on to a criterion for a different disorder. This goes on for forty-five minutes or so, the questions shunting you from one branch of the diagnostic tree to the next until you land on the leaf that is your diagnosis.

First eventually did develop his own diagnostic program. He called it DTREE, but it was a commercial failure. "I learned a lesson," First said. "Doctors don't care much about diagnosis. They use diagnosis mostly for codes. They don't really care what the rules are." When a patient comes in complaining of pervasive worry and jitters, with a little dread thrown in, most clinicians don't take the time to climb around on the diagnostic tree. They don't bother consulting the DSM's list of criteria to diagnose Generalized Anxiety Disorder. They just write the code, 300.02, in the chart (and on the bill) and move on.

"That was my first lesson in how people think about diagnosis," First told me.

First doesn't think the solution is more reverence toward the DSM. Indeed, there may be only one thing worse than not paying attention to the DSM and that is paying it too much heed. "I think people take diagnosis too seriously," he said. The DSM may appear to be a master text of psychological suffering, but this is misleading. "The fiction that diagnosis could be boiled down to a set of rules is something that people find very appealing, but I think it's gotten out of hand. It is a convenient language for communication, and nothing more." The rules are important, but they should not be applied outside of a very particular game.

In this respect, First thinks, "the DSM has been a victim of its own success." If it was merely the lexicon that gave psychiatrists a way to talk to one another, then it might live in the same dusty obscurity as, say, *Interventional Radiology in Women's Health* or *Consensus in Clinical Nutrition* does. If it was treated as a convenient fiction fashioned by expert consensus, and not the embodiment of a scientific understanding of human functioning, then newspapers would not be giving psychiatrists valuable op-ed real estate to debate its merits. If it hadn't escaped its professional confines, it would not be seen as a Rosetta Stone capable of decoding the complexities of our inner lives. If it had not become an epistemic prison, psychiatrists wouldn't be languishing in it, trying to find the biological correlates of disorders that don't really exist, that were invented rather than discovered, whose inventors never meant to make such mischief, and whose sufferers, apparently unreasonably, take medical diagnoses seriously enough to expect them to be real.

First is right about at least one thing. Most clinicians don't care what the DSM's rules are. I know I don't. I rarely take it down off my shelf. I use only a handful of the codes and by now I know them by heart.

At the top of my favorites list is 309.28, which stands for Adjustment Disorder with Mixed Anxiety and Depressed Mood. Here's how the DSM-IV defines it:

A. The development of emotional or behavioral symptoms in response to an identifiable stressor(s) occurring within 3 months of the onset of the stressor(s)

B. These symptoms or behaviors are clinically significant as evidenced by either of the following

1. marked distress that is in excess of what would be expected from exposure to the stressor

2. significant impairment in social or occupational (academic) functioning

C. The stress-related disturbance does not meet the criteria for another disorder

D. The symptoms do not represent Bereavement

E. Once the stressor (or its consequences) has terminated, the symptoms do not persist for more than an additional 6 months

I'm sure you can see why 309.28 is popular with clinicians, and why insurance company claims examiners probably see it all the time. It sounds innocuous, which makes it go down easy with patients (if, as I do, you tell your patients which mental illness you are now adding to their medical dossier) and with employers or insurers or others who might have occasion to scrutinize a patient's medical history and be put off by a more serious-sounding diagnosis. It offers all kinds of diagnostic flexibility. Take Criterion B1, for instance. It is easy to meet; it is easy enough to use the fact that the patient made an appointment as evidence of "marked distress." And that lovely parenthetical in Criterion E makes it possible to re-up the patient even after the six months have elapsed.

But Adjustment Disorder also has a special place in my heart because it was my own first diagnosis, or at least the first one I knew about. I got it sometime in the early 1980s, when I was in my early twenties and the DSM was in its third edition. I don't remember why I wanted to be in therapy or very much of what I talked about with my therapist. I do remember that my father was paying for it. He was probably hoping I would discover that my self-chosen circumstances—living alone in a cabin in the woods without the modern conveniences—were a symptom of something that could be cured. What I was being treated for, however, was not "Back to the Land Disorder" or "Why Don't You Grow Up Already Disorder," but rather, as I discovered one day when I glanced down at my statement on the receptionist's desk, Adjustment Disorder.

I guess the tag seemed about right. I definitely wasn't adjusting; and if it occurred to me that by calling my lifestyle an illness (if indeed that's what he meant to do, as opposed to just rendering the most innocuous-sounding diagnosis possible), my therapist had passed judgment on exactly where the problem resided, I didn't think much of it at the time. But I do remember that I noticed, for the first time, that I'd been going to these weekly appointments in a *doctor's office*. It happened to be in a building adjacent to the office of my childhood pediatrician, but it did not smell like alcohol or have a white-shoed woman bustling about, nor did its business seem a bit related to the shots and probes I'd suffered next door, so the discord stood out. But still the fact of that diagnosis, right there in black-and-white, was undeniable. I was a mental patient.

I was eventually cured of my maladjustment—not by therapy, but by a family coup that resulted in my grandfather's being relieved of the farm he'd inherited from his mother. That happened to be the land on which I'd built my home, and so I was evicted, my cabin eventually bulldozed and the land converted to McMansions, and it became necessary for me to earn a living. Of the many adjustments I have had to make, diagnosing people in order to secure an income was one of the strangest—not only because the DSM's labels seemed so insufficient, its criteria so deracinated, the whole procedure so banal in comparison with the rich and disturbing and ultimately inexhaustible conversation that was occurring in my office, but also, and much more important, because of the bad faith involved. I didn't mind colluding with my patients against the insurance companies; sometimes I actually enjoyed the thought. I brought them in on the scam, explaining exactly what diagnosis I was giving them, sometimes even taking out the book and reading the criteria and occasionally offering them a choice. But the fact that we were sharing the lie didn't make our business any less dishonest.

I know therapists who diagnose everyone with Adjustment Disorder unless the insurance company limits benefits for its treatment on the grounds that it isn't enough of an illness to warrant much treatment—at which point the patient often contracts a sudden case of something much worse, like Major Depressive Disorder. Myself, I prefer to mix things up a little. But mostly I prefer not to do business with insurance companies, so I often don't have to bother with such dilemmas. Of course, that means I get paid less money, since not everyone can afford my rates without a little help from their friends at Aetna, so I end up giving people a break in return for steering clear of the whole unsavory business. Over the thirty years I've been in practice, I've probably left a couple million dollars on the table by avoiding the DSM. It's an expensive habit, but I think of it as buying my way out of bad faith.

And it's not just my rank-and-file colleagues and I who think of the DSM as if it were a colonoscopy: a necessary evil, something to be endured and quickly forgotten, and surely not to be taken seriously unless you have to. I once asked psychiatrist and former president of the APA Paul Fink to tell me how the DSM was helpful in his daily practice.

"I have a patient that I've been seeing for two months," he told me. "And my secretary said, 'What's the diagnosis?' I thought a lot about it because I hadn't really formulated it, and then I began to think: What are her symptoms? What does she do? How does she behave? I diagnosed her with obsessive-compulsive disorder."

"Did this change the way you treated her?" I asked.

"No."

"So what was its value, would you say?"

"I got paid."

It is at least ironic that a profession once dedicated to the pursuit of psychological truth is now dependent on this kind of dishonesty for its survival. But I suppose that any system guided by the invisible hand—financial markets no more than health care financing—is bound to be gamed. And the DSM, whatever its flaws, has proved to be a superb playbook.

Maybe Michael First's claim that psychiatry is somehow the victim of the selfsame diagnostic manual that pulled its chestnuts out of the fire sounds disingenuous to you, too. After all, the DSM-III could easily have been written in the medical Latinese that doctors usually use when they want to leave us out of the conversation, and its authors could have stuck with those original few diagnoses instead of trying to catalog every problem patients wanted help with, from bed-wetting to binge eating, from Frotteurism ("recurrent, intense, sexually arousing fantasies, urges or behaviors involving touching and rubbing against a nonconsenting person") to Factitious Disorder (when a patient, likely conversant with the DSM, has no mental disorder other than the one that makes him make up having a mental disorder), from Nightmare Disorder to Nicotine Withdrawal. Spitzer didn't have to invite his colleagues to nominate their favorite disorders or try to repair psychiatry's reputation with scientific rhetoric. Indeed, it is hard to imagine any outcome of a DSM tailored to give scientific names to the vast range of our travails other than the one Hyman and First decry. The whole point was to get psychiatry taken seriously by proving that mental illnesses weren't just the figments of some psychiatrists' imaginations and that clinicians weren't treating mere problems of living. If the DSM hadn't been written as an authoritative medical guide to all of mental suffering, it would not have restored the profession to respectability. And it surely would not have become a bestseller.

On the other hand, there's plenty of evidence that the framers of the DSM saw the possibility that their book would fall victim to reification. Each edition has carried some version of this disclaimer that appears at the beginning of the DSM-IV.

There is no assumption that each category of mental disorder is a completely discrete entity with absolute boundaries dividing it from other mental disorders or from no mental disorder.

They also foresaw the potential for the book to be taken too seriously—especially by lawyers intent on proving that their client has (or doesn't have) a mental illness. "The purpose of DSM-III," reads that manual's introduction, "is to provide clear descriptions of diagnostic categories in order to enable clinicians and investigators to diagnose, communicate about, study, and treat people with various mental disorders." The use of the book for "nonclinical purposes" must be "critically examined," it says, especially when those uses involve the "determination of legal responsibility, competency or insanity."

But lawyers who wanted to turn the DSM into a book of excuses, each diagnosis a way to get clients off the hook of free will, weren't the only people who had to be cautioned, and the DSM-III-R devoted an entire page to a more general Cautionary Statement. It warned DSM users that the diagnostic criteria reflected only a "consensus of current formulations of evolving knowledge in our field" and that "the proper use of these criteria requires specialized clinical training." Apparently, the necessity of strenuously reminding readers not to take the book too seriously outweighed the possibility of undermining its authority at the outset.

The disclaimers are not unlike the wink-and-nudge signs at head shops announcing that bongs are not intended for use with illegal substances. They also resemble the black-box warning the FDA has required on various antidepressants alerting consumers that the drugs increase risk of suicide in children and adolescents. No one knows how many people this cautionary note has stopped from taking antidepressants, but since 2005, when it was added in bold type inside black lines to the insert that everyone discards along with the cotton in the top of the pill bottle, antidepressant sales have only skyrocketed. Disclaimers don't seem to be taken anywhere near as seriously as the products themselves.

Still, listening to First revel in the technicalities of *criteria sets* and *dimensional measures* and *clinical utility*, it's easy to believe that he'd be glad if psychiatric diagnosis had remained a wonky pursuit of little interest to anyone outside the field. If the DSM only helped ensure that one doctor's study of schizophrenia used the same definition as another's, that a hallway consultation about a patient's condition could be conducted expeditiously, that a depressed patient with a diagnosis of Bipolar Disorder wouldn't get prescribed the antidepressant that might trigger a manic episode, that drug companies could have their indications and epidemiologists their numbers and bureaucrats their forecasts of disability—if only the DSM had stayed small and obscure, First wouldn't be submitting to my questions, which he's doing pretty graciously, and he would be free to get on with the work of sorting and counting and defining that, like Bob Spitzer before him, he finds so compelling. He also wouldn't be so worried about the fate of the DSM-5. Because it's clear to him that the APA's aspirations for the new manual are grander than the evidence warrants. He should know. He authored that line in the *Research Agenda* about how the new paradigm was "yet unknown."

"The research agenda was really on a lark," he told me, referring to the conferences and papers that began the DSM-5 campaign. "I mean, it was pretty obvious there was no paradigm shift at hand." Assembling the experts and finding out what they were up to might set the stage for a new approach in the future, but surely not in time for the DSM-5. The fact that the paradigm would not be shifting anytime soon was fine for a guy who only wants the DSM to help clinicians communicate and make decisions—ends that could be served by tweaking the current model and holding all those pesky questions about validity at bay until the paradigm actually shifted. But the APA leadership, First thought, was not content to wait, which is why they decided to invite so many biological psychiatrists to those planning conferences.

"They had this idea that we had the wrong people doing the DSM, and if we had the neuroscientists and geneticists around, they'd tell us all we need to do to make a paradigm shift," First said.

Despite his doubts, First organized the conferences, attended all of them, wrote summaries of the proceedings, and designed a website on which to post them. He might have been sure those scientists would never find what the APA was looking for, but he soldiered on. He no doubt did this out of loyalty—to his profession and to his discipline. But he had another reason. The APA's aspirations to meet the scientific demands of the day might have been quixotic, its ambitions outsize, but First had an ambition of his own: to lead the effort to produce the DSM-5.

Chapter 5

Michael First wasn't the only old DSM hand skeptical about the prospects for the planning conferences. "When I heard about them, I was amazed," Allen Frances told me. "It was absolutely ridiculous from the beginning. There was no way you could force a breakthrough like that." If scientists had made those seminal discoveries connecting mental disorders with brain function, Frances thought, the paradigm would have already shifted. The attempt to "jump-start science" was part of a "grand ambition that will take many decades to realize."

It was that kind of ambition that Frances attempted to dampen with his conservative approach to DSM-IV. And First had set his sights similarly low for DSM-5. "However much we don't like this paradigm, it's as good as we have," he told me. "So let's find out how to make it more helpful to clinicians." For all their talk about clinician communication, the defenders of the DSM have precious little idea of exactly how it figures in the way psychiatrists talk to one another, and how it can help them do a better job of it. They've spent a lot more time dreaming up new diagnoses than looking into the far less glamorous matter of *clinical utility*. First thought the APA's time and money would be best spent tweaking the DSM-IV's criteria and correcting its obvious errors, while focusing on making the manual maximally useful to clinicians.

Neither First nor Frances seems conservative by nature. Their politics, to the extent they discuss them, appear to be well left of center. But when it comes to the DSM, they see themselves as stewards of a tradition that, even if imperfect, it is important to uphold, possibly because both men have witnessed the consequences of playing fast and loose with the DSM.

Perhaps the most disturbing of these consequences was unfolding as the preliminaries to DSM-5 were getting under way. The trouble began at Harvard's Massachusetts General Hospital, where Joseph Biederman worked as a child psychiatrist. In the 1980s, he developed a stellar reputation as a researcher and clinician working with children diagnosed with Attention Deficit/Hyperactivity Disorder (ADHD). Author of more than six hundred articles, winner of numerous professional awards, a perennial choice as a *U.S. News & World Report* Top Doctor, and an inductee in the Children and Adults with Attention Deficit/ Hyperactivity Disorder Hall of Fame, Biederman was what is known in his industry as a *key opinion leader.*

Sometime in the 1980s, Biederman's opinions turned to a particularly difficult group of his ADHD patients. These were kids who, in addition to being fidgety and distractable, were from a very early age—sometimes, so their parents said, from the time they were born— quick to rage, slow to be comforted, and precocious in all the wrong ways: threatening suicide before their peers even knew what the word meant, acting out sexually before they'd reached puberty. They were defiant and contrary and cranky all the time, hard for parents to parent, teachers to teach, and therapists to treat.

Biederman thought he detected in these children something different from what he saw in other ADHD patients. In particular, he saw what the DSM called a *mood disorder* in their chronic irritability, their prolonged and frequent tantrums, and the profound sadness that set in after the storm. ADHD diagnostic criteria did not include mood symptoms, but there was a small literature reporting a few cases of "hyperactive children" who also had "nervous irritability" and who went on to develop one of the best-known and most feared mood disorders of all: what had been called manic-depressive insanity by Kraepelin and, in the 1980s, was renamed Bipolar Disorder (BD). Doctors generally considered it to be neurological or genetic in origin and incurable, although it could be managed with mood stabilizers, usually lithium.

Biederman thought that he was on the verge of a major discovery: that BD, the onset of which was generally agreed to be in early adulthood, started much earlier. This would indicate that these kids ought to be treated with mood stabilizers rather than the stimulants generally prescribed for ADHD and that they and their parents should be prepared for a lifetime of managing a chronic illness, just as juvenile diabetic patients are.

The appeal of this hypothesis to doctors and parents was immense. It invoked one of the most time-tested diagnoses in the DSM, it gave clinicians something to call these kids' condition besides "bad ADHD," and it pointed in the direction of a new treatment. But there was a problem. According to the DSM-IV, "the essential feature of Bipolar Disorder is a clinical course characterized by the occurrence of one or more manic episodes." And manic episodes have what the DSM calls *Criterion A symptoms*, features necessary, but not sufficient, for the diagnosis—in the case of BD, "a distinct period of abnormally and persistently elevated, expansive, or irritable mood, lasting at least 1 week." But Biederman's patients didn't have episodes of mania—or of anything else for that matter. Indeed, the parents' major complaint was that they never got a break from their children's biliousness.

The DSM also lists *Criterion B symptoms* for most disorders—features that must be in place in addition to Criterion A for the diagnosis to be made. Manic episodes have seven Criterion B symptoms, four of which are required for the diagnosis. And three of those seven symptoms—excessive talkativeness, distractibility, and fidgetiness—also appeared on the list of possible symptoms of ADHD. So it was hard to distinguish the two disorders. Clinicians following Biederman's lead might be only slapping a new label on "bad ADHD," one that moved the patients to a different, but still ill-fitting, category. This kind of ad hoc diagnosing is exactly what the DSM, with its symptom lists, is supposed to preclude.

So Biederman set out to prove that the new label was a winner, that it could reliably gather together particulars once thought to be scattered, and point in the direction of a previously undiscovered natural formation. If he looked only at the chronically irritable patients, he wondered, would their Criterion B symptoms differ from the ones that the rest of the ADHD kids had? If so, then this would be evidence that these kids constituted a different diagnostic group from the others.

Sure enough, when Biederman and his team looked carefully at the Criterion B profiles of the chronically irritable group, they found that they were more likely to have the four symptoms that BD does *not* share with ADHD than children who weren't irritable. The team also looked at levels of impairment among the irritable group—the extent to which the patients' symptoms interfered with their lives, landed them in hospitals, or led to psychosis—and found a similar grouping: the children who were chronically irritable *and* scored high on the four unique Criterion B symptoms tended to be more impaired than the ADHD kids. Taken together, Biederman said, patients with this distinct profile account for around 20 percent of children diagnosed with ADHD. One in five of those patients, Biederman concluded, actually was bipolar and was getting exactly the wrong treatment: stimulants known to aggravate mania.

Biederman's announcement provoked an outcry from his colleagues. They argued that his proposal flouted hundreds of years of observations about the episodic nature of mania. In addition, they pointed out, a recent epidemiological study, conducted by people other than those trained and supervised by Biederman, had turned up exactly zero children with mania. Biederman's own research indicated that his patients were not only more irritable than ADHD patients, but also more withdrawn and prone to sulk—hardly consistent with a diagnosis of mania. Critics also complained that by rejiggering the criteria, he'd lowered the threshold for what was a very serious diagnosis. The Criterion B symptoms that remained after eliminating the ones that overlapped with ADHD—"grandiosity, decreased need for sleep, flight of ideas (i.e., a free-flowing stream of consciousness) and excessive involvement in pleasurable activities that have a high potential for painful consequences"—weren't these really just a working definition of childhood at its most exuberant? And finally, they cited longitudinal studies, which showed that plenty of "bad ADHD" kids indeed went on to develop various mental disorders, but bipolar was not among them—a finding hard to reconcile with the presumption that BD is a lifelong illness.

I'll spare you the ensuing back-and-forth, which is as bitter and rancorous, and as impenetrable, as most academic controversies, and which continues more than fifteen years later. It's not that it hasn't been entertaining, at least at points, as when Biederman was moved to liken his critics to people who insist the earth is flat and circled by the sun, and his own discovery to that of Edward Jenner, whose "smallpox vaccine was ridiculed when initially proposed"—suggestive comparisons for a man studying a disorder with grandiosity among its symptoms. It also illustrates the bruising politics behind the DSM, the way in which changing it is as much a legislative as a scientific process, and the self-validating nature of diagnosis, by which once you've created a diagnostic category, the fact that people fit into it becomes evidence that the disorder exists. But what happened next is of much greater significance, so suffice it to say for now that Biederman proved, to his own satisfaction, that he was correct, that those "bad ADHD" kids really had BD.

Biederman didn't try to change the DSM-IV definition of Bipolar Disorder to reflect his findings. The book had just come out when he began his campaign to convince doctors and parents that chronic irritability was the juvenile form of episodic mania, and a revision wasn't expected for many years. Fortunately for him, however, he didn't really need it to change. The DSM provides, in addition to the seven variations on BD—Bipolar Disorder, Single Manic Episode; Bipolar Disorder, Most Recent Episode Depressed; and so on—a category called Bipolar Disorder Not Otherwise Specified (BDNOS). (There are NOS categories for every major diagnostic classification in the book.) The BDNOS category is designed for "disorders with bipolar features that do not meet criteria for any specific Bipolar Disorder." In other words, if your patient doesn't qualify for the diagnosis, but you still think he's bipolar, you can just go ahead and give the kid the diagnosis anyway.

By the time children get to a doctor of Joseph Biederman's stature, they've generally been through any number of therapists, pediatricians, and psychiatrists. They've been the subject of countless meetings at schools, endless testing by psychologists, and home interventions from social service agencies. Their parents have tried everything—drugs and diets, hug therapy and tough love, private schools and residential treatment and family therapy vacations, prayers, and even exorcisms. And in the end they still have a child who seems unhappy nearly every waking moment, who is likely to fly into a rage at the slightest provocation, who holds a knife to his own throat and threatens to plunge it in if he isn't allowed ten more minutes on PlayStation. They are, in short, devastated and desperate.

That's why, when the important doctor tells the beleaguered parents that their child is irrevocably mentally ill, even if they are aware (which they usually aren't) that he's stretching the truth, they listen. Besides, the news isn't all bad. At least now they know. They have been given a name for their (and their child's) pain. And when the key opinion leader tells his colleagues what he's doing at Harvard for these kids and offers them the opportunity to provide the same kind of explanation and hope to their own patients, they are quick to follow him through the NOS loophole.

And by 1999, parents could even go to their doctors and suggest they do exactly that. That at any rate was the advice of Demitri and Janice Papolos, a husband-and-wife team whose bestselling book *The Bipolar Child* explained that "thoughtful clinical investigators are beginning to realize that bipolar disorder in childhood presents a very different pattern" from the adult version. Unfortunately, they wrote, only psychiatrists conversant with the "latest research findings" would recognize the symptoms—the unsettled infancy, the precociousness and separation anxiety, the nightmares and fear of death and mercurial moods, the sweet tooth and bed-wetting and maybe even the in utero kicking, or any of the forty or so other signs that your child is bipolar that are listed in the book—and issue the proper diagnosis.

By 2001, parents could comfort themselves and their diagnosed children with books such as *Brandon and the Bipolar Bear*, in which Dr. Samuel explains to Brandon why he (Brandon, not Dr. Samuel) dismembered his teddy bear. "You have bipolar disorder," the doctor says. He explains that Brandon has a harder time controlling his feelings because the chemicals in his brain "can't do their job right so their feelings get all jumbled up inside." He tells Brandon that he doesn't have BD because he is bad, nor did he get it from a classmate. Rather, he says, Brandon most likely inherited it.

Websites sprang up, self-help groups formed, foundations were funded, and in August 2002, *Time* devoted its cover to the "Young and Bipolar" and their families, who had been saved by receiving the diagnosis. Soon, the magazine predicted, a "blood test that will allow bipolar disorder to be spotted as simply as, say, high cholesterol" would shorten the period of incorrect diagnoses and fruitless treatments. By 2003, Biederman's opinion had led his colleagues to conclude 6.67 percent of office visits made by children for mental health problems with a diagnosis of BD—up from less than half a percent in 1994.

It was possible that the new diagnostic approach had uncovered a previously unknown epidemic. But as Duke University's chief of child and adolescent psychiatry, John March, told *The New York Times* when the diagnostic increase was reported, "The label may or may not reflect reality." No one questioned that there were many children whose explosiveness and irritability terrified their parents and defied treatment. But did they really have BD?

But March had it backward. The diagnostic label had been redesigned specifically to reflect reality, and reality had followed suit; those explosive children were now bipolar patients, and the sooner parents thought of them (and taught them to think of themselves) as afflicted with a chronic disease, the sooner they could get help. If Biederman had set out to become the Johnny Appleseed of an entirely new disorder—"scary impossible child disorder," let's say—rather than of a new version of an old illness, then the websites and self-help books and cover stories would be offering support for kids diagnosed with that disease, doctors would be arguing about whether or not it reflected reality, and parents would be wondering whether or not their kids warranted the SIC label.

But that's not what Biederman did. Neither did he tinker with, say, ADHD or Oppositional-Defiant Disorder (ODD), or simply suggest that clinicians use a perfectly good DSM diagnosis—Disruptive Behavior Disorder, NOS (312.9) seems well suited—and be done with it. He wasn't determined only to give these children a new diagnostic home. He also had a very specific idea about where they belonged, and if the evidence didn't support his conviction, then he would change the rules by which the evidence was admitted.

It's not clear why Biederman settled on Bipolar Disorder. But it's easy enough to imagine the possible motives: to ensure that insurance companies would pay for the extensive treatment these kids needed, which a diagnosis of ADHD or ODD did not always justify, but BD does; to make his professional mark by changing one of psychiatry's most venerable diagnoses; to confirm a hunch. But the label also reflected another reality: that, as Dr. Samuel tells Brandon, there is "some medicine that could help you feel better." Indeed, just as Biederman was starting to persuade his colleagues to be on the lookout for childhood mania, new treatments were coming to market to supplement the old standby, lithium. Drug makers were touting anticonvulsants such as Abbott Laboratories' Depakote, and rebranding *atypical antipsychotics*—Zyprexa, Seroquel, Abilify, and Risperdal—as *mood stabilizers*, the category to which lithium belonged and surely a less terrifying term.

These treatments were not without their problems. They are sedating—heavily so in the case of the antipsychotics—which means that it is hard to know if they were treating BD or just tranquilizing the children. They are also associated with devastating side effects: cataracts, obesity, diabetes, tardive dyskinesia (a movement disorder characterized by tics and spasticity), which add up to a twelve-to-twenty-year decrease in life expectancy for treated versus untreated patients. And even as the drug companies began to seek (and eventually receive) FDA approval to use the drugs as mood stabilizers and to rechristen them accordingly, they did not study their effectiveness (or their side effects) in children—largely because BD wasn't thought to affect kids.

Biederman and others did run some studies indicating that children's symptoms improved in response to the mood stabilizers. But these were short-term trials, often eight weeks or less, and could not possibly explore the consequences for a developing brain of daily use of a powerful drug. Nor could the studies tease out the question of whether the results were due to the overall sedative effects of the drugs or to something specific to these patients. Neither did advocates of mood stabilizers for children talk very much about the obesity and resulting diabetes that were known side effects of the drugs. None of this ignorance put the brakes on the bipolar express, however. Diagnosis and treatment rates continued to soar—by 2003, prevalence of BD among children had increased fortyfold over a decade and, hardly coincidentally, by 2005, antipsychotic use in children and adolescents had grown by 73 percent in only four years.

In 2007 alone, half a million children, twenty thousand of them under six years old, were prescribed drugs that a decade before would have been prescribed only in the most dire circumstances. Biederman's diagnostic innovation was a runaway hit.

Skeptics eventually raised questions about Biederman's success. In 2006, Gardiner Harris reported on the front page of *The New York Times* that young children on drug cocktails—and often on government disability for their officially diagnosed Bipolar Disorder—were sometimes no better off than they had been before treatment, that their families were now torn apart not by their behavior but by the problems created by the drugs, that the kids were gaining weight and becoming suicidal. Most disturbing, Harris wrote, there was precious little scientific knowledge about this subject. This, coupled with stories such as that of Rebecca Riley—a four-year-old girl who was diagnosed at age two and a half with Bipolar Disorder and prescribed a combination of an antipsychotic, an anticonvulsant, and an antihypertensive, and whose parents were arrested when she died after they gave her an overdose of the drugs—led to a disturbing conclusion: that no matter their intentions, doctors were conducting an experiment on children.

In 2007, Charles Grassley, a Republican senator from Iowa, convened a series of hearings on the relationship between doctors and the pharmaceutical industry. "In psychiatry," *The New York Times* reported in 2008, "Mr. Grassley has found an orchard of low-hanging fruit." Psychiatrists were the lowest-paid specialists in the country, with a median pay of just under $200,000—an income that you and I might find quite acceptable, but which paled next to the $464,420 earned by the average radiologist, and which, the *Times* insinuated, made the $750 to $3,500 speaking gigs offered by drug companies that much more attractive and the unseemliness of the business that much easier to gloss over. In Minnesota, psychiatrists who had taken $5,000 or more from antipsychotic manufacturers had written three times more antipsychotic prescriptions than unfunded doctors, and Vermont psychiatrists were receiving more drug company money than any other specialists in the state—an average of $56,944 each. A Cincinnati doctor reported $180,000 in income from AstraZeneca (makers of the antipsychotic Seroquel) over two years—bad enough, but, as Grassley discovered when he subpoenaed Astra's records, the doctor had actually received $238,000, the unreported part funneled to her through a corporation the doctor had set up to hide the income.

But this was all small beer compared with what Grassley found when he investigated Joseph Biederman. Biederman and an associate had acknowledged a couple hundred thousand dollars in drug company income between 2000 and 2007, but Grassley, with the benefit of subpoena power, reckoned that it was more like $1.6 million, and that another associate had raked in at least another million. Much of this money was for the research that Biederman used to prove that BD existed in kids and that antipsychotics were the best treatment, but the Grassley committee found something out about that, too. Those studies not only were small and inconclusive—as research conducted by just one group of doctors tends to be—but also had one main patron: Johnson & Johnson, whose Janssen Pharmaceuticals makes risperidone (Risperdal), one of the antipsychotics often prescribed for bipolar kids.

This shouldn't have been a big surprise. The Johnson & Johnson Center for the Study of Pediatric Psychopathology was one of the affiliations Biederman listed among his credentials. But if Grassley had only discovered gambling in Casablanca, he had also revealed just how unsavory that business was and how much it favored the house. Biederman's pitch to Johnson & Johnson for funding his center was that it would "move forward the commercial goals" of the company, and when he succeeded at that, he sold his patrons a research project on the promise that it "will support the safety and effectiveness of risperidone in this age group"—something a scientist shouldn't say out loud, even if he thinks it's true, and something he definitely shouldn't write in an e-mail that an ambitious senator might get hold of.

On the other hand, most scientists wouldn't testify in a sworn deposition as Biederman did in this exchange, which followed his testimony that he was a full professor at Harvard:

Lawyer: What's after that?
Biederman: God.
Lawyer: Did you say God?
Biederman: Yeah.

Divine or not, Biederman didn't always get what he wanted. The company turned down his request for $280,000 to fund a study, and it balked at paying him $3,000 for a talk at a medical school. But, as a marketing executive pointed out in a plea on Biederman's behalf, it wasn't such a good idea to poke the bipolar bear. "I have never seen someone so angry," he e-mailed his superiors, describing Biederman's reaction to being denied the research grant. "Since that time, our business became non-existant [*sic*] in his area of control." Should Johnson & Johnson not cough up the three grand, the hapless marketer warned, "I am truly afraid of the consequences." There were, after all, plenty of other makers of equally unproven antipsychotics ready to cozy up to this key opinion leader. (Biederman, who denied any quid pro quo in his arrangement with Johnson & Johnson, was sanctioned in 2011 for having "violated certain requirements" of the university's policies. The university forbade him to engage in industry-sponsored activities for one year, required him to get approval for outside work for the two years immediately following the ban, and imposed a "delay of consideration for promotion or advancement." It did not say how long his elevation to God would have to wait.)

Grassley wasn't stopping with Biederman. He went after Charles Nemeroff, head of the department of psychiatry at Emory University and the beneficiary of more than $2.8 million in drug money over seven years, nearly half of which had gone unreported to the university—a violation of federal law. He revealed that Frederick Goodwin, the psychiatrist who hosted *The Infinite Mind*, an NPR program, had taken money from drug companies on the same day he reported that mood stabilizers were safe and effective treatments for pediatric Bipolar Disorder. (Goodwin responded to Harris in a lengthy note on his website pointing out that he had never concealed his drug company ties and that in his talks to psychiatrists he had discussed lithium, a drug that has been "generic for decades and doesn't make enough money to justify promotion by drug companies.") And Harris reported that Stanford psychiatrist Alan Schatzberg owned nearly $5 million in stock in a drug development company—which might not have raised an eyebrow but for one thing: Schatzberg was slated to become the president of the American Psychiatric Association in May 2009.

Grassley was beginning to set his sights on the guild to which all these doctors belonged. On July 10, 2008, Jay Scully, the APA's CEO, received a letter from Grassley on United States Senate letterhead. The senator had read the stories in *The New York Times*, he wrote, and he was not amused.

> I have come to understand that money from the pharmaceutical industry can shape the practices of nonprofit organizations which purport to be independent in their viewpoints and actions. Specifically, it is alleged that pharmaceutical companies give money to non-profits in an attempt to garner favor in ways that increase sales of their products.

Grassley ordered the APA to disclose how much of its income was drug money. The answer turned out to be a lot—according to the *Times*, nearly one-third of the organization's $62.5 million annual revenue in 2006. Some of it came from advertising, but much of it went to educational programs in which drug companies tutored doctors attending APA conferences in the fine points of prescribing their drugs. The problem wasn't a few rogue psychiatrists who had somehow risen to the top of their field. It was woven deeply into the fabric of the profession. It would have been nearly impossible to justify prescribing antipsychotics sold by any manufacturer to four-year-olds without the BD diagnosis. And the diagnosis would have been impossible without a DSM that Biederman could exploit. As the *Times* had reported earlier, the DSM was not immune to industry influence. The paper cited the report of a team led by psychologist Lisa Cosgrove, which calculated that 56 percent of the doctors who made up the work groups that produced the DSM-IV had financial ties to Big Pharma. Every member of the groups recommending changes for mood disorders and psychotic disorders had received drug money; and, as Cosgrove pointed out, "Pharmaceutical companies have a vested interest in what mental disorders are included in the DSM."

Of course, the drug industry has a vested interest in disease in general, and it has not restricted its creativity to psychiatry. Restless legs syndrome, for instance, a disease invented as an alternative indication for GlaxoSmithKline's underperforming anti-Parkinson's drug Requip, can't be blamed on the DSM. But there is no other field quite so susceptible to diagnostic exuberance as psychiatry. While many diagnoses are made on clinical signs and symptoms rather than on lab tests or other external validators, only in psychiatry are *all* diagnoses made that way. Psychiatry may have been low-hanging fruit for Grassley, but it was even riper picking for the pharmaceutical industry.

"With every new revelation, our credibility with patients has been damaged, and we have to protect that first and foremost," former APA president Steven Sharfstein told *The New York Times* in the aftermath of the Grassley investigation. "The price we pay for these kinds of revelations is credibility," E. Fuller Torrey, one of the country's most influential psychiatrists, chimed in, "and we just can't afford to lose any more of that in this field." These doctors probably didn't know just how closely they were echoing the lament of Thomas Salmon. It was as if nothing had changed in a century. And, indeed, in a crucial way nothing had.

That may be part of the reason that the APA decided that it was time for a radical DSM revision, that even if the paradigm had not really shifted, they couldn't afford to stick with the tried and untrue. Michael First attempted to stop them. He figured he had the juice to criticize the APA's reformist ambitions and still be tapped to head up the new effort. "I thought they would need my skills, so I pushed," he told me.

But he soon realized he had miscalculated. "I stood my ground, but it was becoming more and more clear that I was getting iced out." And in April 2006, when he heard that the APA had appointed University of Pittsburgh psychiatry professor David Kupfer as chair of the task force and Darrel Regier as the vice chair, he was not surprised.

Even five years later I could still hear disappointment in his voice when he told me, after a long pause, about hearing the bad news. He sounded a little bitter as he recounted the DSM-5 leadership's failure to respond to his offer to repeat his stint as text editor, and its refusal to take his ideas seriously, but no more than you might expect from a guy who has seen the opportunity to do what he was born to do snatched away by people who he thought had the wrong idea of how to go about it.

In the meantime, the task force's attempts to get the revision under way were hampered by the shadow of corruption that was passing over the profession. In *The Truth About the Drug Companies*, author and former editor of *The New England Journal of Medicine* Marcia Angell had drawn attention to the unsavory relationship between the industry and the profession. And with a series of articles in prominent journals, she made it clear that the problem was not a figment of sensationalist journalists' imaginations.

Many psychiatrists thought the case against them was overblown. They insisted that drug company money did not influence their prescribing habits or, when it came to the DSM, their deliberations about what would get into the book. They also pointed out that the $4 million or so the industry kicked down every year for the APA's "educational programs" amounted to free money for the organization and its members, providing training that ultimately benefited their patients. But, said Scully, "my board thought that through and instructed me to phase out those programs," deciding, he told me, that "public trust was more important than money."

The board of trustees also decided to purge the DSM-5 of drug money. Task force and work group members would be able to hold no more than $50,000 in drug company stock and had to limit their earnings from the industry to $10,000 annually as long as they served. The trustees didn't say how they had established those criteria for diagnosing corruption. Nor did they seem to have wondered whether this move was really the best solution to the Pharma infestation. After all, the corruption wasn't so much financial as intellectual, the whole psychiatric-industrial consort dancing together to mutual satisfaction. The drug companies didn't have to pay off psychiatrists to create particular diseases, not when whatever disorder found its way into the DSM could be exploited as an indication for a drug; who needs conspiracies when you have capitalism?

For their part, psychiatrists didn't have to be on the take to be eager to turn all the troubles their patients faced into nails for their chemical sledgehammers; they only had to want to give patients relief. And they surely didn't have to be seduced into the medical model at lavish lunches, not when from their first days in medical school they had been, as Freud put it, "flirting with endocrinology and the autonomous nervous system." But then again, while the trustees may have been more worried about public trust than money, they surely were still worried about money, which would continue to flow only so long as the public was convinced that psychiatrists were practicing real medicine.

The trustees also underestimated the difficulty they would have in rounding up psychiatrists willing to take vows of relative poverty in order to spend years arguing over diagnostic criteria. Between those requirements and some others—that no university have more than two members on the same committee, for instance, and that efforts be made to recruit members from professions other than psychiatry and from outside the U.S.—it took nearly two years from the time Kupfer and Regier were named to the time the eighteen-member task force was assembled and appointed the 140 or so experts to the work group. So even as they announced their roster in May 2008, they had to know that their deadline—May 2012, which meant that they'd have to have a draft ready by the end of 2011—already loomed impossibly near.

Michael First was not appointed to the task force. He was not placed on any of the work groups. He was not assigned to consult with the two work groups that requested him as an expert adviser. In 2007, the APA terminated the contract under which he had been the in-house DSM expert, representing the organization around the world. He was not alone in being left out in the cold. "All the people at the top of the previous DSMs were completely excluded," he said. "There was some idea that the old forces would impede the paradigm shift, stand in the way of a new vision."

But the new forces were already losing confidence in that vision, or at least hedging their bets. Setting out the guidelines for making changes, the task force still asserted that "a new diagnostic paradigm must be developed," but it also cautioned that the DSM-5 would "not in itself represent a 'paradigm shift.'" It vowed to maintain continuity with past editions, but it also promised that "unlike in DSM-IV, there will be no a priori constraints on the degree of change between DSM-IV and DSM-V."

The new book, it seemed, would be a departure, but then again, maybe it wouldn't. The APA wasn't going to constrain itself, nor would it commit itself to change. Instead, it would try to have it both ways.

Chapter 6

One of Allen Frances's heroes is Cincinnatus, the Roman dictator who, drafted out of retirement to lead the army, slaughtered the enemy and promptly abdicated to return to his beloved farm. In Frances's version of the story, by the time the DSM-5 effort got under way, he had lost interest in nosology.

"I was bored stiff with the subject," he told me. "I was pursuing another of my life's goals—being a beach bum."

That was not the immediate purpose of his retirement from Duke in 1997, ten years earlier than he had planned. And it wasn't boredom that drove him out. "Psychiatric classification may be the only boring topic in psychiatry," he said. "Seeing patients and teaching never got boring," and Duke offered plenty of opportunities to do that, as well as to travel the world giving talks, to conduct research, to add to his seventy-plus-page CV, to collect awards and fellowships, and, if he'd been so inclined, to burnish his reputation as the most powerful psychiatrist in America. Rather, it was a personal matter: his wife Vera's Parkinson's disease was getting so bad that she needed his full-time care.

According to the doctors, Vera wasn't even supposed to be alive by then. She had been diagnosed in 1988 with brain cancer and given a year to live. "Perhaps not surprisingly, the diagnosis was unreliable and imprecise," Frances said. "And the prognosis was simply wrong."

In the end it wasn't the cancer that took her life. It was the treatment, which had caused her Parkinson's. After it worsened in 1997, they moved, first back to New York, where he had spent the first twenty-five years of his career at Cornell and Columbia (where he worked with Bob Spitzer), and then to San Diego. When planning for the DSM-5 started in 1998, he was nursing Vera, sitting on the beach, reading history, and spending time with his grandchildren, who lived nearby. After Vera died in 2007, he remained uninvolved. But then in 2009 a colleague told him about a proposal for what Frances thought was an unreliable and imprecise diagnosis with a questionable prognosis and a dangerous treatment—so dangerous, in fact, that it got Allen Frances off the beach and into the fight of his professional life.

Frances had already passed up one opportunity to weigh in on DSM-5. In 2008, Bob Spitzer had called with some disturbing news. The previous year, Spitzer, who by then was almost eighty years old, semi-retired, and hobbled by Parkinson's, had asked the leaders of the DSM-5 to forward him the minutes of the task force meetings. (Spitzer says he was just curious.) Initially, the APA agreed to provide them. But then, after a long silence, the organization informed him that because of the need for "confidentiality in the development process," his request had been nixed. Only APA trustees and members of the DSM-5 task force and work groups would be privy to the proceedings. In fact, the APA had insisted that no one could participate in the revision without promising in writing never to reveal what had gone on in their meetings.

Spitzer kept his counsel for a couple of months. But then in early June 2008, the *Psychiatric News* ran a story about the DSM-5. "We are rethinking the fundamental structure of DSM," Regier told the reporter, "which would be a first since 1980, when DSM-III was produced." Not only that, but according to APA president Carolyn Robinowitz, the revision process itself would be different. The APA was committed to an effort that was "open, transparent, and free of bias"—an indirect but unmistakable dig at Spitzer, who was known for his autocratic management style.

"I was dumbfounded," Spitzer told me, "and then appalled." It was bad enough that he'd been put out to pasture and that the APA seemed almost paranoid in its attempt to "not let anyone know what the hell was going on." But the article's disingenuousness in light of his exclusion was intolerable. "I found out how transparent and open the DSM-V process was," he wrote to the *Psychiatric News*. Spitzer recounted his reaction upon discovering that participants had been forbidden to "divulge, furnish, or make accessible to anyone" any "pre-publication materials, group discussions, internal correspondence, information about the development process, or any other written or unwritten information in any form."

> I didn't know whether to laugh or to cry. Laugh—because there is no way task force and work group members can be made to refrain from discussing the developing DSM-V with their colleagues. Cry— because this unprecedented attempt to revise DSM in secrecy indicates a failure to understand that revising a diagnostic manual—as a scientific process—benefits from the very exchange of information that is prohibited by the confidentiality agreement.

Spitzer's complaints, previously published in the *Psychiatric Times*, an independent paper, had already stirred up psychiatrists across the country, and this latest salvo made the national news.

Spitzer tried to recruit Frances's support for his opposition to the gag order. "I told him I completely agreed that this was a disastrous way for DSM-5 to start," Frances said. "But I didn't want to get involved at all. I wished him luck and went back to the beach."

But Frances left San Diego long enough to attend a party for Columbia-affiliated psychiatrists held at San Francisco's Asian Art Museum during the APA's 2009 annual meeting. Among the attendees was Will Carpenter, the University of Maryland psychiatrist who headed the work group for psychotic disorders. Carpenter's committee was considering a proposal for a new diagnosis to be called Psychosis Risk

Syndrome. The disorder would address what some psychiatrists who treated schizophrenia thought was a critical gap in the DSM-IV. Schizophrenia generally comes on in late adolescence or early adulthood, but doctors had noticed that many patients' troubles started long before, with symptoms that looked like signs of the disease only in retrospect, after their first psychotic break. Some of these patients had gone to psychiatrists, often taken as children or adolescents by worried parents. But even if the kids were behaving bizarrely or harboring strange beliefs or having hallucinations, their symptoms did not rise to the level of the DSM's criteria for schizophrenia. This in turn limited the benefits for which they were eligible and the treatments that doctors might consider.

To psychiatrists like Carpenter, who spend their days with patients ravaged by schizophrenia and who could only offer them sedatives of limited efficacy that made them obese and shortened their life spans, the idea of catching schizophrenia early and possibly preventing it was irresistible. If doctors could determine just what those early signals were, then perhaps they could test for them as they already did for high cholesterol or blood glucose, identify those who were at risk, and head off the real trouble before it arrived. In addition, an official diagnosis could attract research dollars from industry and government, even as it helped psychiatry keep up with the rest of medicine, which was increasingly interested in early intervention.

But although researchers thought they had identified the early warning signs—delusions, hallucinations, or disorganized speech that didn't rise to the level of full-fledged psychosis but occurred more or less weekly for a month and led them or their parents to seek treatment—and had followed patients who met those criteria for months or years, they found a *conversion rate* of 25 to 30 percent, meaning that only something like one-quarter of the patients went on to develop a psychotic illness. That's more than in the general population, of course, but still pretty low for a disorder that purports to predict psychosis.

"I had not been closely following the psychosis risk," Frances said.

"But I knew enough about it to know that it was an absolute disaster." Among the things he knew was that to create a DSM disorder, which is to say a disease that can be diagnosed by a checklist of symptoms, is to create a huge opportunity for drug companies to market their products to doctors and patients—especially when the new diagnosis lowers the threshold for being declared ill. It was too easy, Frances thought, to confuse normal adolescent bizarreness—strange haircuts and odd beliefs, high drama, and the occasional emotional crisis—with the new criteria, especially for harried doctors trying to help worried parents. And, most dismaying of all, the drugs most likely to be prescribed for a diagnosis with *psychosis* in its name were heavily sedating, obesity-inducing antipsychotic drugs, such as the ones Biederman had used to treat his bipolar patients.

Frances sought out Carpenter at the party. "Have you thought through these things?" he asked.

The discussion was brief. Frances saw someone else he wanted to talk to. "I had a choice of being with my wife and a friend I don't get to see," he told me, "or arguing diagnosis with Will Carpenter. It was a no-brainer. Basically at that point I just didn't care that much."

But before Frances abandoned the conversation, he spotted another old hand from Columbia, Harold Pincus. He called Pincus over, explained the situation, and asked him to pick up the argument where he was leaving off. "Harold is smarter than me and more articulate and more precise. So I figured it was no great loss."

Carpenter explained to Pincus what he says he would have told Frances if he had stuck around: that there were other ways in which these patients were set off from the rest of the world—"alterations in cognition," Carpenter told me, "and changes in gray matter." He explained to Pincus that the studies followed kids who were in treatment, which might have accounted for the low conversion rates, and might, in fact, indicate that the diagnosis was a good idea. He told Pincus he didn't think drugs were necessarily indicated for these patients, that they could be provided with *psychosocial treatments*—which is what psychiatrists call therapy these days—and *watchful waiting*.

While Carpenter argued his case—unsuccessfully, according to Pincus, who told me, "I still think it's a crazy idea"—Frances set off on a tour of the museum. But the conversation stayed on his mind. It reminded him of other times that he had remained silent while his profession launched diagnostic epidemics on an unsuspecting public. Some, like the childhood bipolar debacle, had had nothing to do with him; the DSM-IV committees had not even taken up the question of childhood mania. But others were the direct result of DSM-IV, and Frances regretted them.

One of the worst of these, in his view, was called Bipolar II Disorder. It was among the few new disorders introduced in DSM-IV. The doctors who had proposed it were trying to fix a problem that had arisen in the few years since Prozac had been introduced: the new generation of antidepressants had a tendency to cause depressed patients to become manic—what psychiatrists call *switching*. Although these patients had never been manic before, closer examination showed that they had had episodes of *hypomania*—times when they had a mood "clearly different from the usual nondepressed mood," but not fully manic, and not lasting as long as a full-blown manic episode. Four days of "elevated, expansive, or irritable mood," a decreased need for sleep, and increases in "distractibility" and "goal-directed activity" were now enough to qualify for what had once been considered a rare and debilitating disease. The lowered diagnostic threshold came along just before the FDA gave the drug industry the go-ahead to market their drugs directly to the public, thus changing forever the meaning of the phrase "Talk to your doctor." Advertisements touting Zyprexa and Abilify and other antipsychotic drugs as treatments for the new disease soon appeared; suddenly twice as many people had bipolar disorders as previously thought, and antipsychotics rocketed to the top of the charts. Some key opinion leaders were suggesting to their colleagues that many of their patients—indeed as much as 5 percent of the population—weren't depressed but rather were on the

"bipolar spectrum," which is why they weren't respo. antidepressants and should be switched to antipsychotics. anti-

"We couldn't have foreseen any of this," Frances said. But he did se.
it happening, and he failed to use his clout as head of the DSM-IV to
speak out against it. He had also remained silent when he was vice chair
of the APA's program committee in the 1980s and the pharmaceutical
industry had all but taken over the organization's training programs.
And there was one other time he had not spoken up, and he now regretted it. Early in his training at the New York State Psychiatric Institute, he
had taken on a patient, a medical student. He had diagnosed him with
pseudoneurotic schizophrenia—"a local concoction invented by the PI
director," Frances remembered, "and one that everyone seemed to us to
have." The effect of this diagnostic fad on the patient, who Frances
thinks now was merely anxious and depressed, not schizophrenic, was
devastating. "We kept him locked up for a year," he said, and the patient
never got back to medical school. "It was the original sin of my career."

As he toured the museum, Frances said, these failures nagged at
him. The prospect of "more kids getting unneeded antipsychotics that
would make them gain twelve pounds in twelve weeks hit me in the gut."
And if Will Carpenter—"a fine man and a great psychiatrist"—couldn't
see the danger, then no one else was likely to. "I was stuck without an
excuse," he told me. "If not me to correct it, who? If not now, when?"

When the tour was over, Frances found Bob Spitzer's wife at the
party. (Spitzer was too ill to attend.) He told her to tell Spitzer that he'd
be joining his crusade. He never returned to his conversation with Carpenter. But Carpenter already knew something momentous had happened. "It was over in seconds," he said, "but it lasted just long enough
for it to be clear that the trigger had been pulled."

Chapter 7

The first time Jay Scully met with his DSM-5 troops, in the spring of 2008, he warned them about what they were getting themselves into. "People are going to write dissertations on what you are doing. Reporters are going to be all over you. It's probably going to be *DSM-5: The Musical*."

The drama started almost immediately. The task force appointed Kenneth Zucker, a University of Toronto psychologist, to head up the sexual and gender identity disorders work group. Among the group's members was another Toronto psychologist, Ray Blanchard. The appointment of two non-American nonpsychiatrists may have helped the diversity statistics, but it infuriated transgendered people, who had a direct stake in the outcome.

Zucker was known for research purporting to show that the conviction that one had been born with the wrong sexual organs was acquired and thus, at least in some cases, malleable. He argued that some young children who expressed the desire to be the opposite sex should be discouraged from acting out their wishes, that girls who wanted to play with soldiers should be given dolls and that boys who wanted to wear skirts should be forced to dress like little men, lest they grow up into people with Gender Identity Disorder (GID). For his part, Blanchard had earned the wrath of the transgendered by suggesting that at least some of them did not suffer from having been born with the wrong sex organs, but rather that they derived erotic pleasure from fantasizing that they were the opposite sex, a fetish Blanchard called *autogynephilia*.

To many transsexuals, Blanchard's suggestion that their condition was nothing more than an abnormal sexual inclination—what the DSM calls a *paraphilia*—seemed to trivialize their suffering, and Zucker's notion that transgender children could be put back on the right track smacked of the bad old days of sexual reorientation therapy for homosexuals. And they had a very practical concern: surgeons and endocrinologists would not provide sex-change procedures (and couldn't get paid by insurers) without an official diagnosis of GID. If Blanchard's and Zucker's views carried the day, the work group might modify or remove a diagnosis that had been crucial to the gains transgender people had made.

Nearly as soon as the appointments were announced, the protests started rolling into APA headquarters. The National Gay and Lesbian Task Force, which had led the charge against the homosexuality diagnosis in 1973, issued a press release charging that Zucker and Blanchard were "out of step" and that the APA was not "keeping up with the times when it comes to serving the needs of transgender adults and gender-variant children." If the irony of pleading with psychiatrists *not* to take away a diagnosis that explicitly pathologized an inborn condition occurred to them, they did not note it in the communiqué.

In late May, the APA sent out a statement pledging a "thorough and balanced" revision that would be "based on sound scientific data but also sensitive to the needs of clinicians and patients." The effort would start with an assessment of "DSM-IV's strengths and problems," move to a "comprehensive review of scientific advancements," and then, using "targeted research analyses and clinical expertise," generate changes that would be subject to scrutiny from the larger professional community before being assembled into a final draft. There would even be a website where the public could eventually take a crack at the proposed revisions. The process would be orderly, deliberative, rational, nonarbi-trary, and, it seemed, prolonged—too prolonged to be getting into par-ticulars at this point.

It was a strange way to make a case for the scientific soundness of the DSM-5. After all, if the revision was going to be scientific, then why would the APA need to be sensitive to the needs of clinicians or patients or, for that matter, anyone else? A revision of cancer nosology based on "scientific advancements" like the increased ability to genotype tumors might conclude that certain patients actually belong in a different diag-nostic category from the one they currently occupied. This might ren-der them no longer eligible for treatment—a development that ought to make doctors sensitive to their patients as they deliver the bad news, but one that should not figure into whether or not the diagnosis is revised. As Joseph Biederman might have pointed out, if Galileo had been sensi-tive to the needs of the priests, we might still think that the sun moves around the earth.

The authors of the APA statement seemed to grasp this problem. After reassuring all the "stakeholders" that they would be listened to, they ended by urging people to recognize that "the DSM is a diagnostic manual and does not provide treatment recommendations or guide-lines." Those complaints had evidently gone to the wrong department. Not that such a department existed, at least not yet, but the APA did promise to set up a committee to look into the matter of GID treatment. In the meantime, perhaps because it was so proud of itself for listening to complaints that were, by its lights, irrelevant, the APA didn't seem to notice that, as it had when it came to the "paradigm shift," it was signal-ing that it would take whatever position was expedient, even if it ended up both asserting and undermining its scientific authority in the same one-page statement.

Scully had barely put out the GID fire when the *Psychiatric News* ran Spitzer's letter complaining about the gag order. He teamed up with Regier, Kupfer, and Nada Stotland, then the APA president, to fashion an immediate rejoinder. Spitzer, they wrote, had misunderstood the intent of the confidentiality agreement. The organization was only trying to protect work group members from any "fear of recrimination" that might pressure them into "premature conclusions and misconceptions," which might "damage the viability of DSM-V." They did not spell out exactly who might seek recrimination, or what form it would take, or why, if the process was scientific, any of that should matter. They didn't explain how sheltering their experts from outside views would help them be sensitive to the concerns of the rest of the world or protect the rest of the world from experts like Joseph Biederman. Neither did they elaborate on the claim that controversy could be harmful, let alone on what it meant to "damage the viability" of the DSM.

But the APA leaders didn't really think they needed to answer such questions. In fact, in their view, it was Spitzer who had some explaining to do. He had failed to acknowledge the long public record, dating back to the *Research Agenda*, and including fourteen books and more than eighty peer-reviewed papers, all of which were in the public domain (even if they had been authored mostly by the same experts who were now being protected from controversy). He had given short shrift to the fact that the APA had "invested a great deal of effort to develop a process allowing appropriate communication while protecting the integrity and value of the DSM-V." And he had misrepresented the agreement by failing to note a parenthetical clause allowing members to divulge material "as necessary to fulfill the obligations of [his or her] appointment." A member who isn't quite sure if he or she would be in violation, they added, "can simply ask." People evidently could say whatever they liked, as long as they got permission.

Two years later, in fall 2010, Scully tried to be philosophical about this drama—"I suppose that's the nature of the scientific process; scientists argue with each other"—but he was leaning forward, bouncing his arms on his knees, like he was having a little trouble staying in his seat. He is a big man, a blue-eyed blond with fair skin that flushes when he's mad, which he was now that I had brought up this subject. He was evidently still smarting from the attack, which he thought was "pretty personal" and totally misplaced. In fact, Scully said, anyone was free to say anything. He didn't mention the part about getting permission.

Neither did Darrel Regier. In our interview the next day, I told him about a work group member, a psychiatrist who would talk to me only anonymously and who had declined to ask permission—for fear, he said, of "reprisal." Regier wanted to know who the doctor was.

I described a conversation I'd had recently with a psychiatrist named Sid Zisook. Thinking he was a task force member, I had asked Zisook if he had reservations about letting me interview him. "I'm not on the task force," he told me. "And if I were, I wouldn't be talking to you."

"Sid said this?" Regier asked. He looked wounded.

David Kupfer had joined us by phone from his office in Pittsburgh, so I couldn't see his reaction. But there was hurt in his voice as he explained that he had "encouraged everybody to talk"—so much so, he said, that colleagues in other specialties were saying, "My God! Nothing like this has ever happened in internal medicine or pediatrics. You guys are pretty brave to put all that stuff out there."

Before I could ask Kupfer if he was calling Zisook a coward, Regier spoke up. "I'm putting myself in Sid's shoes," he said. "I think the secrecy stuff was so well sold by some of our critics that even some of our friends started to believe it."

And it's not only the critics who had victimized the APA. It was also their own people, although not the psychiatrists. "Unfortunately, the lawyers . . . It's a misnamed thing," Scully said. All the lawyers were interested in was "protecting the integrity and value of the DSM-V." The gag order was actually an "intellectual property agreement" designed to prevent anyone from using "material that belongs to the APA" for their own personal enrichment. And this wasn't just any intellectual property, but one that "we're putting $25 million into creating" and whose value could be diluted if some unscrupulous psychiatrist decided to publish his own DSM, or maybe write an embarrassing tell-all musical. This was what the lawyers had failed to make clear, what Spitzer had misunderstood, and what made the wound he inflicted all the more grievous: that the APA, like any corporation, had to protect its brand against pirates and bad publicity.

"We have enemies," APA president Nada Stotland told her troops as they assembled for their 162nd annual meeting in May 2009. Antipsychiatry was alive and well, and its troops would be sure "to use doubts about the DSM to undermine our profession." It was as if only people out to get the APA would question its credibility.

Stotland didn't say exactly whom she had in mind, although she did mention the Church of Scientology, whose most prominent member, Tom Cruise, had publicly scolded Brooke Shields for taking Paxil and then told NBC's Matt Lauer that "psychiatry is a pseudoscience" and "there is no such thing as a chemical imbalance." Stotland probably would have counted those pesky transsexuals among them as well. But it's a safe bet that she wasn't thinking of Allen Frances and Bob Spitzer. On the other hand, she gave the speech the night before Will Carpenter pulled Frances's trigger.

Frances didn't bother with warning shots. In July 2009, he fired off a full-on salvo from his BlackBerry—his sole link to the Internet, which he'd purchased a couple of years previously, and only after "Michael First shamed me into it" by telling him that if he didn't have a link to the Internet, Frances's grandchildren would come to regard him as he had regarded his Yiddish-speaking grandfather. It was the first time he'd used the device for anything other than e-mail.

The three-thousand-word missive ended up in the June 26 issue of the *Psychiatric Times*. Under the headline "A Warning Sign on the Road to DSM-V: Beware of Its Unintended Consequences," Frances wrote that his successors had "displayed the most unhappy combination of soaring ambition and weak methodology." Their attempt to effect a paradigm change was "absurdly premature." They were heedless of the fact that because psychiatry was "stuck at its current descriptive level . . . until we make a fundamental leap in our understanding of what causes mental disorders . . . there is little to be gained and much to be lost in . . . changing the system." They had compounded that error by populating the work groups with experts from "the atypical setting of university psychiatry," whose clinical experience was limited to "highly select patients treated in a research context" and who tended to be far more worried about "missed cases" than about diagnosing people with illnesses who weren't really sick. The task force had given them precious little guidance, leaving the experts free to pursue their pet projects, like Psychosis Risk Syndrome. And they were preparing to field-test the new diagnoses, using them with real patients in the controlled settings of academic medical centers, without having first subjected the new criteria to outside scrutiny and then refined them, as Frances had in the DSM-IV. Conducting a field trial on what amounted to a rough draft of the new DSM would be "flying blind." It couldn't possibly tell psychiatrists anything about how the final draft would perform in the real world.

This was Frances's biggest complaint: that the DSM-5 leaders seemed heedless of the way that the new revision threatened to put psychiatry even more into the "business of manufacturing mental disorders" and that those lowered thresholds and new diagnoses and revamped criteria would touch off diagnostic epidemics. "The result would be a wholesale imperial medicalization of normality," he wrote, "a bonanza for the pharmaceutical industry but at a huge cost to the new patients caught in the excessively wide DSM-V net." Operating in an echo chamber of experts, secretive and sealed off from outside views by its "ludicrous confidentiality agreements," the task force couldn't even see how far off course it had veered. Neither could it grasp how far behind schedule it already was, how time pressure would "soon lead to an unconsidered rush of last-minute decisions." Barring a "midterm course

THE BOOK OF WOE 107

correction"—which Frances thought required the appointment of an external review committee with no ties to the DSM—the DSM-5 would be "an embarrassment and a burden to the field," creating problems that would "haunt psychiatry for many years to come."

The APA didn't waste any time firing back. "Setting the Record Straight" appeared in the next week's issue of the *Psychiatric Times* under the byline of the organization's new president, Alan Schatzberg (the Stanford psychiatrist whose drug company ties had raised Grassley's dander), along with Scully, Regier, and Kupfer. They accused Frances, as they had Spitzer before him, of launching his salvo with "disregard for the facts"; taken together, these were "unjustified ad hominem attacks" to which the APA now reluctantly had to respond.

"The process for developing the DSM-V has been the most inclusive ever," they wrote. More than 400 scientists and 200 advisers had bolstered the 150 experts from sixteen countries who constituted the task force and work groups. Their discussions had not been inhibited by the confidentiality agreements, nor had any of them been stopped from presenting at professional meetings, in journals, and even "in countless interviews to the mainstream press." Indeed, if the proceedings were really secret, they asked, then how could Frances have gotten hold of enough information to fashion his litany in the first place? It wasn't their fault that he had mistaken their drafts as "final decisions, rather than as statements of work in progress." Far from being secretive, the DSM leaders were really the victims of their own transparency.

Frances had gotten one thing right: "The DSM-V work groups were freed from the constraints inherent in DSM-IV's conservative process." The task force had not, however, simply emancipated them from Frances's shackles. They had given the committees marching orders: to optimize clinical utility, to use research evidence to guide their recommendations, and to maintain continuity with previous editions. "We are setting up a process that will allow the new DSM to change with new developments, rather than being reified for a decade or more," they wrote. The authors didn't add "like some DSMs we know."

Neither did they name Spitzer or Frances when they complained that the "DSM-III categorical diagnoses are now holding us back," or that the "DSM-IV system poorly reflects the clinical realities of [our] patients," or that "researchers are skeptical that the existing DSM categories represent a valid basis for scientific investigations." And they left out Frances's name when they suggested that what some might see as a revision in disarray and up against time constraints was really only the rapid process made possible "thanks to new publishing technologies, not even imagined in the early 1990s." The DSM could be nimble, not the lumbering beast Frances had created and with which they were now stuck.

In case the point wasn't clear, and speaking of ad hominem attacks, the APA signed off by reminding readers that Frances had promised them a "full disclosure" at the outset of his screed, allowing that "it is reasonable for you to wonder whether I have an inherently conservative bias or am protecting my own DSM-IV baby."

"It is unfortunate," the APA leaders wrote, "that Dr. Frances failed to take this [promise] to heart when he did not disclose his continued financial interests in several publications based on DSM-IV." As a matter of fact, they went on, he had been informed—at the very same APA meeting at which he had suddenly become galvanized—that his royalties would end upon publication of the new revision. This coincidence, the APA suggested to readers, was something that "should be considered when evaluating his critique and its timing."

Allen Frances had made his way onto the APA's enemies list. Of course, that wasn't how Schatzberg was going to put it. Nor would Will Carpenter, when he ended his own *Psychiatric Times* rebuttal by responding to Frances's charge that the task force was overly ambitious. "Soaring ambition is another matter," he wrote. "Here my empathy is with Allen. If I had directed DSM-IV, I imagine that I would think that anyone trying to improve on my work must be very ambitious indeed." Nor would Renato Alarcon, a work group member, when he suggested, also in the *Psychiatric Times*, that Frances was "letting nostalgia and passion obstruct clarity of vision." Instead of talking about enemies and taking the risk of sounding even more paranoid, they did what their training told them to do when confronted with disturbing behavior. They offered empathy, even pity, and, of course, a diagnosis.

Not that you need special training to approach enmity in this fashion, although psychiatrists may be better at turning supposed insight into a person's character into a weapon. Passive aggression may be particularly unseemly when it comes from the people in charge of our mental health, but claiming that a person who disagrees is ill motivated, that his objections are really the result of malfeasance or dishonesty, that if he weren't deluded by ideology or greed or ignorance, if he weren't somehow pathological, then he'd come to see things the right way—this is a ubiquitous feature of American political life.

And here is a place where science, at least the psychiatric form of it, and politics really come together. Whether among senators or psychiatrists, the exchange of diagnoses generates more heat than light, and the smoke it gives off obscures the trouble that gave rise to the disturbing behavior in the first place. But there was one vulnerability that no one, defender or critic, was discussing, at least not in public. Even Frances muted this concern in the blogs he was thumbing out with regularity, which now appeared in *Psychology Today* as well as the *Psychiatric Times*. He did, however, address it in a letter to the APA trustees that was also signed by Spitzer. "You must understand," they wrote, "that the APA has never held a guarantee on the DSM franchise. There have been serious objections in the past that it is inappropriate for one professional 'guild' to control a document with such wide usage and great public health importance." Frances knew that psychiatrists had been lucky enough to be in the right place—asylums—at a time when the Census Bureau took a sudden interest in counting the insane. History had bestowed the franchise on the APA, and history could take it away—and with it the riches it had brought the guild.

When Frances and Spitzer warned the trustees that to ignore this was to "bet the house," they meant that literally. The APA's financial picture was bleak, the organization battered by hard economic times and the partial purge of Pharma. Income from the drug industry, which amounted to more than $19 million in 2006, had shrunk to $11 million by 2009, and was projected to fall even more. Membership was dropping, off by nearly 15 percent from its highs, and with it income from dues and attendance fees. Journal advertising was off by 50 percent from its 2006 high of $10 million. Only the DSM-IV had remained steady, reliably bringing in between $5 and $6 million annually, nearly 10 percent of the APA's income and just enough to keep the APA in the black. Losing that money could be fatal. The credibility problem first noticed by Thomas Salmon now had a price tag on it.

The APA already had a competitor for its franchise: the World Health Organization. Its International Classification of Diseases had an entire section devoted to psychiatric disorders. In fact, the diagnosis codes found in the DSM are really taken from the ICD. As Michael First, who now works on the ICD, pointed out, "In reality, clinicians in the United States, all of us, don't ever have to buy a copy of the DSM." Most practitioners don't know this, he added—at least not yet. But "the franchise depends on the quality of the book. If they put out a crappy product, people could just say, 'This is so bad, I don't need to use it anymore. I'll just go use the ICD.'" And when we therapists go to do that, we will discover something else that most of us don't know: the ICD, created by a public agency, is available for download from the WHO's website. It won't take up any space on our bookshelves, and, perhaps its best selling point, anyone can browse it for free.

That fact is likely to impress many clinicians who think they have to shell out two hundred bucks when the new book comes out, especially when they discover that the ICD is quick and to the point—no checklists to go down, no long pages about prevalence or family characteristics or recording procedures, which are of much less interest than, say, reimbursement rates, to the average clinician. The APA leaders had to know that all the spin control, all the denunciations, all the confidentiality agreements in the world might not be enough to counter the fact that stalwarts like Frances and First were doubting the soundness of the new book. If a crappy product unleashed a public battle, then the rest of us might discover that the DSM was nowhere near as necessary as it had been cracked up to be. That wouldn't be good for the APA's bottom line.

And here is another way in which the politics of DSM resembles the politics of the larger world. For who can doubt that what politicians are really arguing about is money?

Even when they weren't arguing so openly about dollars—back in the 1970s, before anyone knew that the DSM-III would be a bestseller—the writers of the DSM understood that turning diagnosis into a bureaucratic function left them with only an aspirational relationship to modern medicine. Spitzer may have wrested psychiatry from Freud's grasp and dipped it into the stream of scientific rhetoric, but where he held it most firmly was where it was the weakest. He had left the profession unable to stave off the next drapetomania, except perhaps on the grounds of decency and common sense—important considerations, but not scientific or immune to local mores.

Having eliminated theories about the nature and causes of mental illness, Spitzer had also taken away his colleagues' ability to draw a line between illness and health. A man may be feeling as fit as a fiddle, but a radiologist who spots a mass in his lung or a cardiologist looking at the results of an echocardiogram might have a better idea about his state of health. A woman may be missing her period, suffering nausea in the morning, and feeling lousy all day, but an obstetrician who can read a blood test can reassure her that she is not sick, only pregnant. But no psychiatrist, listening to a patient's woes, can listen to his complaints and offer similarly certain appraisals.

This was not merely an abstract problem for Spitzer. For he was well aware there was at least one group of people who met all the criteria for a mental illness but who, on the other hand, could only be considered sick at the risk of psychiatry's always fragile credibility. Their existence was confirmed not by an enemy of psychiatry playing gotcha, but by one of the DSM-III's own—a Washington University psychiatrist and task force member named Paula Clayton. She was part of the team that had perfected the Research Diagnostic Criteria, the prototype of the DSM-III approach, and she had made an unsettling if unsurprising discovery: people who had recently suffered the death of a loved one often had at least five of the nine symptoms of depression, which meant that if you went strictly by the book, they were mentally ill.

The grief over grief was a scientific and political disaster waiting to happen. How would it look when clinicians began to diagnose mourners with mental illness and declared for themselves a territory that was among the last bastions of religion? And yet if a clinician, suffering from a sudden attack of common sense, was free to decide that the patient wasn't really sick even if he met the criteria, then wouldn't that return psychiatry to the days when clinicians' assumptions determined the line between illness and health, and psychiatry was reviled for its unreliability?

Spitzer's solution was characteristically wily. He carved out an exception to the depression diagnosis and deftly inserted it at the back of the DSM-III. In a section called "Conditions Not Attributable to a Mental Disorder That Are a Focus of Treatment or Attention," a clinician could learn that the recently bereaved may well have all the symptoms of depression, but because "a full depressive syndrome frequently is a normal reaction to the death of a loved one," the patient's condition was better understood as Uncomplicated Bereavement. Clinicians confronted with the absurdities of the descriptive approach were thus given cover to ignore it even as their prerogative to treat the recently bereaved was preserved (although insurers rarely if ever pay for treatment of those non-mental-disorder conditions).

The *bereavement exclusion*, as it came to be known, became part of the diagnostic criteria in the DSM-III-R, where it acquired a time limit: after two months of meeting five of the nine criteria, the bereaved became mentally ill. But certain thorny matters—notably, whether or not a clinician should distinguish among the death of a parent or child, the death of a celebrity, and the death of the family dog—remained up to the individual clinician to decide. Even so, it was a win-win, which may be why no one seemed to notice that the loophole amounted to saying that people who had all the symptoms of a disorder had the disorder—*unless they didn't*. The criteria didn't really add up to a mental illness until a doctor determined that a disorder was present and by this judgment transformed suffering into the symptoms of a disease.

This is, in part, as it should be. Isn't this what we go to doctors for—to learn, from someone who *knows*, the true nature of our suffering, to find out whether that nagging pain is the leading edge of something horrible or just a random twinge, to find out if our persistent malaise is grief or depression or maybe even a malfunctioning thyroid? Even before we ask for remedy, this is what we ask of our doctors: to lay bare the beginnings of our suffering, to elicit our present crisis, to tell us what is going to happen in the end. Without that story, we might not take their pills, and—since so much of our response to medication is the result of placebo effects, and placebo effects in turn depend on the patient's belief in his or her doctor—the pills might not work.

On the other hand, most of us won't accept just any tale about our woes. We want our doctors' stories about us to be based in fact, not opinion. We want them to make sense, which, if they start telling us that grieving the loss of a parent is an illness, they don't. That's why the bereavement exclusion was necessary: without it, the DSM loses its credibility, and the doctors who use it cannot perform their healing magic.

Spitzer did something else to juice the credibility of the DSM-III, something that no one else had done, at least not in a diagnostic manual: he tried to define *disease*. This is harder, and a lot more audacious, than it might seem. Like *life* and *obscenity*, disease is one of those phenomena that you might recognize when you see it—but go ahead and try to define it.

You have to admire Spitzer for making the attempt, for not simply cribbing *Webster's* and then moving on to his list of diseases and the symptoms by which they would be known. But you also have to understand that he really had no choice. So long as psychiatry had no scientific knowledge about which ingredient was missing from the chemical soup roiling inside your head, so long, that is, as diagnosis was still a matter of a doctor deciding that you had a disease and then telling you which one it was, psychiatrists needed to be able to say with certainty how they made that decision, and why it wasn't simply a matter of personal prerogative. They needed a definition that would serve as a gatekeeper to the kingdom of illness, that would reassure the public that the profession didn't intend to claim sovereignty over all our troubles, that would keep homosexuality out and depression in—that would, as Spitzer put it in the introduction to DSM-III, "present concepts that have influenced the decision to include certain conditions and to exclude others." Without that barrier, DSM would not be a medical text but a collection of old wives' tales.

Spitzer understood from the beginning that the commonsense definition of disease—"a progressive physical disorder with known pathophysiology"—simply couldn't be stretched to cover mental illness. He finessed this problem by proposing that *disease* was only one of a number of *medical disorders*—conditions that had "negative consequences . . . an inferred or identified organismic dysfunction, and an implicit call to action." *Mental disorder*, he argued, was "a medical disorder whose manifestations are primarily signs or symptoms of a psychological (behavioral) nature." This was a clever move on Spitzer's part, acknowledging that mental illnesses were not diseases in the usual sense, even as he preserved their place in "real medicine."

But it wasn't clever enough to sneak past the members of the American Psychological Association, who immediately recognized the proposal as a way to maintain physician dominion over mental suffering, and they sent a letter protesting it.

"These guys have some chutzpah," Spitzer groused to the APA's president as he prepared a letter in response. But he didn't dispute the psychologists' conclusion. Indeed, he may have gotten a fight he'd been spoiling for all along. He suggested that the exchange of letters be "made public to our membership, as it would be another way of demonstrating our conviction that psychiatry is a specialty within medicine. It would also make it clear to our profession that DSM-III helps psychiatry move closer to the rest of medicine." If they saw their generals aggressively moving to consolidate their power, Spitzer thought, the morale of the rank and file might improve.

The definition Spitzer finally settled on wasn't quite so chauvinistic as the original. But it had plenty of its own chutzpah.

In DSM-III each of the mental disorders is conceptualized as a clinically significant behavioral or psychological syndrome or pattern that occurs in an individual and that is typically associated with either a painful symptom (distress) or impairment in one or more important areas of functioning (disability). In addition, there is an inference that there is a behavioral, psychological or biological dysfunction, and that the disturbance is not only in the relationship between the individual and society. (When the disturbance is *limited* to a conflict between the individual and society, this may represent social deviance, which may or may not be commendable, but is not by itself a mental disorder.)

Mental disorder occurs, Spitzer seems to be saying, when something has gone wrong in the mental apparatus, and the result is distress or disability. But what is the tip-off that something has gone wrong? The presence of distress or disability, of course. And how can a doctor determine whether it is *clinically significant*? The definition doesn't specify, but one obvious method is to say that the mere fact that a patient's suffering is significant enough to make him or her show up at the clinic suffices. And once the patient has arrived, who gets to decide whether the disturbance is limited to a conflict between individuals and society, whether, say, an impoverished person's distress is caused by poverty or internal dysfunction? Doctors, of course, who might be no more reliable at judging whether a person needs psychiatric treatment than barbers are at judging whether a person needs a haircut.

This definition, an obvious response to the homosexuality debacle, was an attempt by the general to fight the last war, and it doesn't really make diagnosis any less circular. Indeed, it just places the already circular definitions of the individual mental disorders inside the larger circle of clinical significance. And in case you weren't dizzy enough, the DSM-III-R added one more loop: "The syndrome or pattern must not be merely an expectable and culturally sanctioned response to a particular event." For its part, DSM-IV devoted seven of its 886 pages to a list of "culture-bound syndromes," including *ataque de nervios*, an "idiom of distress" common in Latin American groups that an unsuspecting doctor might mistake for an anxiety disorder; *pibloktoq*, an "abrupt dissociative episode" found among Eskimos, in which a person might rend his or her garments, break furniture, or eat feces, but does not suffer from mania or Dissociative Identity Disorder; and *koro*, an "intense anxiety that the penis will recede into the body and possibly cause death" that sometimes afflicts Malaysians but which should not be mistaken for a psychosis or Depersonalization Disorder.

The impetus here is obvious. The gay activism that led to the deletion of homosexuality was on the leading edge of the identity politics that took hold in the 1980s and 1990s. The DSM had to keep up with the times, to reassure the public that psychiatrists were not out to pathologize mere difference or to declare certain identities inherently sick. But how is a physician to know what responses we should expect of ourselves when confronted by unprecedented events like 9/11 or the financial meltdown of 2008? Why is a response that is neither expectable nor culturally sanctioned, but clearly justified, such as, say, occupying Wall Street, any more disordered than blithely taking home multimillion-dollar bonuses for running a company into the ground? And why do doctors get to decide which, if any, of those behaviors is symptomatic of Antisocial Personality Disorder?

Like the bereavement exclusion, these definitions don't really serve to limit psychiatry's prerogative to decide what is sick and what is healthy. Instead, they daub whitewash over the fractures in its conceptual infrastructure. And the result is an edifice that holds up only if you don't place any weight on it.

In this respect, all these loopholes are not unlike epicycles, the little curlicues Ptolemaic astronomers built into the orbits of planets to account for why the heavenly bodies were not where they should have been if they moved, as Ptolemy said they must, in perfect circles. Epicycles, not unlike the codicils and caveats in the DSM, are a way to stave off the challenge of the enemy, intended more to preserve the authority of a profession and the dominion of its paradigms than to get to the truth. Unlike the DSM, epicycles have already gone down in history as the epitome of bad science.

Chapter 8

I f psychiatry's attempt to close the gap between opportunity and knowledge with a definition of mental disorder will always yield bullshit, psychiatry's aspirations to scientific respectability are still not doomed—at least not according to Allen Frances. But you have to be willing to accept one premise: that, as he puts it, "psychiatric classification is necessarily a sloppy business."

But even if the definition of mental disorder is bullshit, Frances thinks, the mental disorders themselves are not. The categories may be arbitrary, their existence impossible to prove, and the lines between them as artificial as the lines between countries, but the fact is that an identifiable group of people do, for instance, have "recurrent and persistent thoughts" that are "intrusive, inappropriate and cause marked distress," that are "not simply excessive worries about real-life problems," that can only be suppressed by some "other thought or action," and that are recognized as "a product of [the patient's] own mind." To say, as the DSM-IV does, that those people have Obsessive-Compulsive Disorder is not, in Frances's view, to make any grand claims about how (or even whether) mental illness exists in nature. It is only to glean from research what unites this population of sufferers and then to capture it in language that helps clinicians communicate with patients and colleagues and that provides researchers with categories for their work in developing treatments. A DSM diagnosis may be a construct, in other words, but it is not *only* a construct.

Neither does using a label require some guiding definition about whose troubles are illness and whose mere suffering. Implementing labels requires only a faithful observation of people who come to doctors' attention, a careful sorting of patients, a scrupulous attention to detail in fashioning the criteria, and then a highly skilled, careful clinician, one to whom the sloppiness of classification is a reason to exercise caution. And if all those conditions are in place, the criteria will indeed detect populations who can then be served by doctors alerted to the contours, if not the exact nature, of their patients' troubles. The diagnostician, to use one of Frances's favorite metaphors, is not so much a pathologist looking for a virus in a blood sample as he is a baseball umpire trained to call balls and strikes—even if an agreement to abide by an ultimately arbitrary tradition is the reason that pitches have those names and the strike zone has the exact boundaries that it does.

That's why Frances was so galled by the ambition that he saw in his successors, and why they seemed so reckless to him: they had failed to account for the fragility of a system that hinges on rules inscribed in language rather than on lab tests encoded in numbers. They were heedless of the possibility that once doctors started speaking the revised language, all kinds of hell could break loose. And even worse, they seemed to have lost track of the people who would be consigned to that hell: the patients.

"A diagnosis is a call to action with huge and unpredictable results," he said. "No decision can be right on narrow scientific grounds if it winds up hurting people."

The Bipolar II epidemic was a case in point. There was no question in Frances's mind that making a new diagnosis was the correct decision on narrow scientific grounds. Research clearly showed that people who became manic after starting antidepressants tended to have a history of hypomanic episodes and that those spells tended to last for less than the week required for a diagnosis of mania. But he failed to consider how many people would get hurt if the diagnostic threshold was lowered, how easy it would be for a harried doctor to render the diagnosis and write a prescription with the pen supplied by the drug company rep who had just taken her to lunch. Real-life psychiatric diagnosis could not take place in a bell jar filled with experts and their pet theories. There would always be unintended consequences. That's what Frances said he was trying to say to the DSM-5 leaders. "I just wanted them to learn from my mistakes."

Even if definitions of mental disorder weren't bullshit, they wouldn't solve the validity problem, at least not by themselves. To declare a boundary between illness and health is not to guarantee that any particular category of illness is real. In fact, definitions could worsen the problem. "One of the reasons that diagnostic classification has fallen into disrepute," Eli Robins and Samuel Guze wrote in 1970, "is that diagnostic schemes have been largely based upon *a priori* principles rather than upon systematic studies."

Robins and Guze were leaders of the team at Washington University that developed the descriptive approach that Spitzer adopted for DSM-III. They recognized that the history of science, and especially of medicine, was littered with examples of prejudice-blinded researchers following their often unacknowledged traditions and principles down dead-end alleys. These beliefs aren't always as dunderheaded as the ones that shaped Samuel Cartwright's understanding of a slave's thirst for freedom or Freud's notions about same-sex attraction. In the nineteenth century, for instance, doctors believed that illnesses should be classified by their signs and symptoms—a conviction that had prevailed since Hippocrates had given birth to Western medicine, and which was not unreasonable, given that doctors had little else to go on. So there was really no reason to doubt that patients with genital sores were suffering from a disease different from what patients with a skin rash had, and patients with general paresis, a form of dementia, had yet another illness. There wasn't even a reason to think that this scheme was based on any a priori principle, that it was anything other than a faithful account of how nature itself sorted diseases.

That all changed when some doctors, notably Louis Pasteur and Robert Koch, began to insist that there was more to disease than met the unaided eye. Beneath the appearances, the pustules and the fevers and the complaints, was a microbial world populated by the real sources of illness. And if the detectable presence of viruses and bacteria was not convincing enough, the successes of pasteurization and anthrax inoculations soon had doctors abandoning those first principles and peering into microscopes to find the germs that caused diseases. Among the first organisms they spotted was a *spirochete*, a spiral-shaped germ they named *Treponema pallidum*, which was present in patients with sores, rashes, and dementia alike. They concluded that *T. pallidum* was the natural formation that united those scattered particulars, which they now recognized as different stage of syphilis. By century's end, doctors were asking questions about bacteria and viruses in addition to signs and symptoms, and seeking cures in drugs that targeted those microbes rather than remedies tailored to those outward appearances. Unfettered by archaic beliefs, they were free to find the truth about what ailed us.

But a century after the advent of the germ theory, as Robins and Guze knew too well, psychiatrists had yet to discover a "schizococcus" bacterium or a "depressenza" virus or anything else that would reduce the profession's dependence on a priori principles, and the disasters of the late 1960s and early 1970s were the result. So the two men proposed a solution that they thought could keep descriptive psychiatry safe from belief, at least until those bugs could be found: a five-step process toward validity that, so they said, required no assumptions, that purely through the accretion of evidence would converge to confirm (or disconfirm) that an alleged disease really existed.

Start with clinical description, Robins and Guze said, with a careful account of how patients present themselves, and establish the criteria that link similar patients. Add laboratory studies—including psychological tests—that will confirm (or not) that those people belong together. Develop exclusion criteria so that a patient who is, say, depressed but also has hallucinations and delusions gets grouped with the schizophrenics rather than the depressives. Do follow-up studies to make sure that the people you've grouped together have similar outcomes, as you would expect if they were suffering from the same disease. And study the patients' families to see if their members share symptoms, which would indicate that there is some genetic link among the patients. By working all of these angles, they argued, doctors would eventually accumulate enough evidence to say which mental disorders were valid and which were only figments of an enthusiastic doctor's imagination.

But nearly forty years after Robins and Guze proposed these validators—four decades in which criteria for inclusion and exclusion were written and rewritten, tests conducted, families studied, and patients followed—Darrel Regier told the *Psychiatric News* that "validity tests . . . have not lived up to the expectations of Robins and Guze." Even after Virginia Commonwealth University behavioral geneticist Kenneth Kendler added another validator—differential response to treatment, on the questionable grounds that a response to an antidepressant, for example, confirmed that the patient had MDD in the first place—the patterns that had emerged were weak and confusing. Indeed, by 2010 Kendler himself was still complaining that "the [diagnostic] categories in use have been heavily influenced by expert opinion, which . . . has been heavily influenced by *a priori* factors."

Psychiatrists had evidently been fooled again. The new a priori—Spitzer's principle that mental disorders could be classified by their criteria—has led them "to consider our major diagnostic categories to be obvious and even 'natural,'" Kendler wrote, when, in fact, they were "fuzzy constructs that shift when viewed in different ways." These benighted psychiatrists had fallen for their own ruse. They had forgotten that the DSM was fashioned by experts, which meant that the diagnostic categories tended to reflect the a priori principles of those experts—which, of course, the rank and file largely shared. "We cannot develop a progressive scientifically based nosology shaped by a single expert-driven conception of psychiatric illness, no matter how wise its advocate," Kendler wrote. Evidently, it is one thing for the public to believe the experts, and quite another, at least in the view of one key opinion leader, for the experts to believe themselves.

But Kendler wasn't ready to get rid of the experts and replace them with, say, a WikiDSM. Nor was he joining with the "critics of psychiatric diagnoses," who, so he wrote, insisted that "there is no truth out there" and who would simply give up on the DSM. Indeed, he became a member of a DSM-5 work group and eventually the head of a committee reviewing its scientific soundness. But like Frances, he thought revisers took on a "heavy and conservative burden." They had to avoid the kind of bruising battles in which "different constituencies in psychiatry . . . vie with each other for influence and control," and, upon seizing power, "reshape the nosologic system in their own *a priori* image." The result, he feared, would be "wide fluctuations between different systems with divergent theoretical perspectives and no net progress."

Kendler didn't point out, because he didn't need to since his intended audience knew it in their bones, that DSM-III was about as wide as a fluctuation can get. Bob Spitzer seized power, wrenched psychiatry away from its Freudian principles, and reshaped it in his own image. He might have gotten away with imposing this profession-saving paradigm shift by sheer force of will, but it was a desperate measure taken in desperate times, and not one you would want to repeat—especially if you want your revisions to lead to a closer approximation of the reality of mental illness and your constituency to have more faith in you than they do in other institutions known more for their thrashings over divergent theoretical perspectives than their net progress, like the United States Congress.

That goal is possible, Kendler wrote, but only if changes are made slowly and carefully. In fact, if you are careful enough, a good outcome is nearly guaranteed, thanks to the process of *epistemic iteration*, a concept Kendler borrowed from mathematics, where it is defined as:

> A historic and scientific process in which successive stages of knowledge ... build in a sequential manner upon each other. ... When correctly applied, the process of epistemic iteration should lead through successive stages of scientific research toward a better and better approximation of reality in a "spiral of improvement."

It's easy to see the appeal of this promise. Kendler himself is the researcher who reported that when Walter Cassidy, the psychiatrist who first proposed diagnostic criteria for depression, was asked why he set the threshold at six out of ten symptoms, he responded, "It sounded about right." If you know that your origins are murky and your tools blunt, and yet you want to claim that you are nonetheless heading toward clarity, then it behooves you to put your money on a "wonderful property of iteration" and its "capacity to get to the real solution regardless of the starting point."

And if you know that your nosology has gyrated wildly through the years, that it has been buffeted by history, its a priori principles brought to light and debunked and hidden away again, if you know that the doubt thus kindled will become your enemies' weapon, if you know that you and your allies must be able to "assure ourselves that each revision of our manuals contains improvements on its predecessor," then what better talisman to carry into battle than epistemic iteration, with its nearly magical power to ensure that even as you are making your mistakes, truth is all along accumulating, that those fluctuations are really only what Kendler calls "*wobbly* iterations," that every day in every way your map of our suffering is getting better and better, and that sooner or later, the experts, well versed in expertise, will produce a DSM that, as Kendler puts it, "asymptotes to a stable and accurate parameter estimate"?

But psychiatry is not mathematics. The way we suffer, unlike the way numbers behave, changes with time and circumstance, and experts' opinions of what ails us change the way we think of ourselves and our travails. Kendler insists that mental illnesses must exist in nature. Rewind the tape of history to the dawn of civilization, he says—about ten thousand years ago, when our biological apparatus would have taken shape but history had yet to make us into who we are—and start again. Record the result, and do this a thousand times. While it is likely that in each iteration you will see psychiatrists arriving at different criteria by which they know our mental illnesses, you will also see the illnesses themselves, just as you are sure to see diabetes and strokes and broken bones.

Of course, just because Kendler says that's what will happen, it's not necessarily what would happen. Indeed, the thought experiment falters when you consider that Kendler borrowed the scenario from paleontologist Stephen Jay Gould. In the original version, Gould rewound the tape to the beginning of earth's history to point out that given all the accidents, the asteroid crashes and ice ages and tectonic shifts, it was very unlikely that human life as we know it would emerge in any of those do-overs. His rhetorical point was that it was folly to assume that the long arc of evolution bends toward anything in particular, that only Whiggishness or presentism or some kind of Voltairian optimism—not to mention a huge dose of species-level narcissism—would allow a person to claim that we are the inevitable culmination of creation, let alone that our endeavors lead inherently toward progress.

"We follow the tape forward until modern science and medicine develop," Kendler writes, but this is the whole lesson of Gould's experiment: We cannot know if anything like modern science and medicine will develop. We cannot simply assume that people will come to identify their subjective troubles as mental, much less place them in doctors' hands. Gould figured that each new spool would be entirely different, not simply an instant replay.

If Kendler has assumed his conclusions here, it is because he has to assume that mental illness exists in the same way as diabetes and strokes, and that the only alternative is to believe "there is no truth out there." He has to believe these things because he is a psychiatrist, and only a notion of historical inevitability can justify the enormous hubris, the inescapable a priori principle of psychiatry: that our psychological suffering is *medical*—which, as our reel has unspooled, means located in bodily processes gone awry. Go to the tape, Kendler seems to be saying, and you will find that doctors' failures so far, including the faulty DSM that urgently needed replacing, are just detours on the road to Parnassus and not a disastrous wrong turn.

Psychiatry is not inevitable. It's not baseball, either. Those wobbly iterations aren't just bad calls that frustrate a batter and raise a crowd's ineffectual, if vocal, ire. They are diagnoses that change people's lives, that render homosexuals unfit for employment, that subject children to untested and powerful drugs, that encourage patients to think of their troubles as chemical imbalances rather than meaningful signs of something gone wrong in their lives. If you go to see a psychiatrist, you probably don't enter the office as if you were going into Fenway Park. You don't think you are about to take part in a game whose rules are arbitrary if venerable and negotiable. You don't expect the number of symptoms that add up to depression to change like the strike zone has or diagnoses to enter the DSM like the designated hitter was added to the rulebook. If you're anything like me, as much as you might like baseball, you expect more from your doctors than that.

You might also think there is a difference between the current DSM and the current *Official Rules of Major League Baseball*—and not just that one costs $95.89 on Amazon, while the other can be downloaded for free and, in its 2011 edition anyway, has an excellent picture of Curtis Granderson crossing home plate on its cover. You might well believe that one compiles the laws of nature and the other the rules of the game, and if you do, it is in part because we all want to believe that someone somewhere can understand and help us when we suffer. But it is also because psychiatrists—with their scientific-looking DSM, with their assurances about epistemic iteration, with their talk of chemical imbalances and their medications to treat them—have spent the better part of the past four decades telling you, and acting like, it is so.

Darrel Regier's August 2009 interview with the *Psychiatric News* was part of a concerted effort to counter Frances's warnings that the DSM-5 was headed for disaster. "The 'disastrous result' in most clinicians' and researchers' minds would be for DSM to continue on the same path it has been on for 30 years," he told the *News*. That's why his task force was proposing "significant revisions," and why the new manual, he wrote in an *American Journal of Psychiatry* article, would "attempt to address the consequences of continuing to use the original . . . hierarchical structure of 'pure' diagnostic categories." Frances and Spitzer's DSM was simply too bad to be left alone.

Regier may have been making a wholesale critique, but he was quick to say that "a wholesale revision was not in the cards." What Regier had in mind was nothing as radical as casting the categories to the wind. Instead, he said, diagnostic labels and criteria would be joined by *dimensional measures*. The problem with the categorical approach was that it forced clinicians into binary decisions. Did the patient have OCD or MDD, ADHD or BDNOS? Too often the result was more than one diagnosis— the comorbidity problem—or a diagnosis that didn't really capture the clinical picture. And then there were the "patients with clinically significant distress and impairment," whose symptoms spanned many diagnoses without reaching a diagnostic threshold in any one. People could be a little depressed, a little anxious, a little obsessive-compulsive, but still in a lot of distress. Wouldn't it make sense to be able to identify, measure, and study these *cross-cutting symptoms* as dimensions of pathology without necessarily attributing them to a particular category?

"The single most important precondition for moving forward to improve the clinical and scientific utility of DSM-V will be the incorporation of simple dimensional measures," Regier wrote. Their "prominent use" would be "one, if not the major, difference between DSM-IV and DSM-V." The revision would focus on measuring the severity of symptoms, both within and across diagnoses. This alone would not entirely spring psychiatry from its epistemic prison, but, especially once researchers could "establish better syndrome boundaries" and "identify continuous measures of the constituent symptoms," he told me in an e-mail, they would be able to determine the "statistically valid cutpoints between normal and pathological." Getting to this goal, of course, would require categories based on "a full understanding of the underlying pathophysiology of mental disorders." But even if this was a long way off, it was important to take the first step now. "Delaying the introduction of dimensional measures in this version of DSM will simply retard both clinical and research progress," he wrote.

But it wasn't as if DSM-IV lacked dimensional measures. Some diagnoses, such as depression, had severity specifiers, in which clinicians rated a patient's disorder from zero to five and reported this as the last digit of the diagnosis code. And the DSM-IV also provided a Global Assessment of Functioning scale, which clinicians were supposed to use to indicate a patient's functioning on a scale of zero to one hundred. But, as we clinicians soon found out, when we rated a patient's functioning too high or his severity too low, insurance companies used these numbers as their own kind of statistical cutpoint—to cut off benefits. So we quickly adapted—inflating the ratings or ignoring them altogether, not telling unless we were asked.

Regier needed a more comprehensive and scientific approach to dimensional assessment than what the DSM-IV offered, but this presented a problem. Very few severity tests for DSM-IV diagnoses had been developed and validated. Nor did he have a huge literature to draw on for measuring cross-cutting symptoms. The National Institutes of Health had created PROMIS (Patient Reported Outcomes Measurement Infor-

mation System) to gather information on h.
were faring, but while this offered a way to det
a person was or how well he was sleeping, Regier
kind of data would be integrated into the diagnos
mensional measures in place for the DSM-5 required a
[sic] approach for instrument development," he wrote, but the group
that had been assigned to dive into that task started its work only in
January 2009. Field trials, in which those tests would presumably be
studied, were slated to begin in summer 2009, so they had had just a few
months to put together their tests. To critics, this seemed like an indication of disarray. "If they really want to do dimensional assessment," Michael First told me, "they should wait the five or ten years it would take
for the scales to be ready."

But Regier did not think it was necessary to have all this nailed
down before the book was published. "We don't expect the DSM-5 to be
perfect or etched in stone for the ages," he told me in an e-mail. This
expectation, after all, was the central trouble with the previous DSMs;
designed to look scientific, they had proven too easy to reify. And even
if the DSM-5 was not going to be anchored in the bedrock of neurobiology, even if it could not fulfill the promise of paradigm change with
which it had been born, still it could achieve one thing: the ratcheting
back of expectations for the revision, and for psychiatric nosology itself.
Diagnostic criteria "are intended to be scientific hypotheses, rather than
inerrant Biblical scripture," he wrote. And the DSM was not scripture.
It was a "living document."

It was a clever rhetorical move. Regier had turned the reification of
the DSM into just another of those "epistemic iterations" that Kendler
wrote about, a wobbly step on the way to the truth. The categorical approach had served its purpose, and now it was time to back away from
it, and from the misguided fundamentalists who took the diagnoses literally. It was time to pirouette on the back of those new dimensional
measures into the "spiral of improvement."

Chapter 9

Throughout the summer and fall of 2009, Allen Frances kept up his attack. He became a regular contributor to the *Psychiatric Times*, blogging, sometimes in every issue, about what he thought the APA was doing wrong. By the time he posted a blog titled "Advice to DSM V," the APA was probably not in the mood to take it.

"There is no magic moment when it becomes clear that the world needs a new edition of the DSM," he reminded his successors. A revision of the ICD scheduled for fall 2012 had reportedly been delayed—and, as he also pointed out, because the codes used by the DSM-5 came from the ICD, a new DSM that preceded a new ICD would soon have outdated codes. Wouldn't it be better to coordinate the release of the DSM and the ICD, and in the bargain give the revision the time it deserved?

Getting out from under deadline pressure was the key to saving the DSM-5, Frances thought, and this now became his mission. Unintended consequences were the unknown unknowns of the APA's revision campaign, and haste only increased their likelihood and severity. Even a good diagnostic change could make unexpected trouble. For instance, he wrote, the DSM-IV had fashioned new criteria for ADHD. They were clearer and easier to remember, and in the field trials the new criteria identified 15 percent more kids with ADHD than the old criteria had—an acceptable result, Frances thought at the time. But once the criteria went into wide use, the actual increase was 28 percent—an outcome he attributed in part to the ease with which doctors, as well as parents and teachers, could apply the simplified criteria.

Of greatest concern to Frances, however, was the task force's failure to take "the most important step in the development of any DSM": to release a complete first draft. Without one, experts outside the work groups could not weigh in on either the proposed revisions or the procedures by which they would be tested, which meant that the field trials might use a faulty methodology to investigate faulty diagnoses comprising poorly written criteria—a compounding of errors that would, he was sure, turn out to be the "fatal flaw" of DSM-5.

This haste, combined with tunnel vision, was particularly distressing, he wrote, because of Kupfer and Regier's ambition. Their vow to make a "bottoms-up" revision meant that "everything was on the table." The experts on the work groups would have free rein to make changes without much constraint from their commanders. The task force, he concluded, had put change over stability, innovation over tradition, and threatened to turn the process into a runaway train that would pull psychiatry "over the cliff." To postpone publication was therefore the "obviously right thing," as obvious as putting on the brakes to slow a speeding car.

Frances wound up his lesson with a confession of his own failings. "It is surprisingly difficult to write clean, foolproof criteria items. I know this from frustrating personal experience. Despite many years of effort and practice, I never mastered this highly technical writing skill." (He couldn't resist adding that "no one working on DSM-V has had any extensive experience in writing diagnostic criteria"—a not-so-veiled reference to the expunging of Michael First.) And the DSM-IV's text, as opposed to the criteria, the sections within each diagnosis that described such matters as the familial patterns, biological factors, and epidemiology of the disorder, was "tired, old . . . in need of exhaustive revision . . . and fails to convey any of the vividness of actual clinical practice," and thus "should be up for grabs." Anyone who said Frances was merely trying to protect his own ego, in other words, had it wrong. He just wanted his successors to change what could be changed and otherwise leave well enough alone.

Frances never misses an opportunity to tell you how dumb or dull or insignificant he and his DSM are. He might mean it. He does seem to subscribe to the conservative notion, made most famous by Edmund Burke, that modesty, born of education and refinement, is the best check on power, at least the kind of power he once wielded. But there is also strategy to his self-effacement. "I take more blame for DSM-IV than we actually deserved," he told me once. "I purposely emphasized the mistakes that we made. But I saw it as a rhetoric that would help them to feel more comfortable hearing, 'Look. I screwed up and I don't want you guys to have the same problems,' rather than 'DSM-IV was such a great document but yours produces crap.' I'm not criticizing you because I think you are a jerk and I'm smart, but I'm criticizing you because I've been through it and this is my mea culpa."

Not that Frances thinks that DSM-IV *was* a great document. It was only what he wanted it to be—a selective polishing of Spitzer's work, the best (or the least bad) that could be done with the tools at his disposal, successful because it was dull and unambitious. But Regier and Kupfer, with their everything-on-the-table ambition, were going to produce crap. He may not have thought they were jerks. But when he semisweetened his advice with faint praise—"The DSM-V task force and work group members are dedicated people doing their best under very difficult circumstances"—and then followed it up with condescension—"They should be given sufficient time to ensure that DSM-V will be a worthwhile contribution"—it was pretty clear that this was getting personal and that he was not going to stop being one of those difficult circumstances.

After defending themselves in the leading journal and both industry newsletters—and in mainstream outlets such as *The Wall Street Journal*, to which Kupfer confessed that "some of us have gotten . . . sick enough about playing defensive ball and being taken out of context"—the DSM leaders went silent. So did APA president Alan Schatzberg, but only after he reassured members that they were the real victims.

"The development process has been so public," he told the *Psychiatric News*, "that anyone can kvetch about one point or another in a blog." Schatzberg did welcome "scholars and clinicians" to engage in "collaborative and collegial interchange" with DSM leaders, but suggested that critics should quit their kvetching, or at least take heed of the unintended consequences of their own behavior. "The news media thrive on controversy," he warned, "and some of these discussions have . . . provided ammunition for those who are anti-psychiatry as a science and opposed to treatment."

But while the APA was hunkering down in public, in private it was scrambling. In the spring of 2009, before Frances began his onslaught, two members of the childhood disorders work group had resigned. One refused to talk publicly, citing fears that the APA would seek retribution. But the second, Duke University professor Jane Costello, made her resignation letter public—"I'm too small a fish for them to bother with," she told me—and it was getting widely distributed. As much as she enjoyed "working with this extraordinary group of people," she wrote,

> I cannot in good conscience continue. I am increasingly uncomfortable with the whole underlying principle of rewriting the entire psychiatric taxonomy at one time. I am not aware of any other branch of medicine that does anything like this. There seems to be no good

scientific justification for doing this, and certainly none for doing it in 2012.

The science simply wasn't available for fulfilling the APA's ambitions for DSM-5, Costello wrote. Indeed, in a line she could have lifted from Harry Frankfurt, she lamented that the more researchers tried, the more they realized that "the gap between what we need to know in order to make revisions and what we do know has grown wider and wider, while the time to fill these gaps is shrinking rapidly." And at least one attempt to fill in those gaps—a research project proposed by Costello and a colleague—had, she said, been rebuffed by Kupfer on the grounds that he needed results sooner than they could produce them. Even worse, the APA could have had their results sooner, but they had been unwilling to pay for the research, leaving her no choice but to turn to the NIMH, whose funding wheels turn slowly—too slowly, it seemed, for the impatient DSM revisers.

All of this she perhaps could have tolerated, but then came the "tipping point": the announcement by Kupfer and Regier that dimensional assessment would be the major difference between DSM-IV and DSM-5.

Setting aside the question of who "decided," on what grounds, anyone with any experience of instrument development knows that what they proposed . . . is a huge task, and a very expensive one. The possibility of doing a . . . careful and responsible job given the time and resources available is remote, while to do anything less is irresponsible.

Costello was "shocked" at the decision. After all, she pointed out, "a drug company that tried to bring a product to market on the basis of inadequately funded research would rightly be censured."

Costello's letter was addressed to the head of her work group, but the response came from Darrel Regier. He spent two of his six paragraphs reciting the failures of the DSM-IV and a third describing the necessity of dimensional measures to remedy them. Costello probably knew all this, but the DSM-IV's inadequacies had become part of an origin story that Regier was already using whenever the revision was criticized. It was as if Costello had been defending the DSM-IV and questioning the need for dimensional measures, rather than acknowledging its limitations while wondering whether or not the revision could possibly meet its goals.

Finally, more than halfway through his letter, Regier began to address her concerns. "There was certainly some miscommunication" regarding proposals such as hers. He didn't say what had been miscommunicated or by whom, but he did point out that at the time she applied for the research grant, the APA did not yet know what kind of data it would need or how it would be analyzed. Since then, he reassured her, the requirements had become clear. And while the APA was indeed not funding projects that cost more than $50,000—a pittance—still there was plenty of data out there. "Billions of dollars" (much of it, Regier didn't add, government money) had been spent in the forty years since the current paradigm had been established. The fruits of this research were available in journals, and some work group members had even made their work available "as a professional courtesy." This data would be the basis for the revision. The APA may have been strapped, but it was also resourceful. And, he reminded her, it was "the only entity with the standing, capacity, and willingness" to undertake a comprehensive revision.

As to the readiness of the dimensional measures, Costello need not worry. "A good number of us involved with this process," Regier wrote, "have extensive experience in supporting the development of the previously mentioned instruments and would not diminish the standards used." Haste will not make waste, he seemed to be saying, because the matter is safely in the hands of the experts—although, he admitted, it was possible that not all the tests would be ready when the DSM that required their use came out. Nor did the APA have, as some had charged, a mercenary intent in developing a host of new tests. "Our intent is to make all such instruments freely available for clinical and research use,"

Regier wrote, "and to copyright them to insure their integrity." So even if the dimensional measures weren't fully developed in time for publication, he promised that researchers would be able to refine them afterward. He didn't explain how clinicians and researchers would make diagnoses in the meantime.

Urgency justified haste; the desperation of psychiatry to meet the scientific demands of the day required desperate, or at least incompletely developed, measures. Regier was not refuting Costello at all. Instead, he was agreeing that the dimensional measures were nowhere near ready while suggesting that this was not the problem she thought it was. A living document is a messy thing, a lesser evil than a faulty document inscribed in stone. And anyway, wasn't it Allen Frances who once said that psychiatric diagnosis is a sloppy business?

The APA didn't make Regier's response to Costello public at first. "Since we considered this a private matter, we did not broadcast this response as her letter was broadcast by some of our critics," Regier explained when he provided it to me. But in private, the kvetching—and the fact that it was coming from people like Costello, Spitzer, and ultimately Frances, rather than, say, Tom Cruise—was causing unrest at headquarters. The APA's board of trustees was growing concerned over the brewing feud. "When there is smoke," trustee (and former APA president) Carolyn Robinowitz told me, "you have to make sure that you take a really in-depth look."

In the summer of 2009, the board appointed Robinowitz to head a DSM oversight committee. The new committee didn't exactly find a fire, but they did find smoldering trouble that was clearly not the work of the APA's enemies. "The board was hearing from Dr. Regier and Dr. Kupfer that things were going pretty much on schedule," she recalled. But then the committee talked to the work group members and discovered that "there was a certain amount of conflict," Robinowitz told me. She was, I thought, straining to be diplomatic.

"Dr. Kupfer wanted to get a flow of ideas and issues," she continued, but the rancor and disorganization within the groups indicated that this method was backfiring. Not that anyone should have expected anything but infighting "when you have a bunch of outstanding researchers strong in their beliefs and strong in their science," but the result was that even the work group chairs thought "their stuff wasn't quite ready for prime time." Robinowitz's panel concluded that "things weren't moving as well as they might be. The process allowed for a lot of input, but it hadn't begun to coalesce as much as it should have by that time."

The oversight committee wasn't only concerned with how far behind schedule the effort had already fallen, now that summer had passed and the promised field trials had not materialized. "We were also looking at the timetable they proposed and everything was tight," Robinowitz said. So the committee recommended that the publication be delayed one year, to May 2013. And, she allowed in fall 2010, the committee might recommend further postponements, depending on what happened in the field trials that Regier insisted would be the proving grounds for the changes. "It's not a contract that we have to execute or there will never be another DSM. I don't think anyone is going to say we've got to go forward if we get crappy results."

In early December, Frances told his growing *Psychiatric Times* following that his "anonymous sources" in the organization were telling him to expect an important announcement soon. Sure enough, a week later the APA issued a press release. The "anticipated" publication date was now May 2013. Schatzberg explained that "extending the timeline will allow more time for public review, field trials and revisions. The APA is committed," he went on, "to developing a manual that is based on the best science available and useful to clinicians and researchers."

The press release didn't acknowledge that the APA had taken

precisely the course that Frances had recommended. And when I put the question to Regier, he claimed that the delay was occasioned only by the "long vetting process and startup time of the work groups," which in turn resulted from the APA's requirement that revisers divest themselves of drug company money. Once again, the APA was claiming to be the victim—not of Frances, but of its own goodness. Regier also insisted that Frances's complaints had "added no content to the discussion," and indeed had "only served to heighten interest" in the revision. Frances, in other words, was *helping* the APA.

Even so, Frances was flirting with danger. "His major critique," Regier went on, was that "nothing has changed in the scientific world since his revision and hence no substantive revision is possible." Not only that, he was also asserting "that his judgment on the pragmatic consequences of revisions should take precedence over any of the experts in a given diagnostic field." He was, in other words, trumping up his personal grievance into a broadside against the institution he once served and in the bargain calling into question the credibility of the APA. The diagnosis was clear: Allen Frances, once America's top psychiatrist, was letting his ego take him on a kamikaze mission directed at his own colleagues. Blinded by pride, he had become his own kind of antipsychiatrist and, even worse, a turncoat.

In January 2010, Frances took his show on the road. After a test run at Duke, he went to Columbia University's medical school to present grand rounds—a medical school tradition in which an eminent doctor describes a case to students. Frances's case was the ailing DSM. "I'm going to be quite critical," he said at the outset of his forty-five-minute talk, but first he wanted to address his own "possible biases"—meaning, it turned out, the charges that the DSM-5 defenders had leveled at him. He was not inherently conservative or opposed to change, he assured the audience, which included numerous DSM-5 work group members (along with

Michael First); his caution over the DSM revision was the exception. He wasn't "trying to save my baby," he told them. "The DSM-IV is not something I feel particularly proud of, and I don't think it was much of a contribution to the world," and as for the $10,000 in royalties that the APA had said was his real motive for agitating for a delay—"Well, it's conceivable that that's why I'm giving this talk," he said, and shared a laugh with his fellow high earners over that paltry sum.

The talk was a concentrated version of the litany he'd been developing over six months of blogging, now for *Psychology Today* in addition to the *Psychiatric Times*. But it was one thing to thumb out a blog on his BlackBerry (or to give a talk on his own home turf) and another to tell an audience such as this one that the DSM-5 was very likely to be "crummy" and a "mess," that the big question was whether or not it would also be dangerous, and that the revisers were so blind to their own faults that only public pressure could avert that disaster.

After the talk, and before he started the Q&A session, moderator Jeffrey Lieberman, the head of Columbia's department of psychiatry and a member of Robinowitz's oversight committee, tried to relieve the tension. "Allen," he said, "I only wish you hadn't held back, and told us what you *really* thought."

Frances reached over and put his big hand on Lieberman's white-coated shoulder. "I did hold back," he said.

David Shaffer, a member of the childhood disorders work group, was the first audience member to speak. He certainly didn't hold back.

"Congratulations, Allen," he said. "It was a daring exercise to list so many strong complaints without having seen what's about to be posted." (The APA had not yet put the promised draft of the DSM on its website.) Even worse, according to Shaffer, Frances had compounded his ignorance by setting up a straw man. "You represented a set of overambitious and vain and silly goals that actually were never stated as such," he said.

As Frances prepared to respond, Shaffer reclaimed the microphone. "One personal thing," he said. He had worked on both DSM-III and DSM-IV, and agreed with Frances that the new revision's "style of management has been completely different." But far from flirting with disaster, the "bottom-up process [had] led to some of the most stimulating debate as I can remember in my career." It was a double rebuke to Frances: he had not only jumped the gun with his criticisms; he had also been wrong to conduct his revision in an autocratic manner, one that had evidently bored Shaffer. It was as if the DSM-IV's troubles were the result of Frances's conservatism. Having been freed from these restraints, it seemed, the DSM-5's experts couldn't help but come up with a better book, or at least have a more stimulating time in the process.

Frances didn't respond directly to Shaffer's complaints, except to agree that "the proof will be in the pudding." And a few weeks later, on February 10, the pudding was served. The APA posted a full draft of the proposed revisions on its website. The draft maintained the DSM-IV's structure, organizing mental disorders into sixteen chapters ("Mood Disorders," "Anxiety Disorders," "Schizophrenia and Other Psychotic Disorders," etc.), but it also featured changes to virtually every part of the book, from the definition of mental disorders at the beginning to the "Listing of Other Conditions" at the end. Doctors would be able to diagnose and get paid to treat Psychosis Risk Syndrome and other disorders, such as Minor Neurocognitive Disorder, that were more harbingers of future trouble than present illnesses. Kids labeled bipolar by the Biederman protocol would now have Temper Dysregulation Disorder, and kids diagnosed with Asperger's Disorder would suddenly come down with a case of Autistic Spectrum Disorder, if they were still sick at all. Pathological gambling would no longer be an Impulse Control Disorder, but instead would become a behavioral addiction, joining Alcohol Use Disorder and Cannabis Use Disorder in the Substance-Related Disorders section, which would be renamed "Addiction and Related Disorders." Pathological gambling would be the only behavioral addiction for now; Internet Addiction had not made the cut, and Money Addiction apparently hadn't been considered. But you would no longer have to be addicted to or dependent on a drug to warrant a diagnosis; any kind of troublesome use was enough. Troublesome sex could also be diagnosed; people who experienced "six or more months of recurrent and intense sexual fantasies, sexual urges, and sexual behavior," in which they spent "a great deal of time . . . planning for and engaging in sexual behavior," would have Hypersexual Disorder. If their attraction was to young adolescents, they would be suffering from Pedohebephilia, and if they got off on forcing people to have sex, they would qualify for Paraphilic Coercive Disorder. Adults would get criteria for their own version of Attention Deficit/Hyperactivity Disorder, and children would need fewer symptoms to qualify for ADHD. The recently bereaved would lose their exemption from the depression diagnosis and would be mentally ill after two weeks of grieving. Where there had once been ten personality disorders, there would now be only five. People who went on Ben and Jerry's sprees would now have Binge Eating Disorder, and people who were worried and sad but didn't meet criteria for either Generalized Anxiety Disorder or Major Depressive Disorder would now qualify for Mixed Anxiety-Depression Disorder. Every patient would get rated for cross-cutting symptoms, and every diagnosis would come with a severity rating, although it wasn't exactly clear how this would be done because these dimensional measures, as Regier had predicted, were still under construction.

Everything was indeed on the table.

The APA would allow the public, kvetchers and scholars alike, to weigh in on the proposals for two months (although, as its website cautioned, while "all input we receive will be reviewed . . . we can not guarantee that your suggestions will be incorporated into any revisions." But it didn't have to wait long to hear from some familiar voices or work hard to figure out where they stood.

"Anything you put in that book, any little change you make, has huge implications," Michael First told *The New York Times* on the day of the release. Those risk syndromes, for instance, carried their own risk, at least the one about psychosis did: "that many unusual, semi-deviant, creative kids could . . . carry this label for the rest of their lives."

And the very next day, Allen Frances listed for *Psychiatric Times* readers "The 19 Worst Suggestions for DSM5." His four-thousand-word evisceration of the draft argued that with its lowered thresholds for old diagnoses and its brand-new, untested diagnoses, the DSM-5 would be like honey to the drug company flies and like gold to lawyers. Psychosis Risk Syndrome would be a "catastrophe," Mixed Anxiety-Depression would become an "epidemic," Temper Dysregulation Disorder was a "nonstarter," Paraphilic Coercive Disorder would be a boon to prosecutors looking to commit sex offenders indefinitely to mental hospitals and to defense lawyers seeking to exculpate their rapist clients, behavioral addictions would provide "a ready excuse for off-loading personal responsibility," and Pedohebephilia would "medicalize criminal behavior." Dimensional assessments, cross-cutting and diagnosis-specific, were "ad hoc, unworkably complex, vague, untested, and premature," not to mention "bewilderingly inconsistent . . . extremely complicated and totally impractical." The proposals confirmed what Frances had feared: that "the DSM5 has been and remains in serious trouble."

"How can such smart and scrupulous people make so many bad suggestions?" Frances wondered toward the end of his diatribe. His answer was that because experts, no matter how well intentioned, would always expand their reach, it was up to their leaders to recognize and resist this "diagnostic imperialism," and that this seemed the last thing that the "DSM5 leadership," defensive and secretive, and still committed to their bottom-up approach, were likely to do. The leaders—he pointedly did not mention Kupfer and Regier by name—had failed to recognize this duty, so they no longer deserved the benefit of the doubt.

Chapter 10

Allen Frances had spoken his piece but no one on the inside had listened, so he redoubled his attack, turning to the rank-and-file psychiatrists who, he assumed, were the people reading his blogs. "The rest," Frances told them, "is up to you." In the dozen missives he fired off to the *Psychiatric Times* between mid-February and the end of May—with acerbic titles like "Biting Off More Than It Can Chew," "Not Ready for Prime Time," and "Psychiatric Diagnosis Gone Wild"—he exhorted his readers to "Just Say No," as he put it in his blog about the sexual disorders proposals. He reminded them of the public commentary period. In April he sent another letter to the trustees that added some new charges—that the field trials (whose design had just been posted) were fundamentally flawed, that the project still lacked oversight, that despite the one-year delay, the revision was hopelessly behind schedule—and urged the trustees to use their "power and responsibility" lest "things drift further over the cliff." Warning that "this might be a last chance tipping point to save DSM-5," he made the letter public and begged psychiatrists to "influence your leaders to take the decisive actions to solve them."

Frances insists he is ill suited, by temperament and experience, to participate in a rebellion, let alone to lead one. "I was of age in the '60s and never protested or went to D.C. to hear Martin Luther King. I was at Jones Beach having a great time," he once told me. He was responding to an e-mail in which I suggested that there was something poignant and quixotic about his battle with the APA. "I am not a quester for truth or a righter of wrongs or a follower of impossible dreams," he wrote. "I am Panza." He implored me to get this right. "[I] would prefer to be portrayed accurately as the lowly brute I am than to be ennobled into some version of David and Goliath."

"I am not battling the DSM-5 leadership in some romantic crusade," he went on. "There was no one else in a position to take on DSM-5 so I was stuck . . . by an unavoidable duty. I started trying to warn them and now I am trying to shame them. Nothing noble or quixotic or poignant."

On the other hand, Allen Frances was once the most powerful psychiatrist in America. You don't need a slingshot to smack your fellow Goliaths in the forehead, and you don't get to be one of them without putting some skin in the game and figuring out how to be forceful. For Frances, or so he says, this came down to one simple tactic. "I never yell," he insisted. "I tease."

He recalled a kerfuffle in the late days of the DSM-IV campaign over Self-Defeating Personality Disorder (SDPD)—which, in what he calls a "nice irony," was the remnant of his own "dumb idea" for Masochistic Personality Disorder. SDPD had been placed in the Appendix of the DSM-III-R, where it presumably awaited "further study," but in the meantime, it had become a magnet for the kind of controversy Frances disliked—not only among psychiatrists, but in the rest of the world, where feminists worried that the diagnosis would lead to laying the blame for domestic violence and sexual assault on the supposed pathology of the victims.

Frances wanted to kick SDPD out of the DSM entirely, but psychoanalytically minded psychiatrists opposed him—largely because, with its insistence that people might be unconsciously motivated to behave against their own best interests, the diagnosis was one of the last vestiges of psychoanalysis in the DSM. They started a last-minute rearguard action. To help quell it, the head of the APA, Melvin Sabshin, suggested that Frances and Herbert Peyser, an advocate for the diagnosis, stage a series of debates at a meeting of the APA Assembly, the representative body within the organization.

"This was the stupidest idea in the world," Frances said. "You don't debate things like this." Not only that, but "Herb was going against the rules. He stubbornly made [SDPD] a political issue." But Sabshin was the boss and Frances found himself doing exactly what the rules he'd made with Pincus had been designed to prevent: bloviating in front of a room full of pontificators.

"Herb and I would debate for a half hour for each of these groups," he told me. "At the end, Herb and I would come out and I'd give him a big kiss on the cheek and a pinch on both cheeks, and I would say, 'Herb, you're absolutely brilliant, it's almost impossible to debate against you. If we were candidates, you'd kill me, because I don't know what I'm doing and you're brilliant.' And then I'd say, 'But I'm sorry you're not going to win, because it's just a stupid idea.'"

Bob Spitzer served as Peyser's cornerman in the debates. "After the third or fourth," Peyser told me, "Spitzer says, 'Herb, the best argument in favor of SDPD is if we keep arguing with Al about it.'" Even if there was a group of people who met the criteria for the diagnosis, who could be reliably identified, who were distinct from other groups of troubled people, and who suffered impairment as a result—even, that is, if the diagnosis qualified in all ways as a mental disorder—"it was clear from the beginning," Peyser told me, "Al was going to win."

And indeed he did, garnering 60 percent of the assembly's votes for his proposal to delete the disorder, without ever yelling.

Teasing, perhaps more than other kinds of joking, only barely conceals the hostility and aggression and the wish to inflict shame that Freud once said was the function of jokes. It is, at least psychologically speaking, a lowly and brute tactic, and, compared with launching a rock at a

Goliath, cowardly. But it can work, so long as the audience, or the butt of the joke, accepts the rules of engagement, as Jeffrey Lieberman did when he laughed—a little uncomfortably, perhaps—with the rest of the grand-rounds crowd when Frances laid his hand on his shoulder and joked with him at Columbia. And Peyser remembers the debates as "delicious," even if his cheeks got pinched and he got trounced.

But at least one man doesn't seem to get Frances's jokes: David Shaffer, the Columbia child psychiatrist who shrouded his hostility toward Frances in gentility rather than humor when he congratulated him for spouting off on proposals he hadn't seen. Shaffer thinks that Frances's "orderly and democratic process" did tame Spitzer's rough-and-tumble—"I liken it to a tobacco auction," he said—but the needling, even nearly twenty years later, still rankled.

"The worst thing about Allen Frances was that he would always find some reason to insult Bob," Shaffer told me. "If Bob said something, he would say, 'Well, that's a typical Spitzerism,' or he would find some other ad hominem thing to say. It was childish and embarrassing."

"David probably misinterpreted what passes as New York Jewish humor for disrespect," Frances said.

And, indeed, Shaffer said he never quite understood the "New York kind of logic" that both Spitzer and Frances seemed to favor. That's not hard to believe when you lay eyes on him. He's as different as can be from those two swarthy, wisecracking New Yorkers—a pale wisp of a man who talks with a soft British lilt and demurely turns his head to the side, looking out his office window toward the Hudson River and the George Washington Bridge when he's reaching for his next words. It's a little hard to imagine a man so mild being married, as he was for fifteen years, to *Vogue* editor Anna Wintour; he's not even particularly well dressed. But he is unabashedly pleased to have a different leadership style in place as he works on DSM-5, and he's pretty annoyed with Frances—not only for his Columbia talk ("a real blot on his landscape"), but also for hammering away at Shaffer's pet proposal for the revision, Temper Dysregulation Disorder (TDD).

Shaffer thinks he was in part responsible for Frances's attacks. "The TDD was my fault," he said.

He's not talking about the new diagnosis. He still believes that was a good idea, and the best way to solve an embarrassing problem. "Biederman was a crook," Shaffer told me. "He borrowed a disease and applied it in a chaotic fashion. He came up with ridiculous data that none of us believed. It brought child psychiatry into disrepute and was a terrible burden on the families of the children who got that label."

It would not be enough simply to put an end to the childhood bipolar epidemic by, say, changing the DSM to restrict the diagnosis by age or introducing chronic irritability as an *exclusion criterion*—a condition whose presence would contraindicate the diagnosis. "These kids are terribly ill," Shaffer said, and if Biederman "hijacked the diagnosis," he did it in part to provide them a "diagnostic home." It was not enough to rescue the orphans from this pharmacological Fagin. They would need a new place to go.

When Shaffer and his colleagues started talking about the rescue effort more than ten years ago, there was one DSM-IV diagnosis that seemed suitable: Oppositional-Defiant Disorder (ODD), "a pattern of negativistic, hostile, and defiant behavior lasting at least 6 months" whose symptoms included "often loses temper," "often argues with adults," and "is often touchy."

"The truth was that many of these kids would meet criteria for ODD," said Shaffer. Without changing the criteria, let alone introducing a new diagnosis, they could be assigned to this category. But there was a problem. "ODD had become tarnished," says Shaffer, by its association with two other diagnoses: Conduct Disorder, the label given to childhood bullies and thugs, and Antisocial Personality Disorder, or what is often called *sociopathy*. Longitudinal studies did not back up the hunch that ODD belonged in the same neighborhood as these diagnoses; kids with

ODD did not go on to become thieves, rapists, or hedge fund managers in greater numbers than other kids. But the bad reputation was impossible to shed, or so Shaffer and his colleagues thought.

"So we had this problem: the criteria of ODD would fit most of the kids who were being diagnosed as bipolar, but we couldn't call it ODD because it was a stigmatized name," he explained. "It sounded like you were heading to be a crook, and people wouldn't go for it." By people, Shaffer said he meant not only the doctors who would be reluctant to deliver that verdict, but also, and more important, parents—who, even if they might want their kids to head for medical school, wouldn't want them to come out like Joseph Biederman. And parents were likely to be unhappy when they discovered that insurance companies tended not to be as generous with treatment dollars for ODD as they were for Bipolar Disorder, which, perversely, has the better reputation of the two because it is a worse disease.

"Our real audience must be the parents," Shaffer said he told his colleagues when they were deliberating over the name for the new disorder. And the name they came up with is what Shaffer thought was his fault. It's not that his proposal didn't make sense, especially for his main audience. "It's an area with a big parent movement," he said. "What they see are kids with terrible tempers. So, I thought, let's give it a nontechnical name. Couldn't we just call it Temper Dysregulation Disorder?"

Shaffer says he couldn't have known that by using such a common word as *temper*, he would be walking into Allen Frances's arguments about "psychiatrizing normal behavior." But it's not as if he didn't have warning. He didn't exactly focus-group the new label, but he did run it by his colleagues. At least one of them objected vehemently. "Ellen said, 'Oh, God, what a terrible name!'"

Ellen was Ellen Leibenluft, a psychiatrist at NIMH. In 2003, she and a group of colleagues tried to tease out the manic from the irritable among kids who were getting snared in Biederman's expanded net. They looked for ways (other than the mania/irritability distinction) in which the two populations differed and proposed a "broad phenotype" that described the nonmanic patients. They called this phenotype "severe mood and behavioral dysregulation" and proposed "multisite clinical trials" to test whether the category was valid—whether, that is, the children would differ from one another not only according to their symptoms but also according to their family histories, the course of their troubles, and their response to treatment. There was already some suggestive, if preliminary, evidence on this last question: "that children with the broad phenotype may respond well to stimulants"—to the old standbys Ritalin and Adderall, in other words, rather than to Bieder-man's pet drug Risperdal and the other antipsychotics.

Leibenluft later wrote that her intention was not to "claim to define a new diagnosis. She didn't mean to establish a new territory in the landscape of mental illness, but rather to strengthen the boundaries of the one that already existed—Bipolar Disorder—and to make sure that certain patients remained outside them. Still, the description of severe mood dysregulation, with its criteria list and its parameters—"markedly increased" and "at least half of the day most days" and its "symptoms have been present for at least 12 months"—looked an awful lot like something that would appear in the DSM. And sure enough, when the DSM-5 proposals hit the Web in February 2010, the disorder, with Shaf-fer's terrible name attached, had been nominated for the big show.

The work group on childhood and adolescent disorders acknowl-edged the doubts their proposal raised. In the paper "Justification for Temper Dysregulation Disorder with Dysphoria," it questioned whether it was "premature to suggest the addition of the TDD diagnosis, since . . . many questions remain unanswered." Most of the research they relied on had been conducted before the idea of TDD had even been advanced, so researchers had had to render "proxy definitions," mining old data for information that, had those researchers been interested in TDD, would have been relevant. And although some clinical trials had been conducted using the research criteria, they hadn't yet addressed the question of which drugs the kids should get, which meant that clinicians might well render the diagnosis and still reach for the Risperdal.

The group also acknowledged that the research had not really demonstrated that TDD was a better-fitting diagnosis than ODD. To the contrary, it had shown that nearly all TDD patients could also be seen as suffering a particularly bad case of ODD, so they could be diagnosed that way, using a severity specifier that would indicate that the kid had the TDD form of ODD—a move that would avoid the uncertainties and wrangling involved in manufacturing a brand-new diagnosis.

In addition, they confessed, "the work has been done predominately by one research group in a select research setting." This was important because the whole point of criterion-based diagnosis is to allow real-life clinicians—as opposed to elite researchers who know what they are looking for and get to look for it in patients preselected for the purpose—to reach the new diagnosis strictly by applying the criteria. The possibility existed, in other words, that TDD would not be a reliable diagnosis and would only add to the confusion about these patients.

Finally, the fact that this one team had generated "relatively little research" also created the potential for the disorder to be "prematurely reified." The work group didn't explain this cryptic comment. Were they worried that doctors (or parents) would make the common error, the one that Hyman and Mirin and every other DSM expert warned about, of thinking that a disease listed in the official manual of mental disorders and used as the basis for research, treatment, and reimbursement actually existed? Or were they only worried that the disorder, with its scant research record, didn't yet deserve to be reified, or, to put it another way, that TDD wasn't even ready to provide fodder for the error that, no matter how regrettable, was indispensable to the industry?

What the justification didn't mention was that the work group was headed by one of those researchers and that Ellen Leibenluft was one of its eight members. Which may or may not explain why the group dismissed its doubts almost as quickly as it raised them. Even if "the scientific data may suggest defining TDD as a specifier to ODD," clinicians "would be unlikely" to use it—not only because it takes a few extra minutes to assess and note severity, but also for the reason David Shaffer noted: ODD's bad reputation. "Indeed," the work group argued, "it is plausible that clinicians assign the diagnosis of BD . . . in part because the BD diagnosis justifies access to a higher level of resources."

Their license to go beyond the science in this fashion, the work group explained, came right from the top, from a task force that had specifically instructed them to weigh "clinical considerations in the decision as to whether to propose a new diagnosis." Questions of clinician time and insurance reimbursement, not to mention any tarnish on the diagnosis, were significant in the clinic. And there were benefits beyond insurance payments: once the diagnosis was established, if not reified, it would jump-start researchers' efforts to fill in the gaps in the data, attracting money to study the new disorder.

If, in their zeal to make sure that children (and, of course, their doctors) had access to resources, it occurred to the work group that their efforts might amount to swallowing a spider to kill a fly, or that there were other, simpler ways to repudiate Biederman (such as adding an exclusion criterion or just calling the cops on the crook, if indeed that's what he was), or if they understood that manufacturing a new mood disorder was like throwing fresh meat to the pharmaceutical industry, or if they noticed that by advancing a diagnosis that wasn't even ready to be reified, they were suggesting a long-term public health experiment whose subjects (children and doctors both) would be unaware of their participation, they didn't say. But then again, hadn't Kupfer and Regier said that this DSM would be a living document?

Indeed they had, and on March 9, the APA made this official when it announced a new "naming convention." The upcoming revision would be known as DSM-5, not DSM-V, and henceforward all new DSMs would likewise be identified with Arabic, rather than Roman, numerals. The new name, like Shaffer's TDD, replaced the arcane with the familiar, but for reasons different from his. "Knowledge of neurobiology will continue to advance," APA president Alan Schatzberg said in the press release. The purpose of the change was not to capture hearts and minds, but to make room for the scientific advances that hadn't happened yet, by turning the DSM into "a document that can respond more quickly when a preponderance of research supports a change." The APA hadn't quite figured out the details, whether, say, it would grant purchasers of the new book a license to download updates as new research developed or just turn the whole business over to Amazon, but one thing was certain: after DSM-5 came "DSM-5.1, DSM 5.2, etc., until a new edition is required." DSM-5, evidently, was going to be beta-tested.

David Kupfer seemed to anticipate the problem hidden in the new convention—that it more or less announced that the foundational text of his profession, the one that provided certainty about matters of vital importance to insurers and regulators and drug companies and patients, was provisional—when he reassured the public that "our primary commitment will continue to be to create a manual that is based on science and is useful in diagnosing and treating patients."

Darrel Regier also telegraphed comfort, first to his colleagues—"By making the DSM-5 a living document, we will ensure that the DSM will remain a common language in the field"—and then to the rest of us: "It will hasten our response to breakthroughs in research." What exactly we were supposed to do before those breakthroughs could occur, he didn't exactly say. The framers of the DSM-5 may have been replacing the Bible with a living document, but they were still asking us to take them on faith.

Naming conventions were definitely on Alan Schatzberg's mind when he delivered his outgoing presidential address to the May 2010 APA annual convention in New Orleans.

Schatzberg reminded his troops that they were still at war. Our "detractors" may be hypocritical—they don't criticize neurologists for talking about minor cognitive impairment, after all, and they don't seem to understand that they are stigmatizing psychiatry out of fear and ignorance and "antipsychiatry sentiment" rather than for anything psychiatry has done wrong. And, Schatzberg continued, psychiatrists themselves were making it far too easy for their enemies by using a "distinctly unmedical" language to name their diseases. "The proposed temper dysregulation disorder . . . does not convey" the seriousness of the condition, and, unlike the cardiologists' recasting of *heart attack* as *myocardial infarction*, it had no "parallel and more medical terminology." Psychiatrists were the victims once again, this time of their own just-folks language.

"Some of the attacks have been by English and history professors," Schatzberg said. "My friends, this does present a problem we need to think about. Everyone feels emotions; everyone reads pop psychology articles or watches pop psychologists on TV; and many come to believe they are experts in psychiatry." It was time to draw the line between the civilians who had those emotions and the experts who knew what they really meant, and the best way to do this might be to shroud nosology in the "Latin and Greek terms" used by other specialties.

"We need to be more medical to be taken seriously," Schatzberg concluded.

Schatzberg had some other bad tidings for his membership. After noting that New Orleans had "risen as the Phoenix from the horrors of Katrina to rebuild itself" (with the help of psychiatrists, he added) and that the theme of the convention was "Pride and Promise: Toward a New Psychiatry," he told them that their finances were turning to ashes. Revenues had shrunk by $10 million, to $55 million, largely because of a recession-related drop-off in drug company advertising in the APA's journals.

Another pool of drug company money had also dried up, thanks to the decision to stop letting the industry fund the APA's education programs. In Schatzberg's reading, this renunciation wasn't quite as noble as Jay Scully had made it out to be, or as unilateral. In fact, Schatzberg said, "the negative attacks on industry have made them gun shy of supporting such programs."

As perhaps befits a man who had made Chuck Grassley's hit parade, Schatzberg regretted this development. "There are a number of new drugs that have been recently released that many of us know little about," he said, "and that cannot be good for either us or our patients." (Apparently, Schatzberg couldn't imagine another way for doctors to learn about new drugs other than from the sales forces of the companies that make them; perhaps he also buys his cars based on what his dealer tells him.) "The strident debate and attacks have obfuscated the negative impact of eliminating industry from our offices," he complained.

As unjust as it might have been, however, the drug company purge seemed irreversible. The APA was going to have to make up that $10 million deficit somehow. The organization won't say how much revenue it anticipates from a new DSM, but you don't have to run a meta-analysis to figure out that a new book would be worth far more at its outset than the $6 million the DSM-IV generated in 2010. Leaders of the APA would not confirm the old suspicion that money was a driving force behind the revision (although one trustee did tell me that "it would be disastrous not to get that income"), but that looming bonanza had to be looking pretty good—if only they could get their hands on it.

Chapter 11

Allen Frances wasn't limiting himself to his blogs, which by mid-2010 were appearing on three different websites and broadcasting a steady tocsin of impending doom. He also published articles in medical journals and on newspaper websites, and gave interviews to all the journalists attracted to the spectacle of a leader of the orthodoxy accusing his fellow priests of heresy. He may not have been a Quixote, but he was surely less a Sancho Panza than a Paul Revere, shouting warnings into the night: the DSM-5 was coming!

In August, Frances sounded his alarm from the op-ed page of *The New York Times*, where he declaimed against the proposal to remove the bereavement exclusion from the depression diagnosis. "Turning bereavement into major depression," he wrote, "would substitute a shallow, Johnny-come-lately medical ritual for the sacred mourning rites that have survived for millenniums." An appointment with a psychiatrist, at least according to this prominent practitioner, was no simple office visit. It was a ritual, and it wasn't even the best ritual available for at least one common form of suffering.

Frances understood by then that his views could be exploited by psychiatry's enemies and that the higher his profile became, the greater the risk that people would get the wrong message. Already some critics of psychiatry had been quick to use him to further their own idea that DSM diagnoses were just-so stories. But that is not what he meant, he said. "Sure, there's a reality out there, but we have an incomplete perception of it. We see through a glass darkly, but that doesn't mean we don't see at all." Uncertainty was inescapable, but it could be reduced—and inevitably would be, he thought. As neuroscience comes into its own, he told me, and "the complexity begins to clarify out of the mist, diagnoses will become better and better constructs, ever closer to a reality that will always be elusive to our limited powers of apprehension."

At stake, Frances insisted, was something more immediate and urgent than intellectual controversy or internecine warfare: the care of patients, particularly those who might be "wavering about treatment and attracted to an antipsychiatry point of view."

"They would not be able to do the calculation," he told me, to say, "'Well, maybe this isn't perfect, but it's still the best way available, and we shouldn't just throw it out.'" Every blog and interview drew back the curtain on psychiatry's inner workings a little further, threatening to make the whole field look like humbug. "I'm reluctant to reveal all the *Wizard of Oz* stuff," he said, "because I don't want people who need help to get disillusioned and stop taking their medicine."

From Plato to Saint Paul to Heisenberg to Baum—it was a typical Allen Frances ramble. And it ended right back in Plato's *Republic*. "The full truth is usually best," Frances said, "but sometimes we may need a noble lie."

Beneficence—the doctor's obligation to act in the best interests of his or her patients—has long been considered a core value of medicine. In its name, doctors have routinely lied to patients, or at least stretched the truth, withholding terrible prognoses from terminally ill people, for instance, or overstating the effectiveness of a treatment. In recent years, another core value has come to the forefront: *autonomy*, the right of the patient to determine the course of his or her treatment. To uphold this principle, at least according to some medical ethicists, doctors need to curtail their beneficence, or at least not use it as a reason to be less than transparent with their patients, so they can make fully informed decisions. And the Internet, much to many doctors' dismay, has opened curtains that they would like to keep completely shut. The two principles continue to vie for primacy, and some of that tension can be seen in Frances's concerns about what the public should know about the nature of psychiatric nosology.

It's easy enough to see this as self-serving, to say that lying can't be noble, at least not when it is used to maintain an authority that might not survive a full disclosure. Plato might well have been appalled to see how the control of information would be used by Machiavelli or Dostoevsky's Grand Inquisitor or Dick Cheney. But you can't really blame Plato for being naive about the attractions of power or for not seeing how useful noble lies could be to people who want to hold on to it. He lived before autonomy and equality were expectations for a good life, before universal justice was the hallmark of a good society, and before a couple thousand years of history had revealed what can happen when people with power—even virtuous people—act in the supposed interests of those with none.

Not that Frances's concern about the effect of diagnostic squabbling on patients was less than beneficent or only about maintaining psychiatry's dominion over our inner lives. "Like most medical specialties, our field depends heavily on placebo effects," he pointed out. And pills aren't the only way to deliver the placebo effect. Even if "the diagnostic label is just a description, and not really an explanation for what has gone wrong," Frances says, still it is crucial to treatment. Delivering a diagnosis gives us solace: that we are not making it up, that the doctor understands, that there are others like us, that there is hope for a cure.

"If you puncture that noble lie," Frances warned me, "you'll be doing a disservice to our patients."

But indiscreet writers aren't the only people who pose a danger. "A doctor saying you have depression, that's part of the treatment—so long as you don't go overboard in promising that everything can be explained through chemical reactions and it doesn't have anything to do with the fact that your wife died last week." This was the risk Frances saw in removing the bereavement exclusion: that doctors would feel free to deliver that verdict to grieving patients, that indeed the DSM would more or less oblige them to do so. And given what Frances calls "the ignorance of philosophy of the average practitioner," not to mention the pressures on him or her to be efficient and to provide relief, doctors might not even know how careful they needed to be about exercising their diagnostic power, how easily it could be ignobly—and globally—deployed. Psychiatric diagnosis, it seems, is more sophisticated than most clinicians realize. Getting rid of the bereavement exclusion would invite not only the overtreatment of patients but, after the inevitable backlash, yet another credibility crisis for the profession.

On the other hand, you have to appreciate the problem that the bereavement exclusion presented to the shapers of the DSM-5.

Some people who weren't enemies of psychiatry thought they smelled a rat even if it wasn't the one that antipsychiatrists smelled. To New York University professor of social work Jerome Wakefield, for instance, the bereavement exclusion itself wasn't such a bad idea. It prevented a person who had all the symptoms of an illness, but who wasn't really sick, from getting mistakenly diagnosed. The exclusion, he wrote, protected patients from "stigmatization [and] inappropriate care" and psychiatry from "inflated epidemiological prevalence rates that undermine the credibility of the diagnostic system." And its caveats—that people who were suicidal or otherwise dysfunctional, or whose symptoms persisted beyond two months of the death should not be excluded—prevented doctors from dismissing severe symptoms as normal reactions and thus ensured that patients who needed treatment could get it.

So far, so good. But Wakefield thought there was a deeper problem. Why, he wondered, did the book "ignore the many other kinds of serious losses that can cause intense symptoms of normal sadness"? Was it possible that not enough people were protected from the potential harms of diagnosis?

Wakefield and a team of researchers that included Michael First designed an experiment to find out. They mined the National Comorbidity Survey (NCS), the NIMH project that demonstrated that 60 percent of mentally disordered people qualified for more than one diagnosis. As it happened, the NCS researchers had asked subjects not only about recent bereavement, but about whether there was "anything else going on" that might have caused them to "feel sad or blue." This created an opportunity for a researcher who, like Wakefield, was curious about whether there was a difference between the bereaved and people who had suffered other losses.

Of the 1,308 NCS subjects with major depression, 157 reported that their symptoms had been set off by a bereavement and 710 said that a different kind of loss had triggered them. Wakefield then examined to what extent those two groups differed along two dimensions: *disorder indicators*, such as how many symptoms of depression they had or how long they lasted; and *symptom group*, which of the nine depression symptoms they reported. It turned out that there was virtually no difference between the two groups in either dimension. Divorce, death of a loved one, financial setback—each was as likely as the others to leave a person sad or apathetic or insomniac, as likely as the others to send a person to a therapist or a doctor for an antidepressant.

Wakefield further divided his subjects into *uncomplicated* and *complicated* groups. Complicated subjects were those with the severe symptoms, such as suicidal thoughts or the inability to function, that would have disqualified them from the bereavement exclusion, and uncomplicated subjects . . . well, you figure it out. Not surprisingly, people in each group resembled one another more than they resembled people in the other group who had suffered the same kind of setback. Loss is loss, in other words. What differs is how we respond to it, not what we are responding to.

Taken together, these two findings—that no matter what the precipitating event is, it has the same effects, and that the main difference is in the intensity of response—indicated that there was no scientific reason to treat the death of a loved one differently from other losses. The experiment was simple, elegant, and conclusive. The bereavement exclusion was arbitrary and incoherent, and if that was so, then the MDD criteria were not able to sort the well from the sick.

In *The Loss of Sadness*, Wakefield and his coauthor, sociologist Allan Horwitz, made it clear that more was at stake than the bereavement exclusion. Even if we accept the inescapable fuzziness of psychiatric diagnoses, they argued, still a nosology must have some kind of integrity, lest the DSM "define every undesirable consequence of sadness as a disorder."

"Psychiatry has made immense strides in recent decades," they wrote, but one thing it had not figured out was how to limit its tendency to "engulf all the problems that life poses." The solution was not to abandon the depression diagnosis, even if the bereavement exclusion constituted a "compelling, clear and major violation of validity." Instead, they wrote, the diagnosis "should be fixed." And the best way to do that was to expand the exclusion beyond bereavement to "other major life stressors" so that clinicians could distinguish between *disorder* and *distress*, and diagnose and treat people accordingly. Forcing clinicians to consider the actual life experience of their patients would limit the damage that their diagnoses could do even as it maintained their ability to help patients.

"There are few signs that changes in the MDD criteria are a high priority for the . . . DSM-V," Wakefield and Horwitz concluded. But that was in 2007, before their book became a minor sensation, and just as a spate of other books and articles complained that depression was getting overdiagnosed and, not coincidentally, antidepressants alarmingly overprescribed. And as the DSM-5 revision geared up, it became clear that researchers concerned about psychiatry's overstepping weren't the only people disturbed by the bereavement exclusion.

"It just doesn't make any sense to me whatsoever," psychiatrist Sidney Zisook told me on the phone. "Maybe it did when I first got into the field, but not anymore."

But Zisook's objection was different from Wakefield's. It wasn't the double standard—the fact that only the grieving were eligible for a reprieve from diagnosis—that bothered him. It was the assumption that bereavement-related depression (BRD), as he called the suffering covered by the exclusion, was somehow different from standard major depression (SMD). If the two were not different in nature, if, in other words, the only difference between BRD and SMD was in their cause, then there really was no difference between them, no reason to distinguish patients according to their recent experience.

In 2007, working with Ken Kendler, Zisook did some data mining of his own. He extracted information from about fifty studies conducted over three decades and comprising more than eight thousand depressed subjects, only some of whom met the exclusion criterion. They looked at the Robins and Guze validators—family history and other demographics, overall health (mental and otherwise), lab tests, response to treatment, and the course and outcome of the patients' troubles. And while some of the evidence was inconclusive—it wasn't clear whether BRD ran in families, for instance—most of the results showed that BRD was no different from SMD. Bereaved people who had the symptoms of depression were no different from other patients who had the symptoms. Wakefield had proved that loss was loss; now Zisook and Kendler had shown that depression was depression, regardless of its cause.

Zisook and Kendler were careful with their conclusions, at least at first. Their analysis only "provides some support, although indirect and limited," they wrote, "that excluding recently bereaved individuals from the diagnosis of MDE [Major Depressive Episode] . . . may not be justified." And pending further research, "the most propitious conclusion may be that, on average, these two syndromes [BRD and SMD] appear to be closely related."

Six months later, however, Zisook and Kendler, along with a third collaborator, published another paper on the same topic. Its data and findings were nearly identical to the earlier report's. But there was something new in the second article. "Because work toward the DSM-V has begun," they wrote, "it is timely to re-examine the DSM's bereavement exclusion."

Reframed as a discussion of what should be done now that the revision was under way, the questions about the bereavement exclusion took on a new urgency and the authors demonstrated a new certainty. First, they pointed out, research had shown that the earlier depression is treated the better, and that antidepressant medication is particularly effective in the earliest stages of a depressive episode. Which means, they said, that the "validity of the bereavement exclusion . . . is not an academic issue." Indeed, Zisook told me, we should also worry about what happens to people who don't get diagnosed.

"I don't think we're doing patients a service by avoiding the label if they meet the criteria," he said. "I think if we say that in addition to their bereavement they are also depressed, we might intervene more aggressively and sooner and save people a lot of pain, discomfort and, who knows, maybe even lives."

"Why should bereavement be singled out as the only stressful life event that excludes the diagnosis of MDE?" they asked. It was a rhetorical question, of course. To Wakefield and Horwitz, psychiatric diagnosis was a potential harm against which we need protection. To Kendler and Zisook, it was a benefit that we should not be denied.

"Idiotic," said Jerry Wakefield, when I asked him what he thought of the proposal to remove the exclusion. "But clever in its own diabolical way—they used my evidence against me!"

Wakefield was not on the mood disorders work group for the DSM-5. Neither was Michael First or Allan Horwitz. Ken Kendler, on the other hand, was, and Sid Zisook was a special consultant to it. Which may or may not explain why the work group decided, even in the acknowledged absence of direct evidence and despite the tentativeness of the conclusions—not to mention the obvious public relations problem—to eliminate the bereavement exclusion. At the very least, the proposal seems to confirm the notion that experts, given the charter to implement their pet theories as diagnostic changes, will tinker, and that their tinkering is likely to be in the direction of more rather than fewer diagnoses.

Experts like Zisook are not unaware of the possibility of overdiagnosis. They're just less worried about what they call *false positives* than about *false negatives*. Leaving an illness untreated is more dangerous, in their view, than making illness out of everyday life. And Zisook may be on the National Advisory Board of GlaxoSmithKline, for whom he once ran a study showing that GSK's Wellbutrin was effective for grieving people, but that doesn't necessarily mean he's shilling for the company by proposing the expansion of the diagnostic net, or even that he will hawk their products to more patients once the exclusion is lifted. "I don't think everyone with major depression needs meds or formal therapy," said Zisook. "I think sometimes watchful waiting is appropriate. Sometimes support and education is appropriate. Sometimes decreasing stress is appropriate." A good clinician knows when to do which. Expertise is what guarantees that a doctor's power is used beneficently.

Zisook places great stock in expertise—and not just when it comes to treatment. "The DSM criteria don't allow for judgment on symptoms," he told me. "I think a really astute clinician will make decisions as to whether a behavior is a symptom of depression or not." Removing the bereavement exclusion won't stop a good doctor from withholding a diagnosis from a grieving patient even if she meets the criteria.

Consider, Zisook said, a patient who is recently widowed and not only sad and withdrawn but also guilt-ridden over all he should have done to prevent the loss of his wife. "That guilt would count toward depression," Zisook acknowledged, but "when I have this patient in front of me, I don't count that as a symptom of depression." Expertise can be relied upon to determine whether guilt is a symptom or just guilt, and whether the criteria add up to a disorder. Astute clinicians, like the crackerjack doctors who staff Zisook's elite university medical center, don't need bereavement exclusions to limit their diagnostic powers. They don't need to slave away at checklists like common clerks.

But Zisook evidently does not want to extend this same latitude to the rank-and-file clinicians, the ones who spend their days seeing patients with a range of psychiatric disorders—not to mention the general practitioners who do most of the prescribing of antidepressants—and who aren't supported by research grants and generous faculty salaries, who don't have an hour or so to spend talking with their patients or administering carefully calibrated diagnostic tests that can be scored by assistants or worrying over the fine points of what it means to say that the miserable person in front of them actually has a mental disorder. Run-of-the-mill doctors, it seems, can't be trusted with a bereavement exclusion, any more than the layman can be trusted with all that *Wizard of Oz* stuff. They must remain loyal to the fundamental tenet of the DSM: that, as Zisook put it, the "criteria are the same regardless of context. If someone meets them, I should give them the label of major depression because that's what they have"—although evidently only so long as the "I" in question is not Zisook or any other clinician too astute to take the DSM too seriously.

"The DSM-IV position is not logically defensible," Ken Kendler wrote in a statement the APA posted on the DSM-5 website shortly after Frances's *Times* op-ed appeared and a public furor broke out.

Kendler wasn't talking about the incoherence of saying that depression is depression unless an elite clinician determines that it is not. He was talking about the way the exclusion contradicted the basic idea of the DSM—that mental disorders can (and, for now anyway, must) be known by their symptoms alone. "The grief exclusion criterion needs to be [either] eliminated or extended so that no depression that arises in the setting of adversity would be diagnosable." And, since "the majority of individuals" who get the diagnosis develop it "in the setting of psychosocial adversity," he added, this curtailing of the diagnosis would "represent a major shift . . . in the nature of our concept of depression."

It's not clear where Kendler got the idea that the only alternative to eliminating the exclusion was to make it impossible to diagnose depression in the presence of a stressor. It couldn't have been from Wakefield, who never said that depression kindled by adversity should go undiagnosed. To the contrary, he was trying to lay the groundwork for a return to a traditional, pre-DSM-III idea of depression: "that sadness in response to loss is natural and normal, and that the indication of disorder lies in the sadness being without sufficient cause in given environmental contexts or being disproportional to actual loss." Depression, according to this abandoned notion, was sick only to the extent that it occurred without regard to a person's life circumstances.

Wakefield was proposing, in other words, that if you want to know if a person is really sick rather than simply reacting to a loss, you have to look at the relationship between the stressor and the person's reaction. You have to try to understand what the loss means to the patient. And if it is out of proportion, then you have to figure that you are in the presence of a genuine illness—something gone wrong in the body (in this case, the brain)—rather than normal sorrow. Indeed, Wakefield was only suggesting that the prerogative Zisook reserved for the astute (but would deny to everyone else by removing the exclusion) was actually an obligation for all clinicians: to pay attention not only to diagnostic checklists but also to the patient in front of them.

Right now, if you are not a psychiatrist or any other kind of mental health worker, or maybe even if you are, you are probably thinking, "Duh!" You're probably wondering how it is possible that something as obvious as this even needs to be said, let alone argued about. But that's only because you have decided to make your living in some other fashion, one that does not require you to satisfy an insurance company or your colleagues in other specialties or yourself—if you take seriously your involvement in the medical-industrial complex—that you are treating "real illnesses." You haven't signed on for a profession whose badly tarnished reputation was once restored by applying the thinnest veneer of scientific rhetoric and polishing it vigorously, and which now has to protect itself from the sullying effects of a proposal like Wakefield's, even if it means taking the absurd position that there is no essential difference between a depression kindled by the loss of a child or parent and a depression brought on by the cancellation of a favorite television show or the death of a pet hamster—or between any of those and a depression that seems to come on out of nowhere.

Good for you, I say. Because if even a man of integrity like Sid Zisook, who is as affable and humane and charming a guy as you might like to meet, and surely the kind of psychiatrist—empathic, articulate, knowledgeable—whom, if you needed one, you'd want to see, if such a man finds himself, in the space of two minutes, totally contradicting himself, talking out of both sides of his mouth, and unwittingly becoming the best evidence of the incoherence of his own position merely by acknowledging that he pays attention to his patients, when smart and compassionate doctors spill buckets of ink over the question of whether or not they should consider what we are going through before they tell us what we are suffering from and what we should do about it, and when the proposal to do so moves Bob Spitzer to say to me, "If we did that, then the whole system falls apart," then you know that you are knee-deep in a setting of psychosocial adversity.

And, indeed, all of us in the mental health industry know this, from the APA trustee who shook his head and told me in a mournful voice, "We're just so stuck," to Allen Frances to Steve Hyman to lunchbucket therapists like me who hold our noses when we put those codes onto the bill. We may not be sophisticated enough to grasp the nobility of the lie that sustains the DSM or to be trusted as its keepers. We may not be astute enough to distinguish between depression and grief. But we all know that the DSM is at its best a clumsy and imperfect field guide to our foibles and at its worst a compendium of expert opinions masquerading as scientific truths, a book whose credibility surpasses its integrity, whose usefulness is primarily commercial, and whose most ardent defenders are reduced to arguing that it should be taken less seriously even as all of us—clinicians, researchers, and copyright holders alike—cash in on the fact that it is not.

Chapter 12

On December 17, 2010, instead of the usual Friday grand rounds, the department of psychiatry at Columbia University honored Bob Spitzer on the occasion of his retirement. Colleagues from past and present paid tribute with recollections and praise. A historian put Spitzer's forty-nine-year career into historical perspective. Allen Frances spoke from the same lectern from which he had railed against DSM-5 eleven months earlier. This time he really did hold back. He scarcely mentioned the revision. He didn't tease Spitzer. He just talked about his contribution, about how he was one of the most important psychiatrists who had ever lived, placing him in the company of Freud and Kraepelin. He couldn't resist reminding the audience about the limitations of the descriptive method, but still, he said, it is "the best we can do, and Bob has been and will remain our master describer."

Like many such celebrations, the proceedings were more than a little funereal—a tone deepened by Spitzer's halting, unsteady ascent to the stage, his quavering voice, his obvious frailty. After warning the audience that his Parkinson's disease had worsened his tendency to burst into tears, he did exactly that. He didn't get everything said that he intended to say. He had a little trouble remembering exactly how many children he had. But between gusts of weeping he told stories and recounted arguments in a way that conveyed both the charisma and the toughness that had allowed him to become the man who saved psychiatry.

That night Spitzer joined some of his colleagues and collaborators and their wives for dinner at a downtown restaurant. Harold Pincus, Michael First, Jerry Wakefield, and Allen Frances were there. The DSM was far from the main topic of the loud and lively conversation. When the subject did come up, it was in a dense shorthand, the code that signals deep agreement, words such as "field trials" and "polythetic criteria" and "prevalence rates" that carried a world of meaning impenetrable to outsiders. Theirs was a shared, private language, much as they thought the DSM's should be.

But when it came to revising that language, they were now the outsiders. Spitzer and Frances had been placed on the enemies' list. First had been pushed aside. Pincus had never been involved. Wakefield (who, as a nonpsychiatrist, was never as inside as the rest) had had his evidence used against him. They were still shouting at one another, still teasing, enjoying conversation as if it were a contact sport. But their shared love of argument, their common language, and the DSM they had fashioned—the one that, in true Talmudic fashion (and it was hard not to notice that these men were all Jews by birth), they were both proud and skeptical of—was now the language of opposition, of resentment, and, increasingly, of powerlessness and cynicism. The event they'd all come together to commemorate signaled not just the end of a career, but the passing of an era.

There was one word in the discussion with deeper meanings that an outsider might have grasped, if only by the seething anger with which it was uttered: "Darrel."

Darrel Regier is not a shouter or a teaser (or, as it happens, a Jew). He is a mild-mannered man, a Midwest-educated bean counter whose time in New York had begun and ended with his medical internship at Montefiore Medical Center in the Bronx, who has no apparent use for irony, and whose ability to insulate his sentences from objection with thick layers of bureaucratese was probably more useful in his ascent to the rank of vice admiral in the U.S. Public Health Service than shouting and teasing ever would have been. After all, it's pretty tough to argue with a sentence like this one, taken from an article he wrote.

Moving forward, I believe the more critical issue for work group members is how to avoid mind-body dualism in which mental disorders are moved in neurological classifications as more precise pathophysiological, neuroimaging, genetic, nutritional, infectious, traumatic or other etiological characteristics are discovered.

Not that Regier lacks the ability to fight. "Darrel knows how to throw an elbow," one psychiatrist told me. Indeed, just a month or so before the gathering for Spitzer, Regier's pugilistic skills had been on full display at a conference on psychiatric nosology held in Copenhagen and sponsored by the Danish National Research Foundation's Center for Subjectivity Research—a gathering originally scheduled for April, but delayed when a volcanic eruption in Iceland closed European airports.

Regier's talk was in many ways a career retrospective. He told his colleagues that he had entered the profession in the early 1970s, in the bad old days when the Midtown Manhattan Study and other pre-DSM-III efforts were turning up inordinate rates of mental illness in the population, and when "the clinical judgment of a psychiatrist was the gold standard of psychiatric diagnosis." The DSM-III had made matters a little better, but not much, he said—the 50 percent lifetime prevalence rates reached in some analyses of his ECA project were still too high and the National Comorbidity Survey, the one that had shown that 27 percent of diagnosable people had more than one DSM-III disorder, were a blot on the nosological record. Diagnosticians may have gotten more scientific, but their methods still yielded results that flew in the face of common sense.

Regier recounted the two epidemiological studies from the 1950s that had yielded much lower (and, Regier thought, realistic) prevalence rates. These projects shared one important characteristic: they relied on doctors to identify the cases in a community. Ask doctors who under their care is sick, it seemed, and you get a much lower number than if you ask randomly selected people about their symptoms. "We had much greater confidence in the clinical assessments of physicians with some longitudinal knowledge of all persons requesting care," Regier said.

So perhaps that old gold standard, clinical judgment, had been too hastily discarded in the name of reliability. Intimate knowledge of a patient's history and circumstances, coupled with sound medical knowledge, seemed to provide a check on diagnostic exuberance, identifying within the group that met the criteria those individuals who were truly ill. But how to incorporate that into a reliable nosology? Or to put it another way, how could epidemiologists cut the vagaries of physician judgment out of the loop while still maintaining doctors as the gatekeepers to diagnosis and treatment?

Regier's solution was to try to establish when a person has crossed the threshold from healthy to sick. In their introductions, Spitzer and Frances had instructed users of the DSM that if the symptoms weren't clinically significant, there was no diagnosis to make; no matter how many symptoms you had, you weren't mentally ill unless your suffering was clinically significant. But that term had never really been defined; establishing the threshold had been left up to the astute clinician. To find a definition that could be consistently and reliably applied to individual cases was to answer this question, or so Regier proposed. It would allow doctors to specify when the criteria signified the presence of illness. And since those cases were sure to be only a subset of all the people who met the criteria, the prevalence estimates would come down from the stratosphere.

Regier thought the answer was hiding in plain sight—in data collected, but lying dormant, in the ECA and NCS studies. Researchers in both had asked subjects about how much their symptoms had interfered with their lives, and especially whether or not they had been so bad that they had gone to see a doctor about them. The answers had not been used to determine whether or not the people were mentally disordered, but in the late 1990s, Regier's team began to dig them out. They fashioned an algorithm, applied it to the data, and presto! Prevalence rates came in at 18 percent—still higher than where Regier thought they should be, but still as much as two-thirds lower than the original findings.

Regier was sure he'd threaded the needle, but others disagreed, sometimes loudly. "To put it mildly," he told the Copenhagen crowd, "howls of protest arose from Spitzer, and later from Jerome Wakefield and others." The first skirmish was at a meeting of the American Psycho-pathological Association in 2002, and two years later, when Regier published the results, a fight broke out in the pages of *Archives of General Psychiatry*. Wakefield and Spitzer pointed out that of the nine questions used to generate Regier's data, seven were about whether people had sought treatment; only two were about how debilitating the symptoms were. But plenty of sick people never saw a doctor, and plenty of people who saw doctors weren't sick. Regier had confused *treatment seeking* with *clinical significance*, they said, which meant he had reduced prevalence by gerrymandering the patient population rather than actually specifying who was sick and who simply met the criteria.

"What is striking about this debate," Regier continued, "is that it became even more personal" when Ronald Kessler, who headed the NCS study, warned in a 2003 *Archives* article that it would be a mistake to use Regier's methods to remove mild disorders from the DSM-5—an agenda Kessler thought he had sniffed out in Regier's research. Kessler wrote that disorders falling short of the threshold Regier was proposing could and often did lead to more severe disorders. A person who confessed to anxiety or depression symptoms on a survey, but wasn't distressed enough to go to a doctor today, might well end up in the emergency room next month with a panic attack or after a suicide attempt. Here again, the problem was a kind of gerrymandering. The way to solve high prevalence rates, Kessler concluded, was not "to define the problem out of existence" by suggesting that mild illness wasn't illness.

It is a little hard to discern what exactly was personal about Kessler's or Wakefield and Spitzer's papers. They are workaday journal articles, all charts and graphs and eye-glazing details leading to careful conclusions. But there's no question that the articles got Regier's goat, at least to judge from his response, which he recalled for the audience in Copenhagen.

> In response to this scientific critique, we thought it would be helpful to highlight the central issue in DSM-5 revisions very clearly and chose the James Carville approach by responding with a letter to the editor in *Archives* entitled, "For DSM-5, It's the 'Disorder Threshold,' Stupid!"

Now *that's* personal.

"Bob did put up quite a fuss at that conference [in 2000]," Jerry Wakefield told me. "But Darrel never forgave him." And ten years later Regier was still settling old scores, or at least revealing scores he'd been keeping for a long time. "I wasn't aware that he had interpreted my remarks that way," Ronald Kessler said when I relayed Regier's comments to him. "I honestly don't know what he means about it being personal." But, he added, it wasn't entirely surprising. "Darrel reacts very strongly to people who disagree with him."

And by the time Regier got to Copenhagen, Allen Frances was on the top of that list.

> Certainly some of the loudest concerns in the blogs and print media are that we will unleash a wave of false epidemics—with the past editor of the DSM-IV claiming credit for creating false epidemics of pediatric bipolar disorder, ADHD, and autism . . . He also proclaims little confidence that the current editors can fix this problem or do better in the next edition.

Regier went on to denounce Frances in a way that seemed more inspired by Joseph Biederman than James Carville. Just look at the history of "progress in the calibration and validation of scientific constructs in astronomy, biology, and psychiatry," he said. "Defenders of the current construct do not yield easily to suggested changes in paradigms."

These debates were not going to end with a pinch on the cheek and a kiss.

But if Frances was playing the pope to Regier's Galileo, did that mean that the paradigm shift was back on? It is possible the DSM-5 leaders couldn't make up their minds, that the APA, like a squirrel in the road, knew enough to know it was in trouble, but not enough to know what to do about it.

There was one way in which a paradigm shift was in the making. It was not the sweeping change to a brain-based nosology for which they so devoutly wished, but it was nonetheless far more than a small technical matter. And it was the subject, beneath the vitriol, of Regier's talk in Copenhagen.

Regier's argument with Wakefield and Kessler was, as his Carvillian title pointed out, about the disorder threshold, about how a doctor determines that a person has become a patient. And here was one place that Regier agreed with Frances. Not that he would use barnyard epithets, or epithets of any kind, but he did not think the solution was to fabricate a definition of mental disorder. "It may be of interest to this audience," he said, after reading aloud the DSM-IV definition, "that almost none of the DSM-V Task Force or Work Group Meetings struggled with these definitional issues as they evaluated the research literature to determine the evidentiary basis for revisions." The committees weren't wasting time on philosophy. "Our plans for DSM-V are to provide a range of cross-cutting measures that will identify continuous measures of emotional, cognitive, addictive, and other domains," he said. "Most of our efforts will focus on the individual diagnostic measurements that permit better assessments of the thresholds between normal and pathological states."

Regier was confirming his intent to forge ahead with the new paradigm. (Don't feel bad if you missed it. If Galileo could have buried his meaning so deeply, his heresy might have been lost on the bishops.) "Since the broad definition [of mental disorder is] almost impossible to test," he said, "most of our efforts will focus on the individual diagnostic criteria and dimensional measurements that permit better assessment of the thresholds between normal and pathological states." The DSM-5 was going to abandon the attempt to define mental illness or to derive clinical significance by proxy measures like treatment seeking. Instead, it would work to overcome "one of the clearest limitations of our current diagnostic criteria . . . the lack of quantitative measures." It would provide the means to "set diagnostic thresholds for disorders." Indeed, it would *require* clinicians to do so by administering tests that would assess the severity of the disorder, as well as the presence of symptoms—anxiety, sadness, obsessiveness, and so on—that might not fit the diagnosis but were nonetheless relevant to treatment. Numbers, not words, were going to guard the gates to the land of mental illness.

Not every psychiatrist believes it's necessary to keep such a tight watch on those gates. Roger Peele, APA trustee and DSM-5 task force member, for example, acknowledged that the "DSM-IV has a label for everyone you might want to treat." But, he added, "ENTs [ear, nose, and throat doctors] don't worry about the fact that everyone is going to have a cold." Peele wished the "APA would get over their hang-up" and stop trying so hard to "avoid implying that everyone has had or will have a mental illness."

Peele is eighty years old. He's tall and handsome and has a sure, long stride and a regal bearing. He's wearing an ascot tucked into an open-collar shirt that matches his blue eyes. But maybe it's his low-cut, old-school sneakers, or his humble office with its government-issue furniture and less-than-commanding views of the Rockville, Maryland, strip malls, or the fact that he works for a county government, but somehow his suggestion that the APA's nosological restraint is a neurotic symptom doesn't seem designed to enhance his power or give the APA permission to unleash its id in unrestrained pursuit of financial satisfaction. Rather, it seems in service of the truth, at least as he sees it: that we all suffer psychological setbacks, that we could all at some point benefit from some time spent with a headshrinker, that the DSM-IV's universal appeal, and its implicit provision for universal treatment (at least for the insured), are good for all of us, doctor and patient alike.

On the other hand, Peele ran for APA president in 2000 and 2009 and lost. The organization might not be ready for this kind of candor or to give up once and for all on the quest for a way to distinguish the sick from the merely suffering.

Darrel Regier certainly isn't. "That's the problem I went into the field to address," he told me at the outset of our interview. To a numbers guy like Regier, concern over the findings of the Midtown Manhattan Study—the infamous 85 percent—is no mere hang-up. The result is a statistical impossibility. We can't all be abnormal any more than everyone who lives in Lake Wobegon can be above average. And if most of those people never seek treatment, then how sick could they be? Moreover, as Regier likes to point out when people accuse the APA of disease mongering, there is no way that the current mental health treatment system, with its 45,000 psychiatrists and half a million psychologists, social workers, and counselors could possibly keep up with all that demand. Bad as it is that the numbers are likely inaccurate, it would be worse if they were not, because then we would truly be awash in mental illness, our treatment resources swamped.

Regier, a lifelong public health doctor, has to think about planning and policies and other unglamorous concerns that cannot be met without knowing how many people are sick and what diseases they have.

That's reason enough to devote a career to finding the elusive threshold, or so it seemed when I asked him to tell me exactly what the problem was with overdiagnosis. I wondered how an elite psychiatrist viewed the question, exactly what kind of harm he thought his profession could cause by labeling us. I wanted to know if he thought that a doctor who tells a widower that his grief is an illness is potentially not only labeling, stigmatizing, and medicating him, but also shaping the patient's understanding of his loss, of himself, of the meaning of his life.

But Regier didn't seem to comprehend my question. He seemed to think I wanted him to explain what *false positive* meant. He might not be the philosophical sort or, after a lifetime of cultivating bureaucratic habits, he might have lost sight of philosophy. He might have only wanted to not get so far away from his talking points with me. Or maybe he thought the answer was self-evident: sky-high prevalence rates are an affront to reason, to everything that scientific medicine, with its aspiration to carve nature at its joints, stands for.

Jay Scully was not so reticent.

We went through the usual reasons that psychiatrists give when they worry about the overdiagnosis problem: overtreatment, stigmatization, the credibility of the profession. But I wanted more from him. I wanted him to tell me why, from a psychiatrist's point of view, it was a bad thing to, as he had just put it, "overpathologize the human experience."

"Because it limits the other potential ways to fix things. It limits the whole spectrum of the human experience," he said. "I mean really bad things happen that are not necessarily psychopathological. You'd have to be crazy to kill your family. Well, do you? Maybe not, but how do we know? Where are the sharp dividing lines? Maybe we never really know."

It was the first time in our half hour together that Scully seemed genuinely interested, reflective, even spontaneous. "So," I asked him, "the false positive problem is the problem of where psychiatry's limits are?"

"Yes," he said. "You know, we always need to be humble."

As I sat with the CEO of American psychiatry, with his $600,000-per-year salary and his large office with its bird's-eye view of the Potomac River and the Capitol, it was good to hear that word. It was good to know he thought that humility was important and to have heard him say, "Our treatment and ability to relieve suffering need work." But he got quickly back on message, and the PR flack was looking at her watch and telling us our time was up, so I couldn't ask him exactly what psychiatrists need to be humble about—whether it's only the gap between suffering and their ability to relieve it, or if he was aware of that other, deeper chasm, the one between opportunity and knowledge, the one that gives psychiatrists the power to say what that dividing line is, and to cash in on saying it, even though they themselves don't really know. Still, I was glad to hear this much.

Because as Montesquieu once said, "The spirit of moderation is what we call virtue in an aristocracy. It supplies the place of the spirit of equality in a popular state." Perhaps medicine is inescapably an aristocracy, and self-imposed moderation the only check on power, the only way to prevent beneficence from becoming oppression. Surely medicine can't be a democracy; we can't vote on whether or not we are sick or elect which illness we have. If we can't depend on definitions of mental disorder or on statistical measures of clinical significance to prevent the DSM from cataloging the entire spectrum of human experience, from turning all mental suffering into illness, then perhaps we are dependent on the sophistication, the restraint, the discretion—in short, the virtue—of our psychiatrists.

This is not a comforting thought. And not only because of the Biedermans and the Schatzbergs and the Nemeroffs out there, whose lack of restraint well exceeds the industry norm. But even for psychiatrists who see no need to supplement their $200,000 annual incomes with drug money, treatment options are deeply circumscribed—not only by the imperfect state of knowledge described by Scully, but also by a for-profit health care system that, with its focus on efficiencies, drives them inexorably toward the drugs about which they have been carefully educated by the makers.

Because Darrel Regier may be the kind of guy who would call his colleagues stupid in public and then complain that the debate had gotten personal, but he has spent an entire career as a public servant hacking away at one of the most daunting problems ever to come down the pike. It is impossible to come away from a conversation with him without believing that he really wants to solve that problem, and for a virtuous reason: to fashion a treatment system that effectively and efficiently relieves suffering. He wants a DSM that can help him and his colleagues to do this. He may be hard to like, but he is not evil.

But he also doesn't seem to understand the spirit of moderation, or why it is incumbent upon an aristocrat to develop it—at least not to judge from what he said at the end of his talk in Copenhagen. Amid his circumlocutions and score settling, Regier had managed to convey one fact: he intended the DSM-5 to move psychiatry decisively in the direction of defining the thresholds of mental illness with numbers.

This alone was not news. But Regier was well aware that people like Michael First and Allen Frances were wondering in public how he could possibly pull this off, how he could, in the little time remaining, create, debug, and standardize measures that would be sufficient to the task. It was a question that made him even testier than usual, or at least it did when I e-mailed him to ask it just a couple of months before he went to Copenhagen. His proposal called for dimensional measures for every diagnosis, I wrote, but in our interview he had mentioned only a small number of tests for a few diagnoses and the information on the DSM-5 website was sketchy. Were there more details that he could give me?

"They [the dimensional measures] will continue to evolve over time," he assured me. When I pressed him for more information, he wrote, "I don't think it will be useful to get into this level of detail on every diagnostic severity measure that we will be considering prior to the publication of DSM-5." Still, he reiterated, even if they weren't quite ready, "these scales will be input for a final clinical judgment about the severity level." But Regier knew, and he knew that his colleagues in Copenhagen knew, that with less than three years to go before publication, dimensional measures were not going to evolve fast enough to be finalized for the DSM-5. Because he was doubling down and staking the DSM-5's claim to a new paradigm on them, he had to explain himself—even if he still didn't have the details.

Regier started by damning his predecessors with faint praise. "It is most remarkable that the simple advance of having some more reliable, explicit diagnostic criteria . . . has made it possible for our research enterprise to advance as far as it has," he said. But those same checklists and categories had been an invitation to the much-lamented reification of mental disorders. Spitzer and Frances had presented the criteria as "essential components of an underlying pathophysiological and psychopathological process." No wonder they had been taken too seriously!

If only the DSM's diagnostic categories had been treated as hypotheses to be proved, rather than as diseases that had been discovered, Regier seemed to be saying, then scientists would have been free to validate them, to measure their severity and establish their thresholds, to find out whether they were really discrete entities or if they merged into one another on one or more spectrums of psychopathology. They wouldn't be saddled with diagnoses that didn't map well onto clinical experience or response to treatment or genetic research or molecular neuroscience, and they wouldn't be cleaning the egg off their faces as those mismatches became evident or as those treatments failed.

Regier was not going to make the same mistakes with DSM-5. His book would not try to freeze mental disorders in amber, leaving a generation of scientists to regret its reifications and yet have no choice but to use them. It wouldn't bury the fact that, as Scully told me, "the DSM will always be provisional" in disclaimers that no one would read.

Instead, Regier told his colleagues, they would be built right into the part of the book to which everyone turned first: the categories and criteria. "Advances . . . will only occur," he said, "if the definitions and diagnostic criteria for these disorders are constructed to facilitate their testing as scientific hypotheses." And once the new book comes out, "the syndrome categories and quantitative thresholds can be tested."

This is evidently what it meant to call the DSM-5 a living document. If the process seemed chaotic, this was only the inescapable ferment of innovation, and if the dimensional assessments weren't quite ready for prime time, or if some of the proposals seemed a little sketchy, or if they ended up leading doctors to diagnose and treat patients who weren't really ill, then that was because they were only hypotheses. If it turned out to be a mistake to, say, remove the bereavement exclusion or to introduce Temper Dysregulation Disorder, or to propose a particular test to measure the severity of a disorder, or to evaluate symptoms that don't have anything to do with a patient's diagnosis, then the troublesome section of the DSM-5 would be scrapped or revised in DSM-5.1. How this would affect patients whose diagnoses came and went, and with them their treatments, their own understanding of their troubles, and whatever identities their diagnoses had bestowed upon them—on this subject Regier didn't obfuscate. Neither did he deflect the question with complaints about its unfairness. He just said nothing at all.

Chapter 13

f Regier was silent about the potential effects of diagnostic caprice, the patients were not. By the end of the summer of 2010, more than eight thousand comments had poured into the DSM-5 website. According to the *Psychiatric News*, 10 percent of them expressed concern that the APA would drop Gender Identity Disorder, and nearly a quarter implored the organization not to delete Asperger's syndrome in favor of an Autistic Spectrum Disorder that may or may not include those currently diagnosed with Asperger's. Four decades after homosexuals demanded to be released from their diagnostic chains, groups of patients were pleading with the APA *not* to set them free.

Regier promised readers more details about the kvetchers, along with an official response, but in the meantime, the *News* offered one explanation for their complaints. Diagnoses, the paper wrote, provided "easy access to health services" like hormone treatments and sex-change surgery and special education programs, as well as therapy and medications.

People who have had to fight with insurance companies or school systems might have disagreed with the "easy" part, but then again, at least for the two thousand people who wrote in about Asperger's, money wasn't the main thing on their mind. As APA president Carol Bernstein wrote in the *News*, since they had been diagnosed, these patients had "developed a strong sense of uniqueness and belonging." They even, she reported, had christened themselves "Aspies." To delete the diagnosis might be to "deprive them of their identity." Even worse, Bernstein acknowledged, those Asperger's patients who were lucky enough to qualify for the new Autistic Spectrum Disorder would suddenly have a diagnosis that would be "more stigmatizing."

The APA seemed caught off guard by the fact that some people liked their diagnoses just fine. "While the work group members conducted a thorough review of the existing data and research literature," Bernstein wrote, the fact that the diagnoses had bestowed an identity on the patients had come as an "additional piece of evidence."

It's easy to see why the work group was surprised. After forty years of fending off their antipsychiatric enemies, after three decades of a diagnostic regime meant to reassure the public that psychiatrists didn't mean to exert control over people's identities any more than doctors parsing leukemia from lymphoma did, the APA had lost sight of what was obvious to Asperger's patients and transgendered people and to anyone who has gotten diagnosed: that a psychiatric diagnosis is a judgment about more than the way your organs are functioning. Once you start to think of your troubles as a disease, your idea of yourself, which is to say who you are, changes.

If anyone from the APA had asked Nomi Kaim about this, they would have discovered not only that it was true, but that it could be a really good thing.

Nomi is twenty-seven. Her wire-rim glasses slip down her nose frequently. She moves her bulky body gingerly, as if she is afraid she will knock something over as she leads me to her favorite spot in the Boston bookstore where we have met. When she describes how much she once disliked herself, it is easy to see why. Not because she is unlikable—indeed, she seems sweet and considerate and acutely concerned for me, asking if my chair is comfortable and our conversation nook quiet enough for my voice recorder, whether my coffee is sufficiently hot—but because she was once exactly the kind of girl whom children will taunt relentlessly: smart and hyperarticulate, but overweight and ungainly and unfashionable, as untalented of body as she is talented of mind.

"I fought to get myself comfortable in high school and before that I fought to get myself comfortable at elementary school," Nomi told me. She saw therapists, took drugs for her depression and anxiety, and finally, mercifully, graduated. She'd been accepted to Bryn Mawr but decided to take time off before she went, hoping that maturity would grant her some more social ease.

The college, she told me, "was exactly what I wanted"—at least when it came to academics. "In classes, I was where I belonged and I felt very fulfilled. But then I had to go back to the dormitory." In the dorm, in the dining room, out on the campus, she felt out of place, overwhelmed by the noise and commotion of a couple thousand students, their loud music and their drinking, their impenetrable cliques. "I hated the whole campus life," she said.

This time around, though, "the fight didn't feel worth it. I was tired of that." She went to the student health service and the doctors arranged for her to move into the school's infirmary, where she lived out her first semester, attending classes but avoiding the parties and the friendships and even the dining hall. When she returned home for her winter break, she pondered her options. "I chose not to go back and fight some more."

Going to college had always been Nomi's plan. "I had only had one path in my head and it was Bryn Mawr," she told me. "I didn't have any other picture of what to do. So I got very depressed."

Her parents placed her in McLean Hospital, a mental hospital associated with Harvard. There she was treated for depression and anxiety with drugs and cognitive-behavioral therapy. She also took part in therapy groups, but the intense contact with her fellow patients traumatized her. "I was just so emotionally flooded and didn't know what to do with it," she said. "I would ask to be excused and take a break and the therapists would say, 'I want you to try to stay with it.' They didn't really get what was going on, either."

What was going on didn't become clear until Nomi's mother, sure that Nomi's lifelong struggles to negotiate the social world were the cause, not the effect, of her mood and anxiety disorders, arranged for her to be tested by a neuropsychologist at McLean. For two days Nomi answered questions and filled out forms and drew figures and solved puzzles. At the end, the psychologist told Nomi she had Asperger's syndrome.

Nomi's mother was glad to finally have an explanation for her daughter's troubles. "She said, 'Well, now we know. Thank God.'"

But not Nomi. "I was like, 'That's not what I was looking for. I don't agree with this.' I mean, it was just so not what I wanted." Bad enough that "it sounded like ass burger," she said; she could only imagine what a bully would do with that name. Even worse, the diagnosis seemed like a pronouncement on the one capacity of which she'd always been most sure: her intelligence. No matter how much the doctors reassured her that Asperger's had nothing to do with her intelligence, still it seemed obvious that "I had this cluster of selective stupidity—social stupidity and practical stupidity," she said. "And stupid was always the biggest insult for me. Kids use it as a weapon. It's something I've always feared."

But that wasn't the worst of it. "All along, I'd been thinking my problems with feeling stupid were connected to mental illness," Nomi recalled. "I was hoping it was a mental illness." With mental illness, "there's always this hope that if I can just conquer this, I'll become normal. But nobody talks about conquering Asperger's. The diagnosis undid all those hopes."

That was before Nomi's mother persuaded her to join the Asperger's Association of New England (AANE), an advocacy group located just outside Boston. It took her a while to figure out that there was a difference between AANE and McLean Hospital. They weren't going to make her stay in the groups if she felt overwhelmed, for instance. They weren't going to make her go to groups at all or ridicule her for her peculiarities or force her to try to fit in. Everyone at AANE had the same kind of troubles, or at least understood what those troubles were. (Many of the group's leaders and staff are parents of children with Asperger's.) Her diagnosis was not a cause for exclusion, but a key into a world where, for the first time in her life, she didn't have to fight to feel welcome.

Nomi thrived at AANE, volunteering in the office and becoming a mainstay of its speakers' bureau. Before we met, I had watched her lead a workshop designed to help people with Asperger's figure out how to live independently. She was a dynamic speaker, reassuring and sympathetic by turns, as she described the way she had learned to organize her life, to maintain a schedule, to stay in touch with family. She gave pointers on how to get disability status from Social Security, to find an affordable apartment, to go to school—all of which she had done after receiving her diagnosis.

Now she's telling me about a benefit she did not mention in her talk: the way the Asperger's label changed her sense of herself. "Spending time in an environment where the diagnosis is embraced as a difference, I started to see my diagnosis differently." The fact that it wasn't a "mental illness," at least not by her definition, had become good news, a "gift" even. There were advantages to not being *neurotypical*, as people with Asperger's sometimes describe the rest of us.

"There are certain things that neurotypical women in particular are obsessed with, shoes and clothes and makeup, that I'm very glad I'm not," she said, adding that it isn't just the girly preoccupations she was pleased to be relieved of. "In general, I'm very content with being completely outside of the popular culture fray." Her diagnosis had helped her to do what is demanded of all of us but comes easier to some than others: to build a self out of the raw materials of nature and nurture.

"If I had to give up my Asperger's," says Nomi, "that would be hard."

Nomi—like everyone thought to have Asperger's—almost didn't have a diagnosis to lose. Asperger's syndrome didn't exist until 1994, at least not officially, and even then it came close to not making it into the DSM-IV. "It was a total add-on," said Fred Volkmar, the Yale psychiatrist who spearheaded the move to include it in the manual.

Less than twenty years ago, Asperger's was not familiar to most American psychiatrists—or to anyone else for that matter. The disorder was first described by an Austrian pediatrician, Hans Asperger, in a 1944 paper outlining a cluster of symptoms that he had observed in some of his patients, mostly boys: abnormal, often pedantic speech; physical clumsiness; difficulty understanding gestures and other non-verbal communication; impaired social interaction; and inflexible interests, often in one narrow subject, such as train timetables. He called the syndrome *autistischen Psychopathen*, or autistic psychopathy.

Asperger's work languished in an academic netherworld, his paper untranslated and mostly unknown until 1981. But then Lorna Wing, a British psychiatrist who had encountered Asperger's work as part of her quest to understand her own daughter's autism, wrote up thirty-four cases that she thought met Asperger's description. They weren't exact matches. Some were adults (the oldest was thirty-five), and many of them, contrary to what Asperger had described, had walked before they talked. And while Asperger wrote that his patients had "an especially intimate relationship with language and highly sophisticated linguistic skills," and were in general more creative (at least in their field of specific interest) and smarter than most people, Wing didn't think her patients were all that sophisticated or creative or intelligent. Their language "gives the impression of being learned by rote," she noted, and "their thought processes are confined to a narrow, pedantic, literal, but logical chain of reasoning." They may have used big words, but they didn't necessarily understand what they meant. They may have been able to tell you the make and model and number of every locomotive on the tracks, but that didn't mean they understood what a train was for. They may have been smarter than the average kid, but, she said, they were "conspicuously lacking in common sense."

Still, however, Wing thought she had only refined Asperger's observations. Her patients and his belonged in the same category, and there seemed to be enough patients who fit the description to warrant further investigation. Among the questions that Wing thought needed to be answered was how patients like hers were related to another group of socially unsuccessful children who had been described by another Austrian doctor. His name was Leo Kanner, and in 1924 he had emigrated to the South Dakota hinterlands, where he got a job as an assistant psychiatrist in an asylum. From there, he worked his way to Johns Hopkins, where he started the country's first dedicated child psychiatry unit. In 1943, just a year before Asperger's paper came out, he published an article describing children much more severely impaired than Asperger's—unable to talk, mentally retarded, prone to rocking and other repetitive activities, and distressed when their rituals were disrupted. But like Asperger's patients, Kanner's were hard-pressed to negotiate the world of others, and he, too, called these patients autistic.

The two doctors were probably unaware of each other, at least at the beginning. They likely both borrowed the term from the same source: Eugen Bleuler, a Swiss psychiatrist who drew on the Greek root for *self* to describe the imperviousness to the outside world characteristic of schizophrenia. (This was the label most likely to be applied to Kanner's patients.) But Kanner's definition, perhaps because it described a much larger group (or maybe because he wrote in English), prevailed, and by the time Wing wrote her paper, it had become the industry standard. The Infantile Autism that made its way into the DSM-III was much more like Kanner's description than like Asperger's: a "pervasive lack of responsiveness to other people," "gross deficits in language development," and "bizarre responses to various aspects of the environment."

On balance, Wing concluded, "the syndromes are more alike than unalike." Both comprised impairments in three dimensions: language, interaction, and play. But where Kanner's kids tended to be unable to talk, withdrawn from or even unaware of the social world, and absorbed in repetitive activities such as rocking, Asperger's tended to be plenty talkative and engaged with the outside world, but in a strange and inept way. Like awkward teens at a prom, they wanted to dance, they even selected a partner, but they just didn't know how to do the steps. This cluelessness, Wing suggested, was only a milder form of the deficits that characterized Kanner's autism.

But, Wing said, this didn't mean that Asperger's syndrome should go unrecognized. A child who talks endlessly about the interstate highway system and nothing else, whose striving to attract people only drives them away, who is tone deaf to the music of human interaction and yet wishes to sing along: this is not someone who should be overlooked or simply dismissed as a little bit eccentric, especially not when there are a lot of such children. For them, Wing wrote, "the term is helpful." It can be used with parents and teachers and bosses "who often cannot believe in a diagnosis of autism, which they equate with muteness and total social withdrawal." It can "help to convince the people concerned that there is a real problem . . . needing careful management and education." Even if Asperger's was only a high-functioning variant of autism, Wing suggested, and even if it was, strictly speaking, *not* a separate disorder, still it deserved its own label.

The argument that pragmatics should trump principle proved persuasive to the psychiatrists fashioning the International Classification of Diseases. When the ICD-10 came out in 1992, it included Asperger's syndrome among the pervasive developmental disorders. This forced the APA's hand: to achieve the goal of harmonization with the ICD, the DSM-IV task force had to at least consider Asperger's for inclusion. "We knew the question was there," said Volkmar, "so we were going to look."

Seventeen years later Volkmar now heads the Child Study Center at

Yale. He's a friendly man with a gentle voice and a brushy moustache on a jolly rubber face that makes people of a certain age remember Captain Kangaroo. He's wearing two pairs of glasses—one on his nose, one on his pate at the ready for reading. It's not clear if he does this for efficiency's sake, or just so he won't lose track of their whereabouts.

Volkmar says he started out uncertain about Asperger's. "I had seen a couple of cases that corresponded with the description, but I was not pro or con," he told me. A literature review and a meta-analysis carried the diagnosis across the bar Frances and Pincus had erected, and the next step was to draft criteria and try them out in field trials. Volkmar recruited 125 clinicians at five sites. They started with patients who seemed likely to get an autism diagnosis and sorted them according to the proposed criteria. Of the nearly one thousand subjects tested, fifty-one turned out to qualify for the Asperger's diagnosis.

"This was totally unanticipated on my part," says Volkmar. But, especially because each diagnosis was confirmed by a second rater, the unexpectedly high number convinced him that it was possible to tell these kids apart reliably—or, in other words, that they were suffering from something distinct from Pervasive Developmental Disorder NOS and Infantile Autism, the labels that would most likely be applied. Even if it was possible that this was only another line in the sand, the statistics were there to prove that it could be drawn accurately and that these kids needed their own section of the beach. Volkmar pushed for Asperger's to be anointed as an official disorder.

Volkmar had to fight for his proposal. He had to overcome the DSM-IV conservatism, which he describes, only half joking, as a "tendency [among work group members] to be on the autism spectrum and not like change." As he put it, "the APA would like not to even have a child section, so they weren't eager to make it bigger by even one diagnosis." He had to flog his evidence—fifty-one cases may have been "the biggest sample that anyone since Asperger had ever pulled together," but it was still a small number. He kept hearing that it would be consigned to the Appendix, or, as he calls it, the "elephant burial ground," and he kept pushing for it to be spared that fate.

There was one last obstacle—one that had nothing to do with the evidence, and of which he was unaware until "someone took me aside and explained": the name of the proposed disorder. The APA was opposed to eponyms, favoring instead plain descriptive language, and this particular name presented a thorny problem. "There were rumors that Asperger had been a Nazi," Volkmar said. People were wary of a diagnosis named for (and first proposed by) a man who sorted children in Nazi Germany according to their pathologies.

Volkmar called Lorna Wing. "Oh my God, no," she told him. "He was a religious man." The reassurance was only secondhand, and it didn't entirely make sense, but when he passed it along, the worries about the name were forgotten. Asperger's syndrome was one of only two entirely new diagnoses—out of ninety-four that were proposed for DSM-IV—to make the cut.

Six years later, in June 2000, *The New York Times Magazine* ran "The Little Professor Syndrome," a long feature by Lawrence Osborne about Asperger's syndrome. Experts described the symptoms. A school director told Osborne that "they simply don't understand social games." A parent called them "perfect counterfeit bills," convincing facsimiles of normal children until they tried to engage others. Fred Volkmar weighed in, saying that "their social interactions are a disaster."

But Osborne had some good news to report. Although, as the school director said, "everything has to be taught to them," it was proving possible to do that. In classrooms, support groups, and doctors' offices, Asperger's patients were learning how to negotiate the neurotypical world. A teacher demonstrated how her students had memorized facial expressions so they could read other people's signals. With techniques like this, according to Osborne, "Asperger's children can at least learn to imitate social behavior that other kids learn intuitively." Like Franken-stein's monster observing human life through a window, they were forced to watch the rest of us from a distance. But unlike the monster, and as Hans Asperger had predicted, they could learn how to approxi-mate what normal people do.

One of Osborne's readers was Barbara Wiechmann, a Brooklyn of-fice manager and playwright. She'd been worried about her son, who was then four, for at least two years. He'd been slow to talk and walk, and, even for his age, seemed terribly clumsy. He didn't exactly play with his toys. He arranged them instead, sorting rather than manipu-lating them in imaginative scenarios. He lined up his blocks neatly on his windowsill, arranged by color, and stacked dog food cans into a neat, perfect pyramid. For bedtime reading, he rejected *Goodnight Moon* or any of the other standbys, insisting instead on the Smithson-ian's field guide to mushrooms, which he'd memorized by the time he was four.

Wiechmann showed Osborne's article to her husband, Michael Car-ley, and told him she thought their son was one of the little professors. Carley wasn't so sure. "Some things made sense, others didn't," he said. But he agreed to have their son tested and continued to read up on the subject. Before the appointment, he went to Cabo San Lucas for a quick surfing vacation from his job with an NGO that was implementing a United Nations drinking water development project in Iraq. "I . . . have yet to stand successfully on a surfboard," Carley later wrote in a mem-oir, "but I've never cared. Water is the only arena where I have felt physi-cally graceful."

His ungainliness wasn't the only limitation Carley was aware of on his trip. After a day of not surfing, he stopped in at a disco. He's no more a dancer than a surfer, and in the crowd of tourists, he wrote later, he felt "like a ghost that no one saw." That feeling was familiar enough, but, in the light of what he'd learned about Asperger's since he read the *New York Times Magazine* article, it took on a new meaning.

As I watched the dictionaries of nonverbal communication flowing back and forth, I was hit fully, finally, that what separated me from them wasn't cultural. It never had been. It wasn't intellectual. It never had been. It was bigger than that.

At that moment, one month before the confirmation of a formal diagnosis, I knew. Staring into that sea of abandon . . . I knew. I realized I had Asperger's syndrome.

A month after his return, and a week after his son received his diagnosis, Carley's psychiatrist confirmed his revelation. With the official diagnosis came relief. "It meant I'm not an asshole. I'm just wired differently," he says. "This is just how I process thoughts and experiences and emotions."

Carley is sitting with his legs crossed under him on the bare wood floor of his sparsely furnished living room, free-associating about his nineteen-year-old single mother, his father who was killed in Vietnam, his "crazy dumb" gallivanting youth, his misadventures with cops on different continents, and the people he's met along the way, who, he says, have been evenly divided on whether he's a "tell-it-like-it-is guy" or a jerk. He talks fast, snapping his fingers for emphasis, and it's easy to believe he had once wanted to be a playwright. He sure has a flair for drama.

That's a skill Carley has put to a different use since he got his diagnosis. Shortly after his visit with the psychiatrist, he took over a loose network of Asperger's support groups in New York, and in 2003, he used his NGO savvy and his forceful personality to wangle money from the Fund for Social Change and turn the network into GRASP, the Global and Regional Asperger Syndrome Partnership, the largest organization for adolescents and adults with Asperger's. Like AANE, Nomi Kaim's group, GRASP works to provide patients and their families with information and resources. But Carley has a larger agenda, captured in GRASP's mission statement.

At GRASP we envision a world where all individuals on the autism spectrum are respected, valued, and fairly represented; where appropriate supports and services are readily available to those in need; and where people on the spectrum are empowered to participate in policy and personal decisions that affect their lives.

Asperger's syndrome, according to Carley, isn't just a diagnostic label or a psychiatric disorder. It is a fundamental part of identity, not unlike race or sexual orientation. His is a civil rights crusade, a quest for cognitive pluralism.

Carley often slips into the language of identity politics as he describes his odyssey from getting his diagnosis to attending his first support group to becoming leader of GRASP. "Knowing that I had the same genes running through my veins as they did," he says, remembering the first groups, "gave me the guts to open up and share that experience. And what's the response? A room full of people saying, 'I've been there, too.' That's biblical."

As important as that experience was to him, his mission now is to make it unnecessary for others to go through it. "This is about us creating a more diverse atmosphere," he told me. "Eventually, Asperger's and autism are going to be thought of as natural extensions of the human condition and not illnesses. We won't even need to separate them."

That's what GRASP is for. "We want to get rid of the shame," he says, "so we've made a very concerted effort to change the iconography of Asperger's"—from an affliction to a gift. And, he thinks, the proposal to eliminate the Asperger's diagnosis in favor of a spectrum disorder is an opportunity to extend what Asperger's patients have secured for themselves to the rest of the autism spectrum—including those much more severely impaired than he. This is an adventure he is eager to undertake, which is why he, along with about half the members of GRASP, is in favor of the change.

"I'm going to butt in here," says his son, who has been sitting quietly beside me on the couch. He's wearing a Minnesota Twins baseball cap, although he swears he's a Red Sox fan. He has his father's squat nose and downturned eyes as well as his diagnosis, but right now he wants to tell me about a way in which they are really not the same kind of person at all. "I'm sorry, but the way we've taken Asperger's has been very different."

Like many fifteen-year-olds, the younger Carley finds his father's passions embarrassing. When his friends ask what his father does, he says, "I don't want to be, like, 'He works with Asperger's.'" He looks at his father across the room. "I want the answer to be something like your old UN job." He tells his father how mortifying it was when Carley took his son's school principal to task over her policy of not disclosing students' diagnoses. "I don't want to be affiliated with it," he says. "I'm running around with my friends. I don't want to bring up that subject." He turns to me. "It's something for home. It's something for me and my dad." That, he explains, is why he wants me to call him CC instead of his real name.

Not that the diagnosis hadn't helped CC. "If I didn't have a diagnosis, I'd be totally clueless," he says. He went to special schools; hung out with fellow Aspies; even had a little counseling; and learned, as his father likes to put it, to play the cards he was dealt.

"In seventh grade, I got the worst grades possible, and I was off the charts in eighth grade"—because, he says, his diagnosis gave him a motive for trying harder. "I have this thing on my back—Asperger's syndrome. It's like getting a high score on a video game. Like, let's see how high I can go."

But that's all behind him now, CC says. His problems have been "ironed out." He is in a mainstream school, where his friends don't know about his diagnosis. His Asperger's is in the background—a "huge achievement," he tells me—and he wants to keep it there.

CC turns back to his father. "I know you hate this, and I would love it if everyone would accept it. But you know there are idiots in this world. They don't look at how other people think. They don't acknowledge any evidence. They just put it down."

And this, he thinks, is only going to get worse if the diagnosis disappears in the DSM-5, and kids like him are suddenly considered autistic. "When you hear the word *autism*, you think of institutionalization, speech delay, diapers. It's a scary word," he says. "It's going to make me want to be even more concealed." CC turns to me. "Would *you* rather say you have Asperger's or autism?"

The difference between father and son may only reflect a difference in their temperaments, whatever their similarities when it comes to Asperger's. On the other hand, Michael knows what it is like to live without an explanation and the acceptance that comes with it, while CC doesn't remember a time when he didn't have the diagnosis. The disorder is so thoroughly intertwined with his sense of who he is that it is invisible to him. He has the luxury to forget about it, to carry on as if it weren't there. He can see that he and others could lose this freedom if the DSM-5 proposal goes through, but he also doesn't want to take to the streets to fight about it.

Their argument reminds me of the clash between young women and their feminist mothers, the kids cringing at their parents' stridency, the grown-ups appalled by their children's complacency (and their ingratitude). It's an argument Hans Asperger, writing in a time and place perilous to people singled out for their pathology, probably wouldn't have dreamt of when he noted how many of his child patients had fathers just like them. It's surely not an outcome that the DSM-IV experts would have predicted: that their diagnosis would go far beyond facilitating services, that it would create a whole new brand of identity politics, and that a strange little boy who might have foundered on the same shoals that once snared Nomi Kaim would grow into this impressive, articulate, self-possessed teenage boy.

But, as Fred Volkmar says, when it comes to new psychiatric diagnoses, "one can always be surprised at the outcome."

Not all the surprises were political. Some were statistical. "You never know what is going to take off and what isn't," Volkmar told me, but it wasn't long before Asperger's took off like no other psychiatric disorder ever had, at least not since hysteria had swept across the salons of Europe in the time of Freud.

When Lorna Wing wrote her paper on Asperger's in 1981, figures on the prevalence of autism were scant. She ballparked it at about 4 or 5 per 10,000, and guessed that maybe half of those were the kind of patient described by Asperger. When Volkmar's team conducted their field trials, there were no better statistics for Asperger's because, of course, the disorder didn't yet exist to be counted. But even if Volkmar's group was impressed enough by those fifty-one cases to push for inclusion, and even if they knew that adding Asperger's would likely add patients to the sick rolls, they certainly didn't think they'd stumbled on an epidemic. At best, they had identified a small if significant number of cases that could be carved out of another small number.

So imagine their (and everyone else's) surprise when Eric Fombonne, an epidemiologist working in England, reviewed twenty-three surveys of autism prevalence conducted between 1966 and 1999, and concluded that the rates were on the rise. Estimates varied wildly—from 0.7 percent in a 1970 study to 21 percent in 1996, but one factor alone seemed to affect the overall trend. Prior to 1989, the average study turned up 4.3 cases in 10,000 people; after that year, the rate was 7.2 in 10,000. Even accounting for all other factors—age, gender, severity, IQ, and so on—the relationship between year of study and rate of autism was statistically significant. Time alone, in other words, was making autism rates rise—and not, so the epidemiologists said, simply because the clock was ticking or because there was what Fombonne called a "secular increase in the incidence of the disorder." Instead, he thought, the increase was the result of "improved recognition and detection . . . together with a broadening of the diagnostic concept and definitions."

People like Volkmar might have thought the territory they had established with the Asperger's diagnosis was sparsely populated, but epidemiologists were reaching a different conclusion. Using the DSM-IV criteria, one group reviewed the medical and educational records of schoolchildren in Atlanta and turned up a rate of 34 per 10,000, a tenfold increase over the few comparable studies that had been conducted in the United States.

Fombonne, in an editorial accompanying the Atlanta study, speculated that even these results were "an underestimate." And subsequent studies proved him right. As of 2002, the CDC reported, 1 in 150 children had an autistic spectrum disorder, a rate that by 2006 had reached 1 in 110, or just over 90 per 10,000. It was around this time that Lorna Wing started referring to the publication of her original paper as "opening Pandora's Box."

The numbers just kept going up. By 2008, the CDC said, the rate was 1 in 88, and in May 2011, researchers writing in the *American Journal of Psychiatry* announced they had found a prevalence rate in a city in Korea of 2.64 percent. For those of you keeping score, that's 264 per 10,000—and 374 for every 10,000 boys—a greater than fiftyfold increase since 1981.

And people were keeping score—including the people at Autism Speaks. "The world's largest autism science and advocacy organization," according to its website, it sponsored the Korean study and, soon after its publication, blitzed the media with the claim that 1 in 38 children was autistic. This, the group said, indicated "the need for improved and wider autism screening among the general population"—a move that, to judge from the last twenty years, could only increase prevalence rates, and with them public attention, sympathy, and, of course, money for their cause.

Opinions varied on what was causing this increase. To those who held mercury-based preservatives in common childhood vaccines responsible, the increasing rates were further proof that vaccination policies were ruining kids' brains. Most explanations, however, focused on the old and elusive question of whether epidemiologists were getting better at detecting a disease that was already there, or if they were charting the rise of an epidemic.

But the researchers in the Korean study offered an interesting alternative explanation. They noted that only 63 percent of the people they had solicited had agreed to participate in the study—a disappointingly low number, far lower than the 80 percent considered optimal, and often achieved, in community surveys. But, they argued, if you consider the tendency among Koreans to think of autism as "a stigmatizing hereditary disorder" that "impugns the child's lineage on both sides and threatens the marriage prospects of unaffected relatives," then this level of participation seems not so bad. In fact, it's remarkable: something had inspired nearly two-thirds of the parents in a Korean city to risk having their families marked as members of a defective gene pool.

The researchers focused their speculation on Korea's "highly structured" educational system, with its emphasis on "behavioral regulation" in twelve-hour-long classes that meet six days a week. Some children's problems would be impossible to conceal in such a setting, but "for quiet, high functioning children with ASDs," they wrote, "this environment may reduce the likelihood of referrals to special education programs." Still, even if they remained invisible at school, these children's problems might have been obvious at home, and the survey "may have provided welcome opportunities" for parents caught between their concern for their kids and their fears for their families' reputation to get information and maybe even treatment. "It could be argued that in this cultural context," the researchers wrote, "parents of children with serious but unrecognized developmental problems would be more likely to participate in research than parents of unaffected children."

This wasn't the first time a researcher attributed increasing prevalence to motivated parents seizing an opportunity. The Atlanta study's authors had been disturbed by a finding that the likelihood that a child would qualify for a diagnosis increased with age—but only until they got to the oldest group of children, who were nine and ten. Did this mean that younger children were developing autistic disorders at an increasing rate? Had they found the leading edge of the epidemic?

The scientists didn't think so. "Lower rates in 9- and 10-year-olds may reflect the use of narrower diagnostic criteria for autism before the publication of DSM-IV," they wrote, "and the increased availability of educational, health and social services for children with autism." Perhaps the older children hadn't escaped an epidemic, but rather had been born too late to benefit from the DSM-IV's relaxed criteria and their intersection with the 1991 mandate issued by the U.S. Department of Education to provide special education services to children with autistic disorders. This, the researchers allowed, was "possibly leading to increases in the number of children classified with autism because of the availability of services."

"Diagnosis of ASDs [autistic spectrum disorders] is an uncertain art," wrote autism expert Tony Charman in an editorial accompanying the Korean study, "and in the end one has to make a clinical judgment of whether the number, quality, severity, and accompanying impairment of symptoms are sufficient to fulfill DSM criteria." As in any diagnosis, the need for judgment about ASDs increases when the disorder is milder; a kid who rocks in the corner and can't talk is much easier to diagnose than someone like Nomi or CC. But milder cases like theirs account for nearly two-thirds of the diagnoses that make up the prevalence rates.

It's no mystery why parents would seek out a diagnosis, as Nomi's and CC's parents did—and, like them, to feel relief when the doctor issues it. After all, it's not as if parents have to be encouraged to worry about how their children are faring socially, or to wonder if they will ever learn to negotiate all the complex and unspoken rules of their little societies, or to think that disaster awaits when they cannot. Even if they haven't read *Lord of the Flies*, parents know just how brutal those

THE BOOK OF WOE   201

politics are, and how ill suited some children are to them. In a market-place of worried parents searching for resources, a diagnosis like Asperger's syndrome is bound to be a hot commodity.

And really, how hard is it to sell people on a disorder whose "symptoms" can bestow what Lawrence Osborne called "extraordinary gifts"? Osborne wasn't talking about special education dollars, but about Glenn Gould and Vladimir Nabokov and Ludwig Wittgenstein, all diagnosed—posthumously, of course—into a Hall of Fame that, depending on which website you consult, also includes Isaac Newton, Emily Dickinson, and Albert Einstein.

Even for those who will fall short of greatness, the diagnosis has its appeal. And its charms are on the increase, at least according to the Aspie who predicted to Osborne that "society will actually become more and more dependent on people with Asperger's to usher it through the difficulties ahead." That was more than a decade ago, and since then, interaction has come to rely less and less on the nonverbal cues that Aspies are so bad at decoding and more and more on the tablets and handhelds, the binaries of emoticons and tweets, that they are more suited to. While the neurotypical among us grow more and more bewildered by the barrage of information fed to us by our devices, the burdens of Asperger's, at least in the view of some of the diagnosed, increasingly become a gift. Even for those who think this is an ominous sign—like the novelist Jonathan Lethem, who speculated that people with Asperger's are "canaries [who] sensed before anyone else that we'd entered a coal mine"—the fit between disease and society is striking, the temptation to claim the label obvious.

This may be the real surprise of the Asperger's outbreak: that it is neither a "secular increase" nor an artifact of counting, but rather a supply-side epidemic. Unlike the childhood bipolar outbreak, this one was not set off by a drug company and its shills, exploiting loopholes in the DSM for profit. This one came right from the authors of the book, who wanted nothing more than to help kids help themselves to social resources. They had built a diagnosis, and the patients had come.

———

Volkmar thinks that the rush to get Asperger's into the DSM-IV might have had something to do with the outcome. "Had we had a little more time, we would have been able to have a better definition and criteria for Asperger's," he told me, which might have made the diagnostic threshold a little harder to cross. But even so, Volkmar is glad Asperger's made the cut. "I don't regret getting it in," he said. "You need to have a label to get services, and this is a population that needs them."

Michael First also thinks it was "premature to add Asperger's, given the limited amount of data," he told me. "You could argue that this was a deviation from DSM-IV's conservative approach."

That's an assessment with which Allen Frances agrees. "We probably were premature in introducing Asperger's," he acknowledged. Childhood disorders, he said, were outside his expertise. "Had a comparable situation arisen on the adult side, I would have been more insistent on the strict application of the DSM-IV rules." It's a lapse that he now regrets. "Had I been smart enough to predict that the diagnosis would be made so loosely, that parents would panic and stop vaccinating their kids, and that school services would be based just on the presence or absence of the diagnosis, then I definitely would have insisted on a stricter application of the rules."

Regret over the Asperger's diagnosis, or at least over the way it had become ubiquitous, was one thing that Frances and the DSM-5 leadership agreed on. David Kupfer told *The New York Times* that the swelling ranks of Asperger's patients were getting to be a problem. "It involves a use of treatment resources," he said. "It becomes a cost issue." You don't want to reify your diagnoses, but on the other hand, if a diagnosis is nothing more than a label that gets services . . . well, there is such a thing as too much success, especially when resources are scarce, costs are high, and public credibility is slipping.

The DSM-5 proposal sure looked like a way to raise the bar for entry.

DSM-IV's Autistic Disorder had listed twelve criteria under three main headings and required that patients meet only six of them, with at least two coming from the first category and at least one each from the remaining two; the Asperger's diagnosis required two from Criterion A's four symptoms and one from the four listed under Criterion B. (One math-minded psychiatrist calculated that there were 1,256 combinations of symptoms that would meet the criteria.) DSM-5, on the other hand, required all three Criterion A symptoms to be met and two of four in Criterion B. But even if it seemed like a no-brainer that moving from a Chinese menu to prix fixe would reduce the numbers of diagnoses, the APA insisted this was not the purpose of the change. "The goal was not to change prevalence," work group member Catherine Lord told me. After all, gerrymandering a diagnosis to solve a public policy, or a public relations, problem—that would be cheating.

Besides, Lord told me, "we think these prevalence rates are accurate." There was a problem with accuracy—not with the numbers of diagnoses, but with what doctors meant when they rendered them. "We want to make the criteria match up better with what clinicians are seeing when they make the diagnosis," she said. The problem with criteria that were too vague and broad was not that doctors could use them too liberally—say, to make sure a kid who was a little odd got special services in school. Rather, Lord said, when they rendered their diagnoses, it wasn't clear exactly what, if anything, the criteria had to do with the conclusion. In fact, the most important factor in determining which diagnosis a kid got, at least according to a study Lord had conducted, was the hospital that did the evaluation. Doctors had reverted to the old pre-DSM-III way: deciding which illness a patient had through some combination of local custom and intuition, rather than by systematically applying the criteria.

But only astute clinicians could be trusted with this uncertain art. The rest of us—the parents who want their kids to qualify, the geeks who want to inherit the earth from the neurotypicals, the people who would prefer having a mental disorder over being a jerk—needed to have their leash yanked. "People use 'Asperger's' and 'autism' colloquially," Lord told me. Tightening the criteria would give the masses "who don't know much about autism less of a feeling that everyone who's socially awkward has autism."

On the other hand, if those people want to call themselves Aspies, that's fine by Lord. "We're not trying to take away that identity," she said. "It's very helpful to some people. It's just not a medical diagnosis." Still, it was clear that the APA could take away what it had given—not the name, but the rights and privileges it had inadvertently granted by enshrining Asperger's in the DSM. And, evidently, when the diagnosis got out of hand, that is exactly what it would do.

Lord reassured me that this wasn't the problem it seemed to be. First of all, she said, "people with Asperger's vacillate between wanting to describe themselves as having a disorder or not." So deleting the diagnosis would actually help people like Nomi Kaim and CC Carley by providing the privileges without the burden and by removing the stink of pathology from their identity. As for those privileges, kids in special education have to get reevaluated every three years, so they are always at risk of losing their diagnoses. Of course, generally that would be because their condition has changed, not because it has disappeared from the DSM. But Lord was quite certain that the only problem patients would face was having to move from one diagnostic home to another. The overall prevalence rates, she said, were very unlikely to come down.

That was a question that would have to wait for field trials of the new diagnoses. But as the APA geared up for its annual meeting in May 2011, it was becoming evident that the field trials were in disarray, and even as their significance was increasing, they might not be able to shed much light on questions like these—even to the very few people from whom the results would not be kept a secret.

Chapter 14

In early May 2011, the APA posted its revised draft of the DSM-5. Asperger's syndrome was still slated for removal, as was the bereavement exclusion. But Psychosis Risk Syndrome (PRS) and Temper Dysregulation Disorder were gone. In their place were two new diagnoses—Attenuated Psychosis Symptoms Syndrome (APSS) and Disruptive Mood Dysregulation Disorder. The ingredients of the new disorders were exactly the same as the old ones. Only the labels had changed.

The renaming strategy had its obvious advantages. It got David Shaffer off the hook for suggesting a name that seemed to medicalize ill temper, even as the criteria continued to medicalize ill-tempered kids. It also allowed Will Carpenter to deflect attention from the research showing that kids whose illness consisted of being on the verge of psychosis rarely went on to get psychotic. On further consideration, he told me, his work group had realized that PRS really wasn't a "prevention concept" at all, but rather "a diagnostic concept," not an illness about to happen, but one in progress right now.

That explanation raised the question of why, if PRS was a disorder in its own right, the work group hadn't proposed it as a "diagnostic concept" in the first place. It also didn't explain why, according to the website, the rationale for introducing the diagnosis was that "young people at risk for later manifestation of a psychotic disorder can be identified," or why APSS was still described as "a risk syndrome for psychosis."

Perhaps the APA's marketing department and editorial department weren't talking to each other.

"People say, 'What's in a name?'" Dilip Jeste, the future president of the APA, told three hundred of his colleagues the week after the changes were posted. "But it seems the name means a lot to lots of people." Jeste was talking about Mild Neurocognitive Disorder, a disorder once known as Minor Neurocognitive Disorder. He explained that many people who wrote into the website had complained to his neurocognitive disorders work group that *minor* was a "trivializing" word. "The people pointed out that if you call something minor, insurance companies will not reimburse," he said.

Jeste wasn't entirely happy with the committee's solution. "It really doesn't make any sense," he said. He wasn't talking about the way that the diagnosis, as he acknowledged a few sentences later, is only an exaggerated version of the normal cognitive decline that sets in after age fifty. But he pointed out that if there was going to be a Major Neurocognitive Disorder, "it should be minor versus major, not mild." He solicited better suggestions from the audience. None was forthcoming.

But there is more than money in a name. Neurocognitive Disorder, however you qualified it, was a reworking of a DSM-IV label that was itself pretty tarnished, and getting more so as baby boomers aged: Dementia. "It's a pejorative term," Jeste said, because it came from the Greek for "losing one's mind." And no matter how much those of us over fifty might grouse privately that we're losing our minds along with our memories, we really don't want our doctors to agree with us, at least not officially, and surely not on our permanent medical dossier, not while the problem is still mild (or minor). Even in the later stages of Alzheimer's, an undeniably major cognitive disorder, *dementia* might carry too much stigma, Jeste added. On the other hand, most people with major neurocognitive disorders eventually did lose their minds. So the work group decided to name the new diagnosis Major Neurocognitive Disorder (Dementia), and then, once the DSM-5 came out, to "let the marketplace decide."

That's probably not how Darrel Regier would have put it. He probably would have said, "Let the hypotheses be tested." Still, the relabeling tactics helped to fill in the blank Regier had left when he didn't get back to the *Psychiatric News* about the fate of the public suggestions. The kvetchers had been turned into a focus group, and, evidently, the diagnoses that didn't meet with market approval would be rebranded.

Jeste's talk was part of the APA's 2011 annual meeting, held in Honolulu. "Attire is 'aloha business/casual.' No suits, ties or fancy dresses," the website proclaimed, and many of the ten thousand psychiatrists in the soaring open-air atrium of the Hawaii Conference Center dutifully sported muumuus and Hawaiian shirts. The theme of the convention was "Transforming Mental Health Through Leadership, Discovery, and Collaboration," but the APA leadership had discovered the necessity of keeping their most prominent collaborator at a distance. The conference's printed program began with a sixteen-page disclosure index in which every speaker divulged whether he or she had taken remuneration from any drug companies (although not how much), information that was repeated at the start of every talk.

Not that the organization thought ties to the drug industry were really a problem anymore. "The APA has a management of conflict process for all [educational] activities," read the manual. "This process ensures that all conflicts of interest are identified, managed, and resolved prior to the educational activity." Even so, disclosure before the lecture remained important because an audience that knew "which relevant financial relationships . . . were present and resolved" could assess "the potential for bias" that might have somehow slipped past the conflict managers.

The disclosures weren't the only way in which the proceedings had been sanitized for our protection. There wasn't a Prozac pen or a Depakote dealy-bob or any other Pharma swag to be seen in the lobbies or lecture rooms, sponsored lectures were not listed in the main program, and overall industry funding of the meeting was less than $2 million, down from its high in 2006 of more than $6 million. The drug companies had been relegated to the basement exhibition hall, where they competed for the busy psychiatrist's attention with the mental hospitals and the booksellers and the job recruiters and the shiny-faced men and women hawking neurofeedback gadgets and even a "physical fitness" kiosk where doctors could sharpen their Wii golf skills.

The APA's attempt to clean up its act had not persuaded its enemies to stand down. The Citizens Commission on Human Rights, the Scientology cadre devoted to tormenting the APA, maintained a steady presence on the curb outside the conference center, handing out flyers that touted an exhibition—*Psychiatry: An Industry of Death*—it was staging elsewhere in Honolulu. On the flyer's other side was a rogue's gallery, complete with photos of Alan Schatzberg, Nada Stotland, Dilip Jeste, David Kupfer, and other industry collaborators. The Honolulu police, when they weren't enforcing the jaywalking laws, made sure the protesters did not harass the guests.

The opposition wasn't all behind the barricades. Psychiatrists outside the ten or so sessions related to the DSM could be heard grumbling about rearranged deck chairs, and anyone who stumbled into the "Clinicians' Impressions of the DSM-5 Personality Disorders" symposium would have heard psychologist Thomas Widiger excoriate the personality disorders work group for courting ridicule and chaos by proposing to wipe out in one stroke five of the DSM-IV's ten personality disorders and, as if that weren't bad enough, "invent[ing] out of thin air" a model of personality pathology that ignored decades of research and then, even more embarrassing, changing its mind repeatedly about how many facets made up a personality and what exactly they were and how they related to one another, before finally advancing a proposal that inspired a virtual mutiny among personality researchers, which in turn persuaded the task force to compel the work group to pull it from the website in favor of a notice to check back later. And, Widiger lamented, even if the particulars weren't yet worked out and even if this was the stupidest idea to come down the pike in a long time, maybe ever, still it was clear that nothing was going to stop this juggernaut, that when the new version was posted it would be just as bad as the old, thus proving, as Widiger put it, that "like with the Borg, resistance is futile."

But overall, the protest was nothing like the chaos that had engulfed the meetings in the early 1970s, when gay activists launched their fusillades against the homosexuality diagnosis, or at the end of the decade, when Robert Spitzer and psychoanalysts squared off over the DSM-III. Whatever dissent the DSM-5 might have been sowing scattered quickly in the tropical breezes, which, combined with the Waikiki surf and the palm trees and the dress code, made the open-air atrium feel more like the lobby at a Jimmy Buffet concert than the site of trenchant debates about the nature of human suffering.

If there was any sign of trouble in Margaritaville, it was in the reminders, repeated by Regier and Kupfer at every opportunity, that all was well. The two DSM leaders hadn't gone the full aloha, settling for open-necked Oxford shirts rather than floral prints on rayon, and they seemed at least a little relaxed. But their stump speeches, with their reminders of all that was wrong with the DSM-IV, their recital of the long effort to fix it, and their reassurances that the revision was "very much on target" for May 2013 had, like the APA's protestations that it was Pharma-free, more than a faint whiff of defensiveness, as if they felt some urgency to bolster the confidence of the rank and file. Among the loyal, only David Shaffer directly addressed the controversy, and then only fleetingly. "I do sense a reactionary element penetrating DSM-5," he said, "and I hope it goes away."

Allen Frances wasn't in Honolulu, but he hadn't gone away. In the past few months, his blogs had increasingly addressed the APA leadership directly, imploring them to change course. Privately, he was sending e-mails directly to the few people inside he thought might listen to him. But, at least to judge by his rising stridency and the frustration creeping into his tone, he was pretty sure they weren't listening.

Michael First, however, didn't have the luxury of being retired. "I still have to work with these guys," he said. "And I'll have to work with them after the DSM-5 comes out." So he was there, working to maintain what he described as "cordial" relations with Regier and Kupfer and others in the DSM leadership as he continued in his role on the WHO panel formulating the new ICD.

First isn't exactly a firebrand by temperament. Where Frances shoots from the hip and peppers his salvos with literary and historical references, First sticks to data and the narrowest possible understanding of whatever question is in front of him. Ask him about a diagnostic controversy, and he'll drill deeply into the research, the specifics of which he will recall nearly perfectly, or he'll go on about the fine points of establishing reliability, or he will talk about the clinical utility of the diagnosis. If the subject were baseball, he'd be talking about on-base percentage versus run production, while Frances would be wondering if the designated hitter rule violated the pastoral origins of the game and tracing the origins of the question back to Thucydides.

As much as he has devoted his career to all things DSM, First doesn't think the book has as much social impact as Frances thinks it does. "Allen and I have a big disagreement about these epidemics he always talks about," he told me. "I tend to think he greatly overstates the role of the DSM." Take ADHD, for example, he said. Frances is sure that simplifying the criteria led directly to the increase in diagnosis and prescription of stimulants to kids. "I completely disagree that what we did in DSM-IV was really responsible for the huge overdiagnosis and overuse of medication. There are all these social factors, and all kinds of reasons why people use diagnoses. The DSM is a very small component."

But whatever disagreements First had with either side, they weren't going to be rehearsed at the annual meeting, at least not in the scheduled sessions, which paid scant attention to the brewing controversies. There was a place, however, where conceptual issues were in play: at a Hilton on the other end of Waikiki, where the Association for the Advancement of Philosophy and Psychiatry was holding a confab, "The Future of Psychiatric Nosology," and where First could be found for the first two days of the meeting. The room's low ceiling and dingy carpet, its stale, stuffy atmosphere, the balky sound system that at random moments broadcast the signal of a local radio station—all contrasted starkly with the towering grandeur of the convention center. As you wound your way down the short, narrow staircase that connected the room to the elevator stop above, you couldn't help but think of the film *Being John Malkovich* and wonder if you had happened upon a real-life 8½th floor.

The thirty or forty people gathered seemed unfazed by their surroundings as they dug into questions such as "What Is It to Be Diagnosed?" and "What Would a Scientific and Valid DSM Look Like?" The group was not without its own rifts—one presenter fired back at his questioner, "If I could be permitted just one ad hominem response, do you treat Posttraumatic Stress Disorder or just cause it?"—but all the participants seemed at home with the apocalyptic tone Jim Phillips, the keynote speaker, conjured in the title of his talk: "Slouching Toward DSM-5." If the mood up the road at the convention center was breezily optimistic, at the Hilton it was angry, worried, even despairing—not least because of the way concerns about the meaning of diagnosis, its impact on identity, and the seeming impossibility of grafting psychological suffering onto the medical model of disease had been relegated to this dingy outpost, as if the APA didn't even understand the conceptual complexity, the profound and far-reaching implications of its own product. By the end of the conference, two psychiatrists in the group announced their intentions to leave the field, largely, they said, because they had come to realize that all other forms of resistance were indeed futile. Whatever future psychiatric nosology might have, it seems, they didn't want any part of it.

Amid all these sweeping critiques and meaty topics—"Metaethics and Mental Illness," for example, or "Epistemic and Nonepistemic Values in Psychiatry"—First stuck to small ball. He described how the APA originally justified undertaking the DSM-5 in order to keep in harmony with the World Health Organization's planned ICD-11, but then the ICD-11 had been delayed, and the U.S. put off implementing the ICD-10, which had come out in 1992 and was the original justification for the DSM-IV, which was therefore still using codes from the ICD-9, but the ICD-10 would finally go into effect in October 2013, which had become the new justification for the DSM-5, but since the DSM-IV had been keyed to the ICD-10, it was not really necessary to revise the manual, only to "crosswalk" the codes. "You might be scratching your head about this," he said. "You might go, 'Huh, I'm totally confused here.'"

He was right about that.

But, First continued, a problem much more important and easier to grasp could be seen in the unevenness of the APA's proposed changes. Take Intermittent Explosive Disorder, for example. "It's one of the few disorders for which there are no changes proposed," he said. "Is that because the criteria for IED are so sound that there is no need to change them?" (IED, which got its initials before the war in Iraq made them piquant, is pretty much what it sounds like—a propensity, mostly among children and adolescents, to become quickly and unpredictably enraged, and then quickly return to normal.) He pointed out that IED is one of those "socially constructed, I-don't-know-what-it-means" diagnoses, one that you would think any major revision would reconsider. But, he explained, no one on the work group seemed interested in IED (or, he added, in two other impulse-control disorders—kleptomania and pyromania). It wasn't anyone's pet project, so the criteria had been left unmolested.*

On the other hand, he continued, consider Specific Phobia, de-

---

*The work group did eventually turn its attention to IED, tweaking some of its criteria and changing the text in the final rewrite.

scribed in the DSM-IV as a "marked and persistent fear cued by . . . a specific object." There was apparently no shortage of experts interested in this one, with the predictable result. First flashed a PowerPoint slide on which he had highlighted the differences between the existing and the proposed criteria. The text was a jumble of cross-outs and under-lines. "Marked and persistent fear that is excessive or unreasonable, cued by the presence or anticipation of a specific object" had become "marked fear or anxiety about a specific object or situation." An en-tire criterion—that the patient recognize the fear as excessive or unreasonable—had been deleted in favor of a requirement that the clinician determine if it is out of proportion to the actual danger (but only after taking into consideration the "sociocultural context"). "Avoidance, anxious anticipation, or distress" had become "fear, anxi-ety, or avoidance."

An expert flaps his mouth in New York or Washington, and chaos breaks out in Peoria—an outcome made more vexing, First pointed out, by the fact that these changes seem to be made for the sake of change, to fix diagnoses that aren't broken. "Why did this happen?" he asked. The answer lies not in science, but in sociology, in what he called the *work group effect*. "If you get a group of people doing weekly conference calls for three years, you are going to get lots and lots of changes," he said. "We're dealing with human nature here. Why would someone clamor for a position where they spend five years of their lives doing a lot of work for nothing? The reward is to get your view of the world embedded in the DSM."

It's Monday, the third day of the annual meeting, and the AAPP confer-ence is over. First has settled into a seat to watch Kupfer and Regier demonstrate how they expect clinicians to use the DSM-5 to reach diag-noses, or at least how they will do it in the field trials. This will also be their first opportunity to show off their long-anticipated dimensional assessment methods and perhaps answer some of the questions about proposals such as the move to eliminate Asperger's.

The room is set up for a couple hundred people. About twenty-five have straggled in. If Regier is disappointed by the turnout, he's not saying. Neither is he waiting for latecomers, although he might privately be cursing the scheduler who put this workshop on at noon, the hour at which drug companies like to put on shows while psychiatrists enjoy their box lunches.

You can't blame him for wanting to get started. For nearly two years, he has been responding to worries about the unreadiness of the new criteria and the unwieldiness of the dimensional assessments with some version of the response he gave me in September 2010 when I repeated those charges: "That's why we are doing a field test," he said, and he added that the trials would begin soon.

A month after that conversation, on October 5, the APA sent out a press release. The field trials had started, it declared, and it described "two rigorous study designs." In one, to be conducted at eleven medical centers across North America, two different clinicians would use the new criteria and the dimensional measures to independently evaluate the same patient. To the extent that they agreed, the diagnoses would be seen as reliable. Videotapes of their work would be reviewed by a third clinician, this one considered an expert, to see if either or both of them had come up with a valid diagnosis. The participants would then rate the usefulness of the new procedures. In the second design, called the Routine Clinical Practice (RCP) trial, 3,900 mental health professionals in private offices would evaluate two patients, also using the new criteria and dimensions. They would repeat the procedure with the same patients a couple of weeks or so later, and the results would be compared. The information generated from the two studies would be fed back to the work groups, who would tweak the criteria accordingly and return them to the field trialists for a second round of testing. "Field trials will give us the information we need to ensure the diagnostic criteria are useful and accurate," Regier said.

The release didn't mention that the field trials were already five months late. But that's not all it left out. It also failed to say what Regier had to admit when I asked him directly the next day: that they really hadn't begun at all. What had started was only a pilot study designed to shake the bugs out of the protocols for the medical center trials. This research had to be finished, its data analyzed, the methodology modified according to the findings, and the clinicians trained before the field trial itself could begin in earnest. He couldn't say when this would happen or, for that matter, when the 3,900 practitioners—a number that would soon go up without explanation to 5,000—in the routine practice study would get their marching orders.

In that October conversation, Regier also told me he didn't understand what all the fuss was about. "I'm surprised that the . . . statement would be considered news. Perhaps we should have a daily tweet." It was as if he didn't know that it was his people who had called it a "news release" or that just the previous day, they had quoted him calling the field trials a "critical phase" in an "important process."

The field trials did eventually get under way. Or at least the academic center studies did, with the first opening for business just before Christmas 2010, and the last coming on line in March 2011—nearly a full year past their scheduled start. But even as we convened in Hawaii, the RCP trial had yet to start, and no one was saying when it would. Allen Frances had made the predictable hay of the slipping schedule, adding it to the litany of what he called disarray and disorganization, his tone—"Missed Deadlines Have Troubling Consequences," in case that wasn't obvious—becoming increasingly high-handed. In the meantime, it was safe to say that the field trials had not yet won over a single heart or mind.

So no wonder Regier is eager to strut the APA's stuff. I'm sure he'd like us to go back and talk them up to our colleagues, maybe even tweet the virtues of the new criteria and the dimensional measures. I am also eager, as I have signed up to be one of the RCP trialists, and this session will be my first chance to see what I've gotten myself into.

"Of particular value to us is feedback from clinicians about how useful these [assessments] would be in your practices," Regier is saying. And the feedback starts right now, he tells us, thanks to the electronic keypads, about the size of a television remote control, on the tables in front of us. "Let's try these out with a question, and you'll see how they work when an entire audience uses them."

The entire audience, which by now has swelled to at least thirty-five, grab their clickers. The question comes into view on the PowerPoint screen.

Which of the following productions was not filmed in Hawaii?

A. *Hawaii Five-O*
B. *Baywatch*
C. *Jurassic Park*
D. *Indiana Jones and the Raiders of the Lost Ark*

"There's supposed to be music," Regier says, and looks at the tech guy, who flips a switch. A steel drum song breaks out on the speakers. Which seems a little more "Hey, mon," than "Aloha," but Regier doesn't seem to mind.

We cast our ballots, and as soon as the calypso stops, percentages for each answer pop up on the screen. *Baywatch* leads the way. "Fifty percent of you know your TV series," Regier says.

Regier explains what is about to happen. Emily Kuhl, an APA staffer, and William Narrow, the psychiatrist in charge of research for DSM-5, will be reenacting a session that occurred some weeks ago. Kuhl will "channel" the patient, Regier explains, while Narrow conducts his "regular clinical interview."

Narrow begins by telling us that the patient's name is Virginia Hamm. The lame joke falls flat in the empty room. Bearded and balding, Narrow is laconic, even shy, and not a natural showman; he looks like he'd rather be almost anywhere else than on this, or any, stage. Virginia, he continues, had come to the clinic and been assigned to a computer. She'd typed in her demographics and described her chief complaint as Obsessive-Compulsive Disorder and depression. She had filled out the Cross-Cutting Measures, Levels 1 and 2—the dimensional measures designed to assess symptoms that are not necessarily part of the diagnosis. She had indicated how regularly she felt "irritated, grouchy, or angry" or "nervous, anxious, frightened, worried, or on edge," how often she heard voices or thought of hurting herself, whether she sniffed glue or drank alcohol, or if she had ever found herself "not knowing who you really are or what you want out of life." She'd clicked through the items on the Altman Self-Rating Mania Scale and the Patient Health Questionnaire—Somatic Symptom Short Form, and the PROMIS (Patient Reported Outcomes Measurement Information System) scales for anxiety and depression. She had confided in the computer about her "getting along with people and participation in society," about her "communicating/understanding," her "getting around and self-care and life activities." After about a half hour of pointing and clicking, she had pushed the last button, sending the information to another computer, this one at Vanderbilt University, home of the REDCap (Research Electronic Data Capture) system, which had tabulated the answers and generated a report, returning it at the speed of light to her clinician. We are holding a printout of the results in our hands, a thick sheaf of papers telling us what is wrong with Virginia Hamm, if not how to cure her.

Narrow is going through the results out loud. "Two point nine on the depression measure, anxiety score is in the moderate range, somatic symptoms score is zero, suicidality is one," he reads from the laptop sitting on the table between him and the fake Virginia. "No problems with cognition or memory. Emotionality · tagonism is above average, disinhibition is belo below average."

Narrow seems a little tentative about what to

mation. He tells us that it isn't exactly diagnostic, because it doesn't correspond to DSM categories, and it isn't exactly a screening device; it is only supposed to help direct the clinician's attention to certain DSM categories. But he is short on the details. It might be that his regular clinical interview, like mine and that of most of the therapists I know, doesn't usually involve a laptop and a fake patient and an audience and a computer printout. Still, he seems more uncertain about what to do next than you'd expect from the guy who is in charge of the research.

He seems particularly unsure about how long this is going to take. "If I start running out of time," he says, "we'll just need to cut this short, but I will try and do as much as I can of the high points of the interview." He looks at a cluster of four or five women in the front row, APA apparatchiks apparently. They seem to know something, and if it had to do with the possibility that a ninety-minute session is not sufficient to demonstrate the clinical trial, I realize that I might have made a mistake—not by coming here instead of going to lunch, but by signing up to do four of these interviews and thus committing six or more non-billable hours to the DSM-5 cause. I wonder what is going to happen when my 4,999 fellow trialists, most of whom, or so I imagine, are busier and charge more money than I, do this math.

"Okay, Miss Hamm," Narrow says. "I'm glad you've consented to do this study for us. It's a very important study and will help us to develop a new DSM." He asks what has brought her to the clinic, and she tells him what she has already told the computer about her OCD and depression. "Why don't we start with the OCD?" he asks. She tells him about how she couldn't throw anything away, especially not newspapers, how year and years of them have at times accumulated in her apartment.

"re most of the rooms filled with things?

"

"Fi lled?"

She s him that she left paths between the piles, but even so, one day her brothers showed up at her apartment and tossed her stash into a dumpster they had rented.

He wants to know what that was like "emotionally."

"I was shocked," she replies. "It's stressful, you know, watching them take my stuff out. But we decided it's better to throw away two good things than to leave ninety-eight things that aren't so good." And indeed, she added, while the brothers had to repeat the purge a number of times, she had gotten used to it.

"So you had to go through some real thought to part with these things?" Narrow asks.

Virginia doesn't respond.

Narrow tries more questions about her OCD, but Virginia, at least the way Kuhl is playing her, keeps her cards close to her vest. She is not terribly insightful, or interesting, or engaging.

"So let's talk about the depression now," Narrow says.

It started in college, Virginia tells him, when she was "finding out that I'm gay" and worrying about what her parents would think, but it wasn't terrible, and she was never suicidal, and she was on meds now, and, especially since two of her brothers had come out in the meantime, her depression was really not much of a problem.

Narrow's regular clinical interview doesn't seem to include taking a swing at any of these hanging curveballs. Instead he delivers a volley of questions about whether she has ever been manic or terrified of germs, or had "worries that go around and around in your mind" (no, no, and no). He inquires into her smoking habits (a pack a day), her drug use (LSD once or twice a year, and marijuana if someone offers it to her), and her drinking (none).

"So what kind of person do you think you are?" he asks. "S' Withdrawn?"

"Well, I'm not outgoing," Virginia says.

Nearly a half hour has gone by since we met

Somewhere paint has dried and grass has grown, and I'm beginning to think that back at APA HQ, where Virginia is Emily and Dr. Narrow is Bill, there is some trouble between them. Because she is not helping him at all. Her monosyllabic answers are draining his monotone questions of whatever vitality they might have had. She might be illustrating a clinical point with her reticence, but Narrow's interrogation isn't exploring it. Nor is it clear what use he's making of the Cross-Cutting Measures or the PROMIS or anything else from the heap of REDCap data, or just how these vaunted dimensional measures are supposed to work. Neither does he seem intent on establishing trust by turning the bits of information he is extracting into the first tendrils of intimacy or, for that matter, on achieving any other therapeutic goal. In fact, for the life of me, I can't figure out what he is up to.

But then again, I'm not a psychiatrist, let alone a psychiatrist at the top of my profession's food chain, and it is the nature of the mental health professions that they are practiced in their own little silos, which means that even after nearly thirty years in the business, I might still not know how a regular clinical interview is supposed to go.

My BlackBerry buzzes. It's a message from Michael First, who has the row behind me all to himself, and who *is* a psychiatrist at the top of his profession. "I'm not sure what the point of this exercise is," it says. I am reassured, if no less mystified.

As if he has read our thoughts (or heard the BlackBerry and realized he's losing his audience), Narrow suddenly stops the Q&A. "I think I'm going to go onto the computer now," he says. "I'll be quick." He turns toward it and taps away. It's not clear whether he's reassuring us or the patient or the women in the front row.

We are looking at a giant version of his monitor on an overhead screen. To the left is a list of clickable diagnostic classifications. He tells us he is going to open the module for Hoarding Disorder—"the most ˒ramatic example that we have," he says, although this was surely damˑ ˒n with faint praise. (It also happens to be a diagnosis proposed for

DSM-5; they've smuggled in an advertisement for one of their new products.) We're looking at questions keyed to the proposed diagnostic criteria for Hoarding Disorder. Narrow clicks on the items that, based on the interview so far, he thinks Virginia meets. The computer asks him if he wants to enter a diagnosis of Hoarding Disorder. He clicks yes and then clicks another box. The page disappears before I can read it.

There is a sudden commotion from the front row; the women are waving their hands and stage-whispering to Narrow. I'm thinking that maybe they're going to remind him that he has left out something important, something that will allow us to see what innovation this rigmarole brings to diagnostics or, for that matter, how it does anything other than provide a near-perfect, if unintended, example of the circles in which psychiatric nosology runs, the way he got to the diagnosis through the symptoms and the symptoms through the diagnosis, how Hoarding Disorder is another line carved in sand, a diagnosis that will no doubt be the object of scorn for the leaders of DSM-6 or DSM-7, fodder for their paradigm-busting cannons, an opportunity for them to justify the new book by decrying the old one's reifications. Perhaps, I think, they're going to stand up and say, "But Bill, you didn't even pretend to be in doubt for a moment about the outcome—which, after all, let's face it, you knew all along, since you watched the videotape of the real Virginia—so you couldn't demonstrate how to get to the diagnosis or what it has to do with emotionality or schizotypy or antagonism or with the PHQ and the ASRM or anything we've seen other than the story about the brothers and the dumpster and the piles of papers, which didn't require a computer to figure out, which indeed may have come to you despite the computer," and then add, sotto voce, how it might not be such a good idea to put all this unreadiness and ineffectiveness on such naked display, not even here in front of this crowd whose sparseness must seem to him, and to Kupfer and Regier, like a blessing.

But it's none of that. "You didn't save it!" one of them exclaims.

Narrow has missed a click and lost all the data he's spent the last twenty minutes entering.

Flop sweat breaks out on his brow. "I'm sorry," he says. "This is only the second time I've done this." He sounds more sheepish than petulant, like a batter returning to the dugout after whiffing in the clutch, explaining to his teammates that he'd faced this pitcher only twice before.

"Should I cut this short?" Narrow asks the women. He's also looking across the stage, where Kupfer has replaced Regier. It's pretty clear Narrow has had enough; he's begging for the hook. But none is offered, so he takes matters into his own hands announcing that he will skip over the modules for other diagnoses and will now turn to the severity measures.

These turn out to be quite simple and, unlike the other ratings, clear in their application, if not terribly revealing. He goes through the criteria proposed for Hoarding Disorder and asks Virginia to rate their intensity and the distress they cause her on a scale of one to five. Then, "because we don't want total dependence on all these forms," he gives his own rating, as we field trial clinicians will be expected to do. "I don't have a lot of experience with this disorder"—and how could he, since it doesn't yet exist, at least not officially?—"but I would say it's moderate. It could be a lot worse. I mean, there's no dead animals in there."

Narrow looks back at the front row. "Anything else?"

"Save it," someone replies.

He's clicking through that procedure when Kupfer takes the lectern. There's little mercy in his move. He doesn't even thank Narrow (or Kuhl) for his efforts. Instead, he tells us to pick up our clickers. "Given the fact that we've spent a reasonable amount of time on the interview," he begins (and I don't hear any irony in his voice), we ought to be able to come up with a diagnosis. A list of choices flashes on the board. The steel drums play. The percentages are revealed. Sixty-seven percent of us have voted for Hoarding Disorder.

It is a regular landslide, unless you are in, say, Turkmenistan. Which, evidently, Kupfer wishes we were. He wants to know why a full third of the room—about a dozen of us—have not voted for the party-endorsed candidate. (I'm wondering the same thing. Assuming the five APA functionaries—15 percent of the electorate—voted the right way, only half of the rest of us voted for Hoarding Disorder, and I had cast votes for Hoarding Disorder on the four clickers I could easily reach.) He thinks the next question might help to provide an answer. How useful were the new criteria in reaching our conclusion? When 65 percent of us answer either *moderately* or *extremely*, he observes that this is pretty much the same percentage of the crowd who voted for Hoarding Disorder, as if this somehow strengthened the credibility of the criteria, as if it did more than indicate how circular diagnostic logic is. Of course they were useful in making the diagnosis; there was no other way to reach it and, *pace* that dissenting 33 or 35 percent, no other diagnosis to reach. (I'm feeling a little guilty about that two-point discrepancy; I cast a vote for *moderately* on one less clicker than in the first poll.)

When 31 percent of voters say they think Virginia had Mixed Anxiety-Depression—a proposed diagnosis that has so little to do with Virginia that I figure it was thrown in just to fill out the multiple choices—I begin to wonder if someone is intentionally committing mayhem. Ten people who want to embarrass Kupfer? A terrorist cell sent in by the proponents of MAD to blow up HD? Acting out by the terminally bored?

Kupfer must be wondering, too, because he invites people to come forward and explain their votes. No one does. He moves on. He asks how useful we found the Cross-Cutting Measures and whether the forms were too long (50 percent) or too short (4 percent; he's lost even the front row). When 53 percent say that the DSM-IV criteria are superior (a meaningless question because the DSM-IV doesn't list Hoarding Disorder), Kupfer is quick to call the result a "nice split." When 30 percent say the new approach is superior to DSM-IV's, and 20 percent say it's equivalent, he points out that this means half of us thought it was the same or better. But this turd cannot be easily polished, and when Narrow ends the presentation by saying, "Of those who said this is worse or much worse, we'd like to hear why," it is hard to imagine that he means it or that either man ever wants to hear about field trials again.

When the session is turned over to the audience for questions, Michael First stands up. He waits in line at the audience mic while a man takes Narrow to task for not asking more about Virginia's substance abuse. "I hope you weren't rating my interview, as opposed to the general approach," Narrow responds.

First doesn't attack Narrow for being unprepared or criticize his technique or ask him just exactly what the point of that exercise was. Instead, he says that as he watched the demonstration, he was wondering how he would have asked the questions and how every other clinician would have asked them; and, realizing that there are as many regular clinical interviews as there are clinicians, he was also wondering how Narrow, in his role as the head of research for DSM-5, was going to deal with that. How will he know, in the likely event of diagnostic discrepancies among clinicians, that they are the result of the criteria rather than the way each clinician asks the questions? How, in other words, will the field trials do the job they are supposed to do—evaluate the reliability of the new DSM?

"Well, that's a very complex question," Narrow replies, and proceeds not to answer it, except to say that they had tried to figure it out in a pilot study and it hadn't worked out.

But First asks the question again. Narrow acknowledges that not only are they not requiring a structured interview, they are not even training the study clinicians on the new diagnoses or "telling them how they should be interpreting these measures." They are simply asking them to familiarize themselves with the website. But, he assures us, this is not a weakness in the design but a strength: the field trials will mirror how clinicians practice in the real world and thus yield more realistic results than the DSM-III and DSM-IV field trials did. Those old numbers, the ones that did so much to restore psychiatry's respectability, Narrow is saying, were overstated, inflated by the pristine conditions under which they were conducted. But now that the APA has cleverly dirtied up the trials, Narrow tells us, he can almost guarantee that reliability will be worse than it was in earlier DSMs.

I have underestimated First. He has managed to unearth the point of the exercise after all: to prepare us all for the lousy outcomes the field trials were evidently designed to yield. As we file out of the room, I ask him what it's like to be a bystander to the proceedings. "Oh, it's absolutely excruciating," he answers, as if that were obvious. Which, come to think of it, it is.

Narrow was correct about at least one thing. As Helena Kraemer, the chief statistician on the DSM-5 task force, told a much larger crowd the next day, "People's expectations of what reliability should be have been grossly inflated." She left no question about who was responsible for this: Bob Spitzer.

Spitzer knew it was not enough to ask two doctors to diagnose a patient, compare their answers, and use the results to pronounce judgment on whether the diagnosis was reliable. That approach wouldn't account for the possibility that the clinicians agreed by chance—by, say, flipping a coin or tossing a dart or just plain guessing—rather than because the diagnostic criteria were well written. Fortunately for Spitzer, in 1960 a statistician named Jacob Cohen had invented a method for calculating the extent to which agreement between two people using the same rating scale is the result of factors other than chance. The statistic had come to be known as *Cohen's kappa*, and Spitzer, working with Cohen, had adapted it for use in evaluating the reliability of diagnoses.

Spitzer and Cohen introduced kappa to psychiatrists in 1967, promoting it as a way out of the reliability mess. At first, they used it primarily to quantify just how bad things were, and this agenda shaped the way they addressed a problem built into the statistic. A kappa of 0 indicates that any agreement is by chance alone; a kappa of 1 indicates that researchers have come to the same conclusion for nonrandom reasons (presumably because the criteria work). But what do the numbers in between mean? How much agreement is sufficient to call a diagnosis reliable (or not)? After all, even a low kappa means that clinicians outperformed coin tossers or monkeys at typewriters.

This has turned out to be a hotly contested question, or at least as hot as anything in statistics gets. In 1974, Spitzer proposed an answer. Kappas of around .40, he said, indicated "poor" agreement, .55 was "no better than fair," .70 was "only satisfactory," and more than .80 would be "uniformly high." But as California professors Stuart Kirk and Herb Kutchins noted, Spitzer "could have employed *very good*, *good*, *not so good*, and *bad*," and they pointed out that there was a reason he didn't. Spitzer's 1974 paper was an attempt to put numbers to the widely noted poor reliability of DSM-II diagnoses, "belittling the reliability of the past," as Kirk and Kutchins put it, in order to set the stage for the transition to a criterion-based future.

Having established kappa as the arbiter of reliability and having promised success for his new diagnostic approach, Spitzer then had to show that descriptive diagnosis would achieve high kappas. And the DSM-III field trials did exactly that, in no small part because the patients were preselected for the likelihood that they would qualify for the diagnosis and the researchers were drilled on the criteria—and on a clinical interview that left little to chance or imagination. Now that his ox was in danger of being gored, Spitzer had also come up with some new ways to evaluate kappa—no longer was .70 "only satisfactory"; now it was a "high kappa [that] indicates good agreement." And by this standard, the DSM-III field trials were a success, far outpacing results using the earlier manuals and, in many cases, well exceeding the .70 threshold.

If psychiatrists noticed that the fix had been in from the start, they didn't say so—most likely because the numbers gave the profession exactly what it had been looking for. But just as Spitzer once denigrated the past to clear the way for the DSM-III, Kraemer was now claiming that Spitzer's results were patently ridiculous. "I think it will be a miracle if we get a kappa of .80," she said. "In fact, if someone comes to me and tells me we've got one, I'm going to tell her to go back and make sure there hasn't been some kind of screwup."

Kraemer didn't seem worried about the implications of repudiating the very same statistics that the APA had been using for thirty years to stake its claim to scientific respectability or, for that matter, of calling Bob Spitzer a screwup. But she was telling us what numbers we could expect and what they would mean—and she was singing a much different tune from Spitzer's.

Most of the kappas, Kraemer predicted, would come in somewhere between .40 and .60—the same reliability Spitzer characterized as "no better than fair." But doctors in other fields were satisfied with reliability like this, she said. There didn't seem to be any of those doctors around to object to this—say, an endocrinologist who could testify as to whether it would truly be a miracle if he and a random colleague agreed most of the time on whether a patient with high blood sugar had diabetes—but Kraemer seemed to anticipate the danger, and she tacked. "Until you can do X-rays, until you can do scans, until you can do tissue samples," she said, psychiatric diagnoses could only "aspire to be as good as medical diagnosis." In the meantime, she added, even if the kappa was only between .20 and .40—numbers that Spitzer didn't even deign to characterize—"it will be acceptable."

First was back at the audience microphone. I knew better than to think he would ask exactly how (and to whom) these numbers were acceptable or whether lowering expectations was really such a good idea, given how central reliability had been to reestablishing psychiatry's credibility, or how the APA was going to convince the public that sharply reduced reliability was actually an improvement over the earlier product.

Still, his question, a version of the one he had asked Narrow, was plenty barbed. Let's say you end up with a kappa of .10 on the field trial, he said—a result that wouldn't clear even Kraemer's very low bar. "Presumably they are going to use this information to make the DSM-5 better before it is released." But, he continued, given the impossibility of sorting out the way clinicians used the criteria from the criteria themselves, "how can people find out where the problem is, and how do you know how to fix it? How will they even know where to look?"

"This is why I use the analogy of field testing and airplanes," Kraemer replied. "The airplane crashes, the question is why did it crash and what are you going to do about it? There's a lot of information they"—I think she meant the APA, not the National Transportation Safety Board—"can look at, but it's not a matter of analyzing the data to find out exactly what's wrong." Kraemer seemed to be saying that the point wasn't to sift through the wreckage and try to prevent another catastrophe but, evidently, to crash the plane and then announce that the destruction could have been a lot worse.

To be honest, however, I wasn't sure. She was not making all that much sense, or maybe I just didn't grasp the complexities of statistical modeling. And besides, I was distracted by a memory of something Steve Hyman once wrote. Fixing the DSM, finding another paradigm, getting away from its reifications—this, he said, was like "repairing a plane while it is flying." It was a suggestive analogy, I thought at the time, one that recognized the near impossibility of the task even as it indicated its high stakes—and the necessity of keeping the mechanics from swearing and banging too loudly, lest the passengers start asking for a quick landing and a voucher on another airline. But whatever Hyman meant, I was now pretty certain that he wasn't thinking that the solution was to fly the plane into the ground on purpose, to put the wounded craft out of its misery before it plummeted to earth of its own accord.

First yielded the mic and went back to the end of the line for another round. The next questioner wanted to know why dimensional assessments (an earlier topic of the panel) hadn't been in DSM-IV. "Actually, you can turn around and ask Michael," Kraemer said.

"The answer is that there *are* dimensional measures," First said. He named them: the severity scales for various disorders, the one-hundred-point scale to rate overall functioning, and a numerical scale to rate the psychosocial stressors a patient was facing. "But the reception among clinicians has been a resounding 'We're not interested.'"

His answer was game, and accurate, but it didn't really matter. He had lost the match. As Kraemer had just made all too clear, she was up there with Regier and Kupfer and he was down on the floor, just another guy in line—and one who, she had just implied, was responsible for the mess they had spent the last ten years trying to clean up.

"We'd better get smart about measuring what we do and proving its value," psychiatrist Lawson Wulsin told another audience at the annual meeting, "or we are going to lose." Wulsin was the liaison between the DSM-5 task force and other medical specialties, so even if the APA's plane-crash logic made any sense to him, he had to know that his non-psychiatrist colleagues weren't going to fall for this strategy, especially not if it hinged on claiming that, at least when it came to diagnosis, the rest of medicine was just as unreliable as psychiatry.

But it was too late to change course. Spitzer had chosen kappa as the pole star and used it to steer psychiatry off the shoals. He gave his profession numbers to cite as evidence that it was sailing in the same seas as the rest of medicine. So the proof of the DSM-5's success would also have to be in numbers. With the field trials only just under way, it remained to be seen if the leaders of the APA had really gotten smart about proving they could measure what they do and sell us on its value.

Chapter 15

Y ou have to understand," Allen Frances is telling me. "What Bob Spitzer was interested in, no one else was. I certainly wasn't. Because we were all discovering the meaning of life in every patient."

It's July 2011. I've known Frances for nearly a year, a year in which I've had no luck getting him to explain to me how a man comes to scorch the earth he once strode, how, for that matter, he came to walk it in the first place, how you get to be America's top psychiatrist without just a smidgen of ambition—and, while he's at it, to help me understand how he can simultaneously believe that DSM disorders are not real but that the book nonetheless deserves its authority, how he can both prize the truth and champion the noble lie, and how these contradictions can fit in one life. We've exchanged hundreds of e-mails and sent each other books in the real mail. We've spent four or five days together, the last two with his wife, Donna Manning, and his two teenage grandchildren. I've slept on his living room floor, watched *Gunsmoke* on his bedroom TV, eaten at his table, sat squeezed between the grandkids in the backseat of his convertible, buffeted by the wind on an excursion down to Big Sur. He's ribbed me mercilessly about, among other things, my "naiveté" in thinking that the unfolding debacle of the DSM-5 is about anything more than the rank incompetence of its architects, that in insisting that deep historical forces are at work, I am playing Abbott to the

APA's Costello. He has even given me the Herb Peyser treatment, leaning across the table and pinching my cheek (he spared me the kiss) when I tried to explain to him the dance between editor and writer that had landed his "bullshit" comment in the lead of my *Wired* story—a pinch affectionate and hostile in equal parts and, most of all, devastatingly effective in stopping my explanation cold, the sudden silence thick with rebuke.

For a year he has evaded the question. He's demurred on tactical grounds—"If it seems like this is coming from a personality quirk," he told me, "then the message will get lost." He's protested that he's "just no good at introspection," and when floating like a butterfly has failed him, he's stung me with the accusation that I care about all the wrong things, that these questions are worthy of *People* and not a serious book about the DSM. But as we wind through the California hills early on a July morning, top up, no grandkids, he poses my question perfectly: "You mean, how could a person be interested in the drama of human emotions and psychology and at the same time spend seven years of his life trying to be precise about things at the descriptive surface?" This gets him to reminiscing about the old days with Spitzer at Columbia, and I'm thinking that maybe this year of getting teased and scolded and lectured has all been a prolonged hazing, that I have passed some kind of test, that he is finally going to untangle some of these contradictions.

"The meaning of life," I repeat. "And what was that?"

"That I'm an even bigger schmuck than I think I am."

It's all a little hard to swallow, this brilliant, erudite, effortlessly dominating man insisting that he is stupid and feckless, and evading an account of his own motivation in the bargain. But then again, this is the man who put a disclaimer at the front of the DSM as a prophylaxis against people taking the book too seriously, who thinks that insisting mental disorders don't actually exist even as you enumerate them will somehow make people stop acting as if the disorders are real. He might really think that humility is enough to erase power, that what

Montesquieu really meant was that when aristocrats exercised modesty, it somehow stopped them from having more money than everyone else.

"The least important person on the field is the general," Frances is saying. "The battle is won by an individual soldier deciding to stand, and having his buddies follow him." He's wrested the conversation back to the subject he wants to talk about the most: the small but determined claque of DSM-5 resisters that has recently coalesced around him, attracted, it seems, to his irresistible combination of gravitas and dissent. The soldier in question is a Floridian named Dayle Jones. She's a counselor, a blogger for the American Counseling Association (ACA), and a member of the committee revising the ICD, and she has been assembling her own case against the DSM-5, trying to warn the 115,000 members of her organization that the new manual will be a disaster for them. "She could be, when all is said and done, the most influential person in all of DSM-5," Frances says. The APA may be free to ignore him, he explains, but Dayle Jones has been telling the ACA members that they can get the ICD at no cost, and the APA is surely "going to listen to 115,000 buyers."

The general might be unimportant (and reluctant), but that doesn't mean he isn't leading the battle. "I'm doing several things to help [Jones]," he told me, but "it's better that they're not seen as coming from me." He thinks the APA is more likely to listen to Jones and her organization, and to the other dissenters, if they are not seen as affiliated with him. Or with me, evidently. "She will be an important character in your book," he says. But I should steer clear for a while. "It won't look good if she's doing this from your press box. This should just be a concerned lady from Florida. I don't want anything to happen to queer what I'm trying to do."

For a guy who has no interest in power, he sure knows how to use it.

Still, when he says, "My narcissism couldn't survive the teenage insight that we are all insignificant and transient worms, that no one has much stuff to strut," it's impossible to dismiss that as just another facile gloss from Machiavelli or Sun Tzu. And even if he has copped to exaggerating the flaws in DSM-IV for rhetorical purposes, there doesn't seem to be anything tactical in his acknowledgment of the error that launched the mission we are on today, the one that has gotten Frances dressed in his Sunday best, and both of us up and out of the house by six. "This was one royal fuckup," he says, and he's on his way to try to set it straight.

Our destination is a meeting of lawyers. The royal fuckup was the kind that only they could love, an opportunity buried deep in the interstices of the DSM text, ready to be excavated and exploited—in this case by prosecutors who, aided by psychiatrists, can use it to keep certain sex offenders locked up well beyond the end of their sentences, indefinitely or maybe even forever.

That wasn't what Frances and the rest of the DSM-IV crew had in mind when they decided that meeting Criterion A for Pedophilia—"over a period of at least 6 months, recurrent, intense sexually arousing fantasies, sexual urges or behaviors involving sexual activity with a prepubescent child"—was not enough to diagnose a patient with a mental disorder. The offender also needed to meet Criterion B: "The fantasies, sexual urges, or behaviors cause clinically significant distress or impairment in social, occupational, or other important areas of functioning." This was only the boilerplate clinical significance criterion that had been added to many diagnoses in DSM-IV, and all Frances and First had intended by it, as they wrote in a 2008 *American Journal of Psychiatry* editorial, was to remind clinicians that, as they put it in the DSM-IV, "the symptom criteria alone are insufficient to define mental disorder."

But that's not how Linda Bowles, a contributor to the conservative Christian news site WorldNetDaily, took it. To her, it was just more evidence of the secular humanist conspiracy to further the gay agenda. "While we have been preoccupied with the dangers posed to our children by inanimate objects, namely guns," she wrote in the summer of

1999, "they were under a much more dangerous assault from animate objects, namely psychologists and psychiatrists." The blitz had begun with the deletion of homosexuality from the DSM, she continued, and had gotten worse with Criterion B, which she read to mean that "no matter how heinous the sexual perversion, if the pervert does not feel shame or remorse, he does not have a psychiatric problem."

Bowles's accusations rocketed around the right-wing blogosphere, picking up endorsements from the head of the National Association for Research and Therapy of Homosexuality, the medical wing of the pray-the-gay-away movement, and Charles Socarides, the psychiatrist who had led the opposition to the deletion in 1973, along with radio scold Laura Schlessinger. It also made its way to the APA, whose lawyers wrote to Bowles demanding that she "acknowledge the 'APA's clear opposition to pedophilia.'" The APA also issued a press release reiterating its stance that "an adult who engages in sexual activity with a child is performing a criminal and immoral act which never can be considered normal or socially acceptable behavior."

But as any scandal-scarred politician will tell you, vigorous defenses against charges of turpitude are mostly self-defeating. If you run an organization of helping professionals, you don't want to have to prove that your members aren't really human missiles intent on blasting us all into a secular humanist hell. To forestall the necessity of further defenses, Frances and First recalled in their editorial, they removed the clinical significance clause from the diagnosis when the DSM-IV-TR came out in 2000. In its place was the old DSM-III-R version of Criterion B, according to which if someone "has acted on these urges or is markedly distressed by them," he qualifies for the diagnosis.

This was the royal fuckup: the offender no longer had to be "impaired" to warrant the diagnosis. All he had to do was act. In the original DSM-IV version, the offender also had to have children as his primary sexual object. The attraction was the "impairment," the thing that made his behavior disordered rather than simply repellent or unusual. But in the DSM-IV-TR, this requirement was gone, and since, according to Criterion A, "fantasies, sexual urges, or behaviors" were symptoms of Pedophilia, all the offender had to do to warrant the diagnosis was to commit the offense. This meant that, starting in 2000, a person who had sex with a child was ipso facto mentally ill.

Now, that may seem obvious to you. But that's only because of how reflexively we attribute all our peccadilloes and quirks (or, more likely, those of other people) to mental rather than moral defect. The DSM, with its reach into daily life, has given us an ample vocabulary for expressing this intuition. But in fact, technically speaking anyway, this is not the case. Or at least it's not supposed to be. It is surely not what First and Frances believe.

"Fewer than half of child molesters have Pedophilia," First told me. "Often the child is a victim of convenience for an antisocial person." Without "an underlying pattern of arousal," as he put it, there is no mental disorder, at least not in the sex department; there is only criminality. That's what First and Frances meant the DSM-IV-TR to say, in any event—that having sex with a kid was always criminal, but not always a symptom of Pedophilia, or of any psychiatric diagnosis for that matter.

But to a lawyer, or at least to a prosecutor in a state with sexually violent predator (SVP) laws, which allow diagnosed sex offenders to be kept in "treatment units" even after they have served out their sentences, a diagnosis based on behavior alone is an opportunity to protect (and score political points with) a public disgusted and frightened by sex offenders. The DSM-IV-TR diagnosis had turned into a different kind of opportunity for mental health experts, spawning a cottage industry of doctors ready to testify that the offender has indeed offended, and that this behavior is the symptom of a mental illness. Their practice is not limited to pedophiles. Because Sexual Sadism, Exhibitionism, Voyeurism, and Frotteurism all have the same behavior-only criterion as Pedophilia, rapists, flashers, peepers, and humpers all can be put away until they are "cured"—which may well mean forever. (And if the behavior in question doesn't meet the criteria for one of those diagnoses, the forensic psychiatrist can always resort to Paraphilia NOS.)

"I don't care about the rapist being in jail," Frances said. "Most of them deserve to be there." But they also deserve to get out once they have paid the prescribed penalty. Some rapists—the sadists, for instance, who can't get aroused without inflicting pain on a nonconsenting person—might be suffering from a mental disorder that requires involuntary commitment, but indefinite incarceration based on behavior alone, in Frances's view, "is preventive detention and double jeopardy. It's a violation of due process. It's unconstitutional." (The Supreme Court disagrees. It has ruled that so long as the state can show that they are not punishing mere criminality but treating a mental defect ascertained by an expert, they can keep the offender locked up.) That's what he cares about, that and the fact that this "colossal swindle"—forensic experts teaming up with prosecutors to deprive people of their civil rights—was made possible by his DSM. "I hate the fact that we've made this mistake," he said. "We didn't understand the SVP laws. We blew it."

"I don't wallow in my own guilt," he added, "but I do like to clean up my own messes."

Which is why he testifies in civil commitment hearings, trying to explain that sexual behavior without that underlying pattern cannot be a symptom of a mental disorder, and that the convict might only be a criminal. And it is why we are on our way to this meeting, where he will reiterate that distinction to defense lawyers to help them figure out how to convince judges and juries that mental illness is one thing and evil quite another.

The mess he's trying to clean up was caused by two tiny words: *and* and *or*. Had Criterion A read "fantasies, urges, *and* behaviors," he points out, it would be much harder for those enterprising psychiatrists and prosecutors to detach behavior from psychology and condemn prisoners to endless detention. This was exactly the kind of unforeseen consequence of which the DSM-5 crew seemed heedless. "If an *or* for an *and* could create mayhem," he says, "what unintended harm could be wrought by the paradigm shifters?"

The paradigm shifters had long ago stopped responding to Frances. But he was no longer their only nemesis.

His fellow critics included at least one person who was as surprised as anyone to find herself on the same side as Frances. Paula Caplan, a psychologist affiliated with Harvard, had been a consultant to the DSM-IV personality disorders work group, a position from which she had tormented Frances as relentlessly as Frances was now tormenting Regier. Her main complaint back then was about Self-Defeating Personality Disorder. While Frances thought it was poorly conceived and had little empirical support, Caplan thought it was just plain sexist. Frances thought Caplan's critique was "too polemical" and warned her that since the proposal was sure to be rejected, there was no need for "heated controversy."

Frances's dismissal seemed only to inflame Caplan, who submitted her own DSM-IV diagnosis: Delusional Dominating Personality Disorder (DDPD). Among the fourteen proposed criteria were "a tendency to feel inordinately threatened by women who fail to disguise their intelligence" and "the presence of . . . delusions that women like to suffer." DDPD was, she wrote, "most commonly seen in males," often in "leaders of traditional mental health professions, military personnel, executives of large corporations, and powerful political leaders of many aims." It was a "modest proposal," she wrote, "an antidote to . . . the institutionalized sexism in the mental health system."

"I really wasn't sure what to make [of] your 'delusional dominating personality disorder,'" Frances responded. "How serious are you about it?" Much as he thought the proposal was a provocation, the reason he gave for rejecting it out of hand was the standard DSM-IV demurral:

that there wasn't enough evidence for DDPD even to be considered. But when Caplan asked for funds to develop that evidence, Frances refused. "It is disruptive to constantly tinker with the classification," he wrote, adding, in case she didn't get the hint, "if this sounds discouraging, I'm afraid it is meant to."

After Caplan quit the work group, she wrote *They Say You're Crazy: How the World's Most Powerful Psychiatrists Decide Who's Normal*, a broadside against DSM-IV, in which she cast the affair as an instance of the good-old-boy politics that powered the DSM. So even if Caplan did give Frances a shout-out for "bravely com[ing] forward with a mea culpa," it was very unlikely that she was in cahoots with him when she came up with a modest proposal for the DSM-5: Toxic Psychiatric Drug Syndrome. In her letter to the task force, she also made some recommendations: that the APA "join an initiative to hold Congressional hearings about psychiatric diagnoses," that it add a black-box warning to the actual DSM-5 emphasizing that the diagnoses were not to be used as "the basis for any professional or legal decision that may limit the liberty, or discriminate against, any individual," and that, "because of . . . ongoing significant problems in the process," publication be indefinitely delayed.

The APA swatted away Caplan as summarily as Frances had, although without his personal touch. They used a public relations firm, which arranged a conference call between representatives of "consumer groups"—Caplan was positioning herself as a champion of people given unwarranted diagnoses and prescriptions—and the DSM leaders. Caplan heard that there would be twenty others on the hour-long call, so she tried to coordinate with the others on the questions that would be asked, but the hired guns refused to disclose the participants or forward a list of proposed questions to them. On the appointed day, according to Caplan, after Carol Bernstein assured the callers that the APA needed "the expertise of patients, families, and their advocates," Kupfer and Regier, along with a task force member, used the first half of the call to give their talking points. Participants who wished to ask questions were then instructed to dial a code, and after a silence during which a queue was constructed, six were allowed to ask a single question each; their phones were muted as soon as they delivered it. The APA representatives stuck to their script and, after promising (but refusing to schedule) further discussion, said good-bye.

The new bosses were no different from the old bosses, Caplan concluded. They might give the "impression of openness to debate," she wrote in her *Psychology Today* blog, but in real life, critics like her would be "largely ignored," their evidence "shoved aside," and the world's latest most powerful psychiatrists would once again "put in the next edition of the manual whatever they pleased."

If Caplan was railing against the psychiatrists' process, the British Psychological Society was going right for the content of what displeased them. In a twenty-six-page manifesto released in June, the BPS accused the APA of "the continued and continuous medicalisation of . . . natural and normal responses." These responses, the BPS went on, "undoubtedly have distressing consequences which demand helping responses, but which do not reflect illnesses so much as normal individual variation." Attenuated Psychosis Symptoms Syndrome (APSS), for instance, "looks like an opportunity to stigmatize eccentric people, and to lower the threshold for achieving a diagnosis of psychosis," leading in turn to more drug treatments. The overall thrust of the manual, the BPS complained, was to identify the source of psychological suffering "as located within individuals," rather than in their "relational context," and to overlook the "undeniable social causation of many such problems."

The APA could hardly deny any of this. As Regier had told the consumer groups on the conference call, the manual's new organizational structure was designed to reflect "what we've learned about the brain, behavior, and genetics during the past two decades." It doesn't get much more "within the individual" and outside the "relational context" than that. And, as proposals like APSS and the elimination of the bereavement exclusion made clear, one of the purposes of the DSM-5 was to make sure that no one who was suffering would be deprived of the benefits of diagnosis.

On the other hand, the APA couldn't ignore the British Psychological Society or treat it as a mere "consumer group." But that didn't mean they would acknowledge the actual criticisms, as Regier made clear in his official response. The BPS had cited a "well known member of the 'Critical Psychiatry Network,'" he wrote, one "that has largely adopted the Thomas Szasz approach to mental illness." These critics, Regier reminded his readers, think "we shouldn't consider any mental disorder, including individuals whose psychosis renders them mentally incompetent, to have a brain-based illness." Antipsychiatry was once again deluding people into thinking that the APA was making grievous errors.

Compounding the BPS's ideological excess, Regier went on, was plain ignorance.

What seems to be missing is an appreciation of mental disorders as the result of gene-environmental interactions that would trigger abnormal neuronal function in the brain. Why the brain should be exempt from pathology when every other organ system is subject to malfunction is left unaddressed.

To question the APA's insistence that psychological suffering was always the result of brain pathology was to deny that the brain could malfunction at all.

"It should be recognized that mental disorders are by no means a modern construct," Regier wrote. "Psychiatric disorders have existed since the beginning of recorded history."

Regier didn't offer any evidence for this extravagant claim, nor did he try to square it with his insistence in other venues that psychiatric disorders were constructs that clinicians reified at their own peril. But then again, he probably thought he was saying something nonextravagant (and self-evident): that mental suffering has always existed, and that throughout recorded history it has only been awaiting psychiatrists like him to elucidate the gene-environmental interactions that triggered the brain pathology that causes it. But to think there could be psychiatric disorders before there were psychiatrists, to think the only way to understand our suffering is as an illness to be cured by doctors, is to ignore the fact that for thousands of years of recorded history, people thought that mania and psychosis and depression and anxiety were the mark of the prophet, or manifestations of sin or witchcraft or devil possession, or just the nature of life in a fallen world. It is also to overlook the failure of psychiatry, at least so far, to prove that it is the proper venue for understanding and treating what we have come to think of as mental illness. And to think, after all the failures of the DSM to develop an accurate taxonomy, that this time it will be different, that only naysayers and dead-enders and other benighted miscreants could possibly believe that recasting sin or possession or witchcraft as illness is anything other than the mark of progress—well, that is the province of people who, as Herman Melville once wrote, despite "previous failures, still cherish expectations with regard to some mode of infallibly discovering the heart of man."

These people, Melville observed, are like the mathematicians who "in spite of seeming discouragement . . . are yet in hopes of hitting upon an exact method of determining the longitude." But other scientists maintain this optimism, including, Melville wrote, "earnest psychologists." He probably didn't mean to slight psychiatrists. It's just that he wrote the novel in 1857, which is long after the beginning of recorded history, but only a few years past psychiatry's emergence as a profession, and long before it began to try, despite seeming discouragement, to enshrine its infallible understanding of mental suffering in the pages of a book.

———

Melville's observation comes in his last novel, *The Confidence-Man*. In it, a colossal swindler embarks on a riverboat on an April Fool's Day and proceeds to take advantage of the passengers' credulity and greed. It's a novel about trust—the reader's as well as the passengers'—which Melville advises his readers to place not in psychologists, no matter how earnest, but in novelists, who, he says, can give us the same knowledge of the twists of our nature that a "stranger entering, map in hand, Boston town" has of the city's crooked streets. But Melville, ever the ironist, won't let us forget that we place confidence in the novelist at our own peril. He is anything but earnest; whatever truth he depicts emerges from the elaborate lie of a fictive world. Even his publisher was in on the joke: *The Confidence-Man* hit the streets on April 1.

The APA has books to sell, too. But it doesn't have the luxury of calling attention to its own fictions and chalking them up to art. It can't say with Melville that "he who, in view of its inconsistencies, says of human nature . . . that it is past finding out, thereby evinces a better appreciation of it than he who, by always representing it in a clear light, leaves it to be inferred that he clearly knows all about it." Neither can it afford Melville's arch awareness of the fallibility of all claims to knowledge about the human heart, about the dangers of placing our confidence in anyone's book about us. So don't look for the DSM to be published on April Fool's Day. And, despite the fact that it is full of fictive placeholders, don't expect the APA to suggest that booksellers shelve it with the likes of *The Confidence-Man*.

Which doesn't mean psychiatrists are above the open and intentional use of fiction, at least not when it comes to inventing mental disorders. Indeed, storytelling was central to at least one DSM-5 proposal: to add a diagnosis called Hebephilia to the sexual disorders chapter. Don't feel bad if you've never heard of Hebephilia, which is what Ray Blanchard—the Canadian doctor who incurred the wrath of the transgendered—calls the attraction of grown-ups to kids in early adolescence. According to Blanchard, lead author of a paper calling for including Hebephilia in the DSM, even among professionals there is a "general resistance or indifference to the adoption of a technical vocabulary for erotic age-preferences." Clinicians are more likely to have heard of "granny porn" than of *gerontophilia*, Blanchard said, and hardly anyone uses *teleiophilia* to talk about "the erotic preference for people between the ages of physical maturity and physical decline"—this despite the fact that, as Blanchard noted with some apparent bitterness, "the word *normal* has been off-limits for describing erotic interests for decades."

Blanchard wanted to overcome this resistance, at least when it comes to hebephilia, because he thought it was a "discriminable erotic age-preference." Some men, in other words, have that underlying pattern of arousal necessary to making a diagnosis. They are turned on by kids on the threshold of adulthood more than by anyone else. He can say this with some authority because he and his colleagues examined 2,591 men, most of them convicted sex offenders, in order to determine what aroused them.

This is where the storytelling comes in. The scientists provided the men with audiovisual aids—large pictures of naked young people, ranging in age from five to twenty-six, displayed on a triptych in front of them, and, piped in through headphones, fictional narratives of sexual situations involving people whose ages roughly corresponded to the pictures on display. The men sat in easy chairs, looked at the pictures, and listened to the tales, one of which started this way:

Your neighbors' 7-year-old girl is staying overnight at your place. You tell her it is time to get ready for bed. She asks if you will come and tuck her in. When you go to her room, she is already between the covers. You bend over to kiss her on the forehead, but she wraps her arms around your neck and pushes her mouth against yours.

Giggling, she throws back the covers to show you she is naked. You sink to the bed, tenderly pressing your lips against the little groove between her legs.

Okay, it's not Melville. It's not even *Fifty Shades of Grey*. But the researchers weren't asking the men for their critical opinion of the stories. Actually, they weren't asking the men anything at all, at least not in the usual meaning of that word. They were asking their penises. Sex offenders, especially convicted sex offenders (who were Blanchard's subjects) lie. But penises do not—mostly, however, because they do not talk. But Blanchard had a solution to this problem: the volumetric plethysmograph, or, as I like to call it, the Penis Whisperer.

The way it works is that the subject sits down in an easy chair. He slips a glass cylinder over his penis. After he pulls a sheet over himself "to minimize his embarrassment," a rubber cuff at the open end of the tube is inflated until it seals against the shaft of his penis. A hose attached to the bottle leads to a pressure transducer, which registers the slightest change in air pressure in the sealed cylinder—like, say, the kind that would be caused by a swelling penis. By mapping the behavior of the bottled-up penis onto the pictures and stories provided to its owner, researchers could chart the true course of a man's desires.

But before they could say much about whether the readings meant the men were hebephiles, the scientists had to know which phallometric stimulus category the objects of desire belonged in. To do this, they relied on the Tanner scale, an instrument that uses criteria like breast size, scrotum color, and pubic hair texture to rate the development of each photographic subject on a five-point scale. Having split the pubic hairs, Blanchard and his team were able to use the plethysmograph readings to prove that some men indeed show a strong preference for pubescent kids as defined by Tanner (breasts: 2.67; pubic hair growth: 2.33 [girls] 3.33 [boys]; genital development 3.83), most of whom were between eleven and fourteen years old. From this consistent response, they

THE BOOK OF WOE 245

concluded that "hebephilia exists and . . . that it is relatively common compared with other forms of erotic interests in children." Which meant that the DSM-5 should either expand Pedophilia to include "erotic attraction to pubescent . . . children, or, alternatively, add a separate diagnosis of Hebephilia."

But wait a minute! you're probably saying to yourself—that is, if you weren't so creeped out by this research that you stopped reading. Did it really take doctors poring over pictures of naked kids, showing them to men while whispering erotica into their ears, and charting their penises' responses to prove that men can be attracted to kids in the bloom of youth? Have they not heard of Humbert Humbert? Or read *Death in Venice* or Plato's *Symposium*? Or maybe just grazed the ads of the most recent issue of *Vogue* or the celeb photo spreads in *People*? Have they been to a shopping mall recently? Did they really just crash through an open door and claim to have arrived where no one had gone before?

Well, yes. And that's not all, nor is it the part that Melville might most appreciate. Having infallibly determined the longitude of men's penises, Blanchard and his team went on to make what Melville called "a revelation of human nature on fixed principles"—that the attraction, when it is to kids at a certain Tanner stage, is an illness.

But for all his charts correlating penile response to stimulus category and his charts of mean ipsatized penile response and his tables of Z-score transformations of the extremum of the curve of blood volume change, Blanchard never says which fixed principle allows him to conclude that what most states consider statutory rape, and most people consider flat-out wrong, is a mental illness. He doesn't even bother talking about clinical significance, let alone philosophical notions (and, if he did, he'd have to explain how it goes against natural selection for men to be attracted to girls whose bodies are advertising fertility in nature's neon lights). He seems to think that the charts and tables speak for themselves, that because he has figured out a way to measure it, a doctor's pronouncement that hebephilia exists, coupled with our belief that it is repellent, ought to be enough to convince us that if this feeling is in a human heart, then it can only be the symptom of a disease.

Not that it is such a hard sell, this idea that a person who commits a heinous act is sick, at least not to a public confident that doctors know what is and isn't a disease. Diagnoses are explanations of the otherwise incomprehensible, and to judge from the rates of Bipolar Disorder among children and antidepressant use among adults, from the relief that diagnosis brings to people like Michael Carley and Nomi Kaim, from the speed with which Jared Loughner and Anders Breivik were deemed schizophrenic, and from the opinion, at least in some quarters, that a better mental health system would somehow prevent mass shootings in schools and movie theaters, the market for representing our troubles in psychiatry's clear light is strong.

This confidence—the belief that doctors know all about our suffering—is precious to the APA. It's what they lost forty years ago, and what Spitzer worked so hard to restore with a book that looked scientific. It's what the organization is really selling when it sells the DSM. Without this confidence, who will buy the book? And without the book, who will believe the psychiatrists? And without belief, how will their treatments work?

That's why it's one thing for Steve Mirin and Steve Hyman to acknowledge the book's shortcomings to each other or for Kupfer and Regier to insist that its categories aren't really real, and quite another for the complaint and criticism to come from Frances or Caplan or the British Psychological Society. Criticism from the inside can be tolerated and sanitized and turned into a marketing campaign about the living document. But criticism from the outside must be repelled with all necessary force, for it threatens to let the rest of us in on what psychiatrists already know: that there is no fixed principle for their revelations.

So you really have to wonder why, in the course of revising the DSM, the APA put that confidence at such great risk. Why would they suggest turning statutory rape into a mental disorder, or bereavement into depression, or adolescent eccentricity into psychosis? For that matter, why would they propose, in a country where a third of the population is morbidly obese and where food has become the latest preoccupation of the affluent, to turn "eating, in a discrete period of time, an amount of food that is definitely larger than most people would eat in a similar period of time under similar circumstances," and "eating until feeling uncomfortably full" or "when not physically hungry," and "feeling guilty after overeating" into Binge Eating Disorder? Why would they propose, in a political and economic climate that offers no end of worries and occasions for despair, that people who are anxious and blue, but whose symptoms do not rise to the level of either Major Depression or Generalized Anxiety Disorder, should not be deprived of a diagnosis but instead should be said to suffer from Mixed Anxiety-Depression (which is a pretty clunky name until you consider its acronym)? Why would they propose with a straight face to a society of iSlaves that there is such a thing as Internet Use Disorder? Don't they grasp just how fragile confidence is?

I can't really answer that question. But I will point out that the APA wouldn't be the first American corporation to overplay its hand. It's happened to the best of them—General Motors, Kodak, Xerox, and all those other companies that suffered disruption and failure when they failed to remember what the confidence man must never forget: that confidence is always built on air, and that when it becomes known that what you are offering isn't what you've cracked it up to be, your brand might lose its allure, and your company might lose its franchise.

Chapter 16

Early in August 2011, an "Important Notice" appeared on the DSM-5 website. It was from the DSM-5 field trials team and addressed to DSM-5 field trials participants. "Have our e-mails been reaching you?" it asked.

As it happened, I hadn't heard from the team since the end of February, when I got a note from Regier and Kupfer professing their "delight" at my acceptance as a clinician in the field trials and promising more details soon. In the meantime, however, I'd heard (from Bill Narrow) that my *Wired* article about the revision hadn't played any better at the APA than it had with Frances. So when no news had come by July, I figured that maybe the delight had worn off and that the DSM leadership had come to the same conclusion as Donna Manning had—that allowing me into the field trials was like "letting the plague rat onto the ship." (I think she meant this in a good way.)

But the silence turned out not to be about me at all. "We are . . . test piloting the training materials," the team explained after I e-mailed in July asking for an update. They added that they hoped to have them out "in a few weeks."

A few weeks later, however, the only thing the APA had out was the Important Notice, which offered a new explanation for having been incommunicado. This time the problem was about me, sort of.

The most common reason for this is because our emails are being blocked by your email server's Spam filter. If you have not received any recent (i.e., within the past 2 months) email communications from the APA regarding field trial participation, please be sure to check your Spam or junk mail folder and look for any communications from us.

I wondered if the team had capitalized "Spam" out of deference to Hormel Foods, one copyright holder to another. I also wondered why they didn't just put the information that we had supposedly missed right into the notice. I can't say with certainty that the team was resorting to the excuse that all of us have used at one time or another to explain our dilatory e-mail habits, but I was sure of one thing: there were no messages from the APA trapped in my spam filter. Neither had any e-mails made their way to Michael First or Dayle Jones, both of whom had also signed up—or, according to Jones, to any of the would-be volunteers she knew.

In early September, when I still hadn't gotten the errant messages, or anything at all, I e-mailed Eve Mościcki, the APA researcher in charge of the clinician field trials, asking when I might hear from her team and when the trial might begin. The next day her office sent an apology and the password I needed to log in to the REDCap website. I also received a separate apology directly from Mościcki. She explained, "We have learned that some security settings automatically delete our e-mails and the recipient never sees them." She didn't say why the APA couldn't figure out how to do what every Viagra dealer and Nigerian scamster seemed to know how to do. (I did pass along my skepticism to Mościcki, pointing out that no one seemed to have received anything and suggesting that the problem might be at her end. "Thanks for your candid note," she wrote back. "Much appreciated.")

I went to the Vanderbilt site. My password and login didn't work. Ten days, and many e-mails later, I was finally able to sign in. Just a day after that, the APA finally figured how to get an e-mail blast past all those spam filters. It was another note from Kupfer and Regier, congratulating me, once again, on being accepted into the program. They didn't acknowledge that it had been five months since they first did that, and a full year since the APA announced the start of field trials. They did, however, give me my official title—Collaborating Investigator— and assigned a new significance to this "unique opportunity": it would be, they promised, "one of the most important psychiatric research studies of this decade." And if that wasn't reward enough, they were also offering fifteen continuing education credits, my name in the DSM-5, and a free copy of the book, whenever it came out.

One part of my training had already begun. As Bill Narrow had explained at the APA meeting, and as the team reminded us, we Collaborating Investigators were supposed to "familiarize" ourselves with the revisions by poring over the website, paying attention to the diagnoses we were most likely to render.

This was a tough assignment. The changes were many and complex. Here, for instance, is the DSM-5 proposal for Generalized Anxiety Disorder (GAD), a diagnosis most of us collaborators were likely to use, as it stood in June 2011.

A. Excessive anxiety and worry (apprehensive expectation) about two (or more) domains of activities or events (e.g., family, health, finances, and school/work difficulties).

B. The excessive anxiety and worry occurs on more days than not, for 3 months or more.

C. The anxiety and worry are associated with one or more of the following symptoms:

   1. restlessness or feeling keyed up or on edge
   2. muscle tension

D. The anxiety and worry are associated with one (or more) of the following behaviors:

1. marked avoidance of activities or events with possible negative outcomes

2. marked time and effort preparing for activities or events with possible negative outcomes

3. marked procrastination in behavior or decision-making due to worries

4. repeatedly seeking reassurance due to worries

E. The disturbance causes clinically significant distress or impairment in social, occupational, or other important areas of functioning.

F. The disturbance is not attributable to the direct physiological effects of a substance (e.g., a drug of abuse, a medication) or another medical condition (e.g., hyperthyroidism).

G. The disturbance is not better accounted for by another mental disorder (e.g., anxiety about Panic Attacks in Panic Disorder, negative evaluation in Social Anxiety Disorder, contamination or other obsessions in Obsessive-Compulsive Disorder, separation from attachment figures in Separation Anxiety Disorder, reminders of traumatic events in Posttraumatic Stress Disorder, gaining weight in Anorexia Nervosa, physical complaints in Somatic Symptom Disorder, perceived appearance flaws in Body Dysmorphic Disorder, or having a serious illness in Illness Anxiety Disorder).

And here is the old one:

A. Excessive anxiety and worry (apprehensive expectation), occurring more days than not for at least 6 months, about a number of events or activities (such as work or school performance).

B. The person finds it difficult to control the worry.

C. The anxiety and worry are associated with three (or more) of the following six symptoms (with at least some symptoms present for more days than not for the past 6 months). Note: Only one item is required in children.

1. Restlessness or feeling keyed up or on edge
2. Being easily fatigued
3. Difficulty concentrating or mind going blank
4. Irritability
5. Muscle tension
6. Sleep disturbance (difficulty falling or staying asleep, or restless unsatisfying sleep)

D. The focus of the anxiety and worry is not confined to features of an Axis I disorder, e.g., the anxiety or worry is not about having a Panic Attack (as in Panic Disorder), being embarrassed in public (as in Social Phobia), being contaminated (as in Obsessive-Compulsive Disorder), being away from home or close relatives (as in Separation Anxiety Disorder), gaining weight (as in Anorexia Nervosa), having multiple physical complaints (as in Somatization Disorder), or having a serious illness (as in Hypochondriasis), and the anxiety and worry do not occur exclusively during Posttraumatic Stress Disorder.

E. The anxiety, worry, or physical symptoms cause clinically significant distress or impairment in social, occupational, or other important areas of functioning.

F. The disturbance is not due to the direct physiological effects of a substance (e.g., a drug of abuse, a medication) or a general medical condition (e.g., hyperthyroidism) and does not occur exclusively during a Mood Disorder, a Psychotic Disorder, or a Pervasive Developmental Disorder.

The APA didn't make it easy for us to see the differences by placing the diagnoses side by side or creating a chart or, for that matter, just using their word processor's Track Changes command as Michael First had in Honolulu. And there were many changes. Six months of worry had become three. Fatigue, difficulty concentrating, irritability, and sleep troubles were out, while avoidance, procrastination, reassurance seeking, and "marked time and effort preparing for activities or events with possible negative outcomes" (think Mrs. Dalloway) were in. The threshold had been changed from three out of six Criterion C symptoms to one out of two Criterion C and one out of four Criterion D symptoms. "A number of events" that are the subject of worry has become "two or more do-mains of activities or events." And so on.

The good news was that I hadn't ever committed the old criteria to memory, so at least I wouldn't have to unlearn them. I was, however, going to have to get accustomed to using criteria to make the diagnosis in the first place. That's not something anyone I know in this business actually does. Mostly we're content to find a label that matches people in some vague way and then get on with the business of helping them fig-ure out what's going on in their lives that landed them in our offices.

There are exceptions, of course. Take the psychiatrist I will call Dr. Benway. He's a respected practitioner in my neighborhood to whom I had referred a young woman I'll call Charlotte. She was thirty-two years old, the daughter of Chinese immigrants, and recently divorced. I'd been seeing her for a little more than a year, and she had just begun to talk about the way her father used to crawl into bed with her and, as the rest of the family slept, force her to have sex with him. She hadn't told anyone about this before, and she was unraveling in the way people often do when they start to take apart the finely built edifice behind which they've hidden their shame and fear and rage. Charlotte was also in the midst of a huge project at work, one that she needed to complete if she was going to keep her job. So it was not a good time for her to be anxious all day and sleepless at night. She had asked me if I could help her get a prescription for Valium from someone other than her family doctor, to whom she did not want to have to explain herself, and that's where Dr. Benway got involved.

Returning to me after her visit, she told me that he had given her an antidepressant and a mood stabilizer for her depression and suggested that she try a stimulant for her ADHD; he told her they would explore that possibility more when she returned to him the following week. "Do you think I have ADHD?" she asked.

I told her I did not think she met the criteria.

"Then why would he say that?" she asked. "And why did he prescribe

Zoloft and Abilify? Do you think I have depression?" She told me about the psychological tests she'd filled out as part of her paperwork for Dr. Benway, the ones that asked her about different thoughts and feelings she'd had over the last weeks or month. Then she asked, "What is my diagnosis anyway?"

I tried the therapist's usual evasions, asking her why she wanted to know and what it meant to her to have her professional parent figures disagreeing about her and what it was like for her to think her therapist didn't know what he was talking about. But she wouldn't be dissuaded. This was the first time Charlotte had ever been demanding in this way—direct and forthright and confident—and even if it was a demand I was poorly equipped to meet, I felt that I had to meet it. So I fessed up.

"You don't have one," I said.

"Why not?"

I explained that therapy, not unlike medication, was really targeted at symptoms, not illnesses, and to the extent that we were surely trying to get at what lay underneath the symptoms, the DSM's labels and criteria were not particularly helpful toward that goal, that they renamed her suffering without explaining it.

I didn't tell Charlotte I'd stolen that line from William James. I also didn't tell her the other reason I hadn't given her a diagnosis. But I did tell Dr. Benway, because when I called him (to pester him on her behalf to prescribe the Valium so she could sleep, and maybe to chide him for the cocktail he'd mixed for her), the first thing he asked was what her diagnosis was.

"She doesn't use insurance," I said. "So she doesn't have one."

This could have been Dr. Benway's moment to go Gregory House on me, to reveal the sign I had missed and the diagnosis it led to, to question how I could possibly treat someone in the absence of a diagnosis. He didn't do any of this, however. I'm not sure why. It may be because our clinician communication—about Charlotte's current functioning, her anxiety, her insomnia and difficulty concentrating, her mood swings—didn't seem hampered by the fact that we weren't using the language scientifically proven to make our conversation reliable. It may be because when he explained the cocktail he'd prescribed—the way the Abilify/Zoloft combo could "put a floor under her" without agitating her and how adding Ritalin to the mix might just get her neurotransmitters all nicely balanced—I didn't point out to him that his opportunity to medicate Charlotte exceeded anyone's knowledge about any of that. Truce, standoff, going along to get along: Dr. Benway's silence about my diagnostic negligence and mine about his diagnostic exuberance could have been any of those. But somehow I think it might be something else entirely—that we both knew the truth of what I had said: In the absence of an incentive, who would bother with a diagnosis?

But now that I am a Collaborating Investigator, perhaps I should consider giving Charlotte a diagnosis. The DSM-5 with which I am supposed to familiarize myself offers all sorts of possibilities. GAD, for example, with its *marked*s and *excessive*s providing all kinds of wiggle room for the insurance-dependent, is, despite its many changes, an obvious choice. Major Depressive Disorder has been left mostly alone (other than the absence of the bereavement exclusion, and, no matter what the new criteria said, if presented with a grieving patient, I'm going to pretend to be astute and not add the insult of a diagnosis to the injury of a bereavement), and if Charlotte doesn't reach its five-of-nine threshold, there is always what has been called Dysthymia in DSM-IV and what the DSM-5 proposes to call Chronic Depression, a two-of-six offering. Adjustment Disorder with Mixed Anxiety and Depressed Mood calls for no more than six months to elapse between the psychosocial stressor to which the patient is adjusting poorly and the onset of symptoms, but if I decide that the stressor is Charlotte's disclosure of the incest and not the incest itself, then that diagnosis would work just fine.

But there's another possibility in the DSM, one that doesn't ask me to look for the symptoms of ersatz diseases, but to pay attention to what Charlotte actually brings into my office: herself. Because Charlotte may be anxious and depressed and failing to adjust, but she is also the kind of person who arrives late for her appointment and then, as the clock approaches the end of her time, says, "You're not going to throw me out of here now, are you?"

I tell her that we have to stop at the usual time, regardless of when we started. "Why does that feel like being thrown out?" I ask her.

"I can't believe it. I killed myself to get here on time. Really, almost. I drove like eighty miles an hour. I can't help it if the traffic was bad," she says. "And anyway, what's so important that you have to do?"

I don't answer.

Her voice rises. "You don't care about me, any more than a whore cares about a john," she says. "And why would you? This is just your job. But why would anyone listen to me if it wasn't their job? Look at me." She sweeps her hand along her body, like a salesman demonstrating his product. "I'm fat and ugly and disgusting." (She is actually trim and pretty, but this isn't the moment to tell her that.) She has been fiddling with her hair the whole session, but now she's tearing at it with such force that I can hear it ripping from her scalp and see strands falling onto the couch. "And you just pretend, and you're not very good at it. You can't wait to get rid of me."

Which, at that moment, you wouldn't blame me for saying, is sort of true.

That's how Charlotte wants me to feel: like she feels, unloved and uncertain of herself and the others around her. And now that she's landed her blow, she's pulling even more frantically at her hair. "Okay, I get it. I'll go," she says. "And you don't want me to come back, do you?"

She rummages angrily in her purse, pulls out her checkbook, scrawls the check. But she is not only rebuking me. She's also imploring me to assure her that her outburst hasn't made me want to kick her out or punish her for being mean. Having made herself unlikable, she's waiting for me to tell her that I like her.

Now, I might not go that far, but on the other hand, I didn't kick her out of therapy. I'll take a lot. Not because I'm a saint, but because this is what she is paying for: not indulgence exactly, but acceptance, the peculiar kind of love conveyed when I stand back from the action and participate in it at the same time, when I watch Charlotte flail and let her land her blows and respond to the pain she inflicts without taking it personally. And what I'm seeing when Charlotte is launching her attacks on both of us is not a disease. Neither is it an assortment of symptoms. It's who she is, her character, forged out of the crucible of the family, that strange little enclave where we raise our young, each on our own, behind closed doors or in homes where, if you were lucky, there were the resources and the courage and the love that it takes to send a person into the world more or less intact, but if you were not lucky, if your parents were like Charlotte's, so distracted by the exigencies of life in a strange new country, or so adept at ignoring what they could not afford to acknowledge, that a father could see his daughter as a sexual object and a mother could turn a blind eye—a lapse made even more unlikely, and yet somehow more inevitable, by the fact that the mother and her mother's mother, as Charlotte found out recently, also grew up in incestuous families—if all those stars lined up and crossed you, then you too might have come to think that the disgusting thing that was happening was happening because you were disgusting, so disgusting that no one would care what was being done to you, you too might have figured that the best you could do was to shut up and take your lumps, and you too might have been seething all the time you were submitting. You might have been left desperate for love, and sure that you'd found

it, until one little thing—an encounter with the tyranny of the therapist's clock, his exercise of power over you, his disregard for your
wishes—leaves you raging and unable to do anything but pour out the
rage in a way that gets you rejected, unable to stop yourself, even as you
watch yourself tumble, for maybe the millionth time, through that trap
door in yourself and land in your own self-hatred.

Or you could be like the man whom Charlotte had married—Joe, I'll
call him. I met the two of them together when they came to see me
about two years before the conversation I just described took place. Actually, they weren't supposed to see me as a couple. Joe—eight years
older, tall, good-looking, a wealthy businessman who wore his success
on his monogrammed, gold-cuff-linked sleeve—had been referred by
his lawyer, who thought it would look good to the judge if he was in
counseling when his case came up. Of course, the lawyer didn't put it
that way. He just said something like "This guy could really use to be
seen, if you follow my logic."

It was hard to argue with that. Joe had been arrested after he'd
punched a parking lot attendant in the face. He thought the worker
had shown insufficient respect when he'd told Joe he couldn't park
where he wanted to. "Like it really mattered. Fucking moron!" Joe told
me soon after he sat down, and before I'd had a chance to ask about the
incident.

"That's why you coldcocked him?" I asked. "Because he was a moron?
Or just because he told you what to do?"

"Look, the space was empty. If he had bothered to think about it, if
he wasn't just going by some other stupid fuck's stupid rules, then he
would not have been hassling me," he said. "It's what's ruining the country, the way people just follow rules without thinking, without figuring
out if they should make an exception."

"And he should have made an exception for you?"

"Of course he should have. I could have fit my car in there without
any trouble. I know how to drive, for chrissakes. Any swinging dick can

get into a car and step on the gas. But I've been trained. I did one of those week-long courses for Mercedes owners."

Five minutes with this guy and I was already hating him. I changed the subject.

"Whose idea was it for Charlotte to come today?" I'd been surprised to discover her in the waiting room, the two of them perfectly dressed and groomed, flipping through back issues of *Home & Garden*. I was even more surprised when she followed him into my office.

"Both of us," Joe said.

"But you didn't tell me you wanted to bring your wife with you when you made the appointment."

"Why? Is that a rule of yours?"

I guess I hadn't changed the subject after all.

After I didn't answer, Charlotte spoke up. "Actually, it was my idea to come. Joe was so upset about getting arrested and all, and then it got worse when he heard he had to come here. I thought there were certain things you needed to know, because you'd get totally the wrong idea if all you knew was that he'd punched some random dude. I thought you needed to know that Joe is a special guy, and how well he can treat people." She put her hand on his knee.

"Don't you think Joe can speak for himself?" I asked.

"Of course I can," he said. "But I thought you would need proof that I wasn't that kind of man."

"Okay, well, it is a rule of mine. Not that spouses can't be here, but that if you are here as a couple, then we're going to be talking about your marriage or something like that. A joint business, a problem with your kid, a disagreement about your in-laws, or that you just can't get along. But not as a character witness. My understanding," I said to Charlotte, "is that Joe is here because he's had this fight and this arrest," and then I turned to Joe to say, "My guess is that this isn't the first time someone who failed to appreciate you took it on the chin, Joe."

"So what are you saying?"

"That if what you want to do is to figure out why this kind of thing happens to you, other than the fact that everyone else in the world is a moron, and what you can do about it besides punch their lights out, or why you are so afraid that everyone is going to dislike you, then I'm your guy. But if what you want is for me to help you or your lawyer win a case, or to make you feel like you deserve to be able to assault people, then I'm not. Because I'm sure there are reasons you feel that way, but I don't think you deserve that."

Joe stared at me for a second, probably the same way he stared at the kid in the parking lot. He stood up, pulled a money clip out of his pocket, tore off a hundred-dollar bill, and dropped it on my desk. "This ought to cover it," he said. "I'll tell my lawyer to find someone who can help." Without a word, Charlotte stood up, too, and the two of them breezed out of my office. I can't say I was sorry to see them go.

When she called me about a year later to tell me Joe had left her for a twenty-two-year-old woman and she needed to see me ("Because you were right," she said. "You nailed what an asshole he was"), Charlotte was in the kind of agony that goes along with being a self, with having no choice but to be at the center of your world, and of finding nothing there but fear and self-loathing. But even as she began to get over Joe, and to understand that there is only the slightest difference between fitting another person like a hand fits a glove and sharing a pair of handcuffs, the anxiety and depression didn't go away. They seemed less and less related to what had happened with Joe, more like the inevitable if regrettable outgrowth of who she was.

So I could diagnose her with GAD or MDD—she more or less fit those criteria—just as I could have diagnosed Joe, had he stuck around, with Intermittent Explosive Disorder, for he was surely a walking IED. But diagnoses like these don't quite seem to do Charlotte or Joe justice, especially not when it seems so clear that what they suffered from wasn't anything like the kind of illness that comes and goes like the common cold, or comes and stays like diabetes. Troubles such as theirs seem to arise out of their troubled selves. And as it happens, there is an entire section in the DSM devoted to describing those troubles, which the book calls *personality disorders* and defines this way:

> A Personality Disorder is an enduring pattern of inner experience and behavior that deviates markedly from the expectations of the individual's culture, is pervasive and inflexible, has an onset in adolescence or early adulthood, is stable over time, and leads to distress or impairment.

The ten personality disorders listed in the DSM come last in the book. They also have their own diagnostic duchy, known as Axis II (as opposed to Axis I, where the rest of the disorders reside). This segregation, the book explains, "ensures that consideration will be given to the possible presence of Personality Disorders . . . that might otherwise be overlooked when attention is directed to the usually more florid Axis I disorders." But I think the real reason lies in a more fundamental difference between the two axes. An Axis I disorder is what you *have*. An Axis II disorder is what you *are*. (Personality disorders share Axis II with mental retardation.)

Despite this crucial difference, personality disorders look like the other disorders in the DSM. Borderline Personality Disorder (BPD), for instance, the diagnosis Charlotte would qualify for, is a five-of-nine affair, with criteria like "frantic efforts to avoid real or imagined abandonment" and "markedly and persistently unstable self-image or sense of self." Narcissistic Personality Disorder (NPD), another five-of-niner (including "grandiose sense of self-importance," "sense of entitlement," and need for "excessive admiration"), matches Joe pretty well. (And it's not at all rare to find a borderline married to a narcissist.) But you can't miss the Freudian echoes in these disorders. *Borderline* refers to the border between neurosis and psychosis, and *narcissistic* is a nod to Freud's observation that some people treat the world as a mirror that they must shatter when they don't like what it reflects.

But even if the names weren't a dead giveaway, it would be impossible to conceal the fact that personality disorders are a throwback to the Freudian conviction that our suffering reveals the neurotic shape into which our timber is twisted by the psychosexual catastrophes of childhood and the impossible demands of society, and that treatment always involves a reckoning with those forces and the person they have made us.

The presence of personality disorders in the DSM preserves this old, officially out-of-fashion idea that personality underlies our difficulties. The book never comes out and says so, but Allen Frances wrote the personality disorders section of the DSM, and he'll tell you unabashedly that this is the case. "I think this is the best way to see and treat most disorders," he said. (Although it's not the best way to get paid for treating them. Insurance companies don't generally reimburse for those diagnoses, so even if you think that's what you're treating, you can't tell them that.) But Frances was trained in those olden days, before the demands of science required psychiatry to distance itself from Freud by divorcing its account of our afflictions from their causes. It is as if the psychiatrists of his generation, the ones who saved their profession by meeting those demands, could not quite let go of the idea that who we are matters, and kept that thought alive on Axis II.

As Freud himself might have predicted, smuggling psychoanalysis into a DSM that claimed authority by purging it has created an internal conflict that yields no end of trouble.

"I have never really been a doctor in the proper sense," Freud wrote. That may be why in all his talk of neuroses and psychoses, complexes and symptoms, defenses and resistances, he remained uninterested in carving the psyche at its joints by naming its afflictions. He mostly ignored Kraepelin (who was a contemporary of his) and his parsing of mental disorders from one another. (Although he was pleased to pick up one of Kraepelin's patients, Sergei Pankejeff, and turn him into the Wolf Man, title character of one of his most gripping case studies.) We all have parents, we all live stretched between instinct and conscience, between memory and desire, between brutality and civilization, so we all suffer degrees of the same illness; to have a personality is always to at least flirt with neurosis.

So in the Freudian view, all personalities are more or less disordered. Which is exactly what led to those 85 percent prevalence rates, to the reliability crises, and ultimately to the suspicion that psychiatry may not belong in medicine. As problematic as the DSM's response has become when it comes to Axis I disorders, with its categories and criteria and axes, its *at least three months* and its *three out of six symptoms*, it still works, as long as you limit your definition of *works* to *achieves reliability under ideal conditions*. But personality disorders have never worked even in that limited sense. "They have the lowest reliability of any major category in the book," Frances, who served on the DSM-III personality disorders work group, told me. (The kappas were .56 to .65.) And he's been saying so for a long time. Within a few months of the publication of DSM-III in 1980, he was telling readers of the *American Journal of Psychiatry* that "the personality disorders are not at all clearly distinct from normal functioning or from each other," which is why they were significantly harder for clinicians to distinguish reliably than Axis I disorders were.

In that paper, and in one he wrote two years later, Frances suggested an alternative approach to personality disorders. "Rather than being diagnosed within one or another distinct personality type," he wrote, "the patient might be rated (perhaps on a scale of 1 to 10) for each personality characteristic." People don't have BPD so much as they are anxious about abandonment, impulsive, and entitled—qualities they share more with people who might qualify for, say, NPD than with people whose personalities are less troublesome. Long before Darrel Regier proposed dimensional diagnosis for DSM-5, Frances was suggesting exactly that, at least for the personality disorders.

When he started work on DSM-IV, Frances said, a dimensionalized personality disorders section was one of his goals. He said that he recruited Thomas Widiger as the DSM-IV research coordinator in part because he was a "committed dimensionalist" and that he urged the work group to come up with an alternative to the categorical approach. "We worked hard to forge a consensus that could inform a simple DSM-IV proposal," he said. "But we failed. We couldn't reach agreement on how to rate the factors." The process devolved into those pointless arguments he'd wanted to avoid—"the distinctions without differences that bedevil the field."

Widiger remembers it differently. He's not so sure Frances hired him for his dimensionalist expertise—"I believe I was chosen to be the research coordinator because I was hardworking, conscientious, familiar with meta-analyses, and had collaborated with Allen many years before DSM-IV," he told me, adding that only two of the one hundred projects he worked on concerned dimensions. And, he says, the problem was not really the result of contention among the troops but a failure of the general to bring them together. "There were advocates of different models," but the same was true when DSM-III was written, "and that didn't stop Spitzer from coming up with a compromise among them. If you recognize that the field needs to shift to a dimensional model, you can easily address the differences of opinion."

Twenty years later, Widiger was still mystified by Frances's waffling, especially in light of his long history of advocacy for a dimensional approach. But Frances was committed to making changes only in the presence of incontrovertible evidence. By that principle, if the work group couldn't resolve its own arguments, the only conclusion was that dimensions weren't ready for the DSM, at least not his DSM. No matter how wrongheaded he thought the existing model was, no matter how long he'd been advocating for a different one, in the end he had to settle for the tepid observation, made in a section tacked on to the introduction to the personality disorders, that dimensional models were "under active investigation," and for a paper, published just before DSM-IV came out, suggesting that it was only a matter of time before personality disorders were diagnosed dimensionally. The nosological conservative had been hoist with his own petard.

Widiger thought he was going to get another chance. He was the sole personality disorders expert in the research planning conferences organized by Michael First in 2000. First was also an advocate of dimensions. "Patients have just one personality," he wrote in a paper that set the DSM-5 research agenda for personality disorders. "It might be more consistent . . . to indicate that a patient has one personality disorder, characterized by the presence of a variety of maladaptive personality traits." He went on to suggest a seven-point plan for implementing a dimensional approach in the DSM-5.

First pointed out that much of the work had already been done. Just as Spitzer had drawn on years of research into diagnostic criteria in fashioning his first proposals, so too would-be DSM reformers could turn to any number of dimensional models of personality as a starting point. There was Cloninger's Tridimensional Personality Questionnaire and Timothy Leary's (yes, *that* Timothy Leary) Interpersonal Circumplex, the Big Five and the 16-PF, the DAPP and the SNAP and the SWAP. They differed in many ways, but they were all attempts to find the basic building blocks of personality, and then to show how individuals emerge as different agglomerations of those factors. The 16-PF, for instance, identifies sixteen source traits that are derived from 42 clusters, which were refined from 171 groups, which in turn were reduced from the four thousand or so adjectives in *Webster's* that describe facets of personality, and the Big Five, also known as the Five Factor Model, claims that all those adjectives can be placed under one of five domains—*openness to experience, conscientiousness, extraversion, agreeableness,* and *neuroticism.* An individual personality, according to this theory, is the unique mix of these common qualities.

No matter how they are counted and named, these factors are, of course, all reifications. There really is no such thing as extraversion, even if you know it when you see it, any more than there is such a thing as Major Depressive Disorder. But these personality models have all been used extensively. Researchers have developed tests and subtests and rating scales that can locate people along the dimensions of each model. They've tied the resulting profiles to religious belief and political affiliation, to drug use and child abuse, to learning styles and patterns of memory. And, of course, they've applied their models to the personality-disordered, showing how those patients' troubles can be reliably attributed to the lack or excess of particular factors.

While the competing personality theories have generated as much intramural conflict as you might expect, First saw the proliferation of models as an opportunity for nosology. All that active investigation had yielded a huge body of concepts and measures from which a revision could be fashioned. And if the DSM could incorporate this data into its diagnostic regime, he thought, it could return something vital to the personality researchers who generated it: a "uniform classification of general personality functioning" that would bring the same kind of order to the field that the DSM-III had brought to the general classification of mental illness.

As much as everyone had to gain from this outcome, First didn't think it would be easy to bring about. "That is why I pushed to have the personality research conference take place first," he told me. "I thought if they got started working on it within the next year, before work started on the rest of DSM-5, then maybe they would have it worked out in time."

That meeting took place late in 2004. Tom Widiger, who had been part of the 1999 planning conferences, chaired it. Regier, he said, had asked him to find a "common ground" among competing personality theories and to fashion a model for DSM out of them, and he leaped at the chance to finish the work he felt Frances had abandoned. He searched for the commonalities among them, and eventually determined that the eighteen leading theories, and all their different schematics of personality, converged on four domains, each of which had its own spectrum. According to Widiger's distillation, we are all more or less extraverted or introverted, constrained or impulsive, emotionally stable or unstable, and antagonistic or compliant. People whose personalities were disordered could be thought of as, for instance, too extraverted or too compliant or not stable or impulsive enough, and thanks to the plethora of tests available, their location in those domains could be specified. Charlotte and Joe could thus be diagnosed without recourse to woolly concepts like *borderline* or *narcissism*; instead they could be described in terms of those factors without pretending that they had separate illnesses.

While he knew this compromise was not a shoo-in for DSM-5, Widiger was pretty sure that he had given the APA a way to catch up with the "basic science research on general personality structure" and that, given the hunger for a new approach, it had a good chance for "eventual adoption." The paradigm shift, at least when it came to personality disorders, was finally at hand. It wouldn't be a move to a nosology based on biomarkers (although there are intriguing connections between genetics and neurochemistry on the one hand and personality traits on the other). It wouldn't entirely solve the problem of reification, but it would at least rid one section of the DSM of diagnostic categories that everyone agreed really didn't make sense and replace them with dimensions, which nearly everyone agreed were a better way to conceptualize mental illness. The personality disorders work group—with Widiger at its helm, or so he and many others thought—would lead psychiatry into the future.

"The devil, of course, could be in the details," Widiger wrote at the end of his "common ground" paper. The details he had in mind were scientific, and, given his prominent position in the field, he figured he would be heading the team that would work them out. But the details that arose were not scientific at all. In 2005, he and a colleague began to plan another conference about dimensions in DSM-5. Three months into those conversations, Widiger discovered that he would not be invited to that conference. And then, late in 2006, psychiatrist John Livesley, who had attended the conference, called to tell Widiger that he had just seen the list of people who would be on the DSM-5 work group. Widiger had gotten the Michael First treatment—an acknowledged leader in the field, who had done yeoman service for the APA, who most people thought would get the job, had been unceremoniously exiled. "Nobody on the work group ever asked for my input or informed me about what was going on," Widiger said. He was left to figure it out from what was posted on the website.

The first proposals Widiger saw appeared in February 2010. They represented, according to the work group, a "significant reformulation." Diagnosis would no longer be a matter of checking the criteria against the patient. But neither would it be a shift to a purely dimensional approach. Instead, they proposed a "hybrid" model that required clinicians to go through a four-step procedure. First, they would use seven criteria, including *identity integration* and *cooperativeness*, to determine whether the patient had a personality disorder, which was defined as the failure to develop "a sense of self-identity and the capacity for interpersonal function." They would then determine which of five types of personality disorder (antisocial/psychopathic, avoidant, borderline, obsessive-compulsive, or schizotypal) the patient had. To figure this out, they would not use criteria, but instead match the patient to prototypical descriptions of the disorder. Then they would see which of thirty-seven trait facets—social withdrawal, for example, or recklessness—nested in six trait domains, such as negative emotionality and disinhibition, best described the patient. If the patient didn't fit one of the types, they would diagnose her with a personality disorder, and the facets and domains would be used to describe the disorder further. And finally they would determine how badly disordered the patient's personality was by rating it on a scale of one to three along four dimensions for two different areas of functioning.

Don't worry if you didn't get that. Some hybrids are elegant (think of Priuses or Gala apples). Others are more like mules. Even if the personality disorders proposal makes sense (and I'm not sure it does), as a clinician I can assure you that it is way too complicated and time-consuming for anyone to actually use. More important, however, the proposal had little if anything to do with all those validated theories and their measurement instruments that Widiger had labored so hard to integrate into a single model. The trait facets and domains seemed to bear little relationship to the long history of research that had once made personality disorders seem so promising as a game-changer. And the types—well, it was at least clear where the committee had found them: in the DSM-IV. But they didn't explain why they had adopted only five of the original ten personality disorders.

Actually, they did try to explain. Andrew Skodol, the work group chair, reported that they had conducted a literature review and eliminated the five diagnoses that the least amount of research had been done on. They argued that the lack of studies indicated that these diagnoses had insufficient "empirical evidence of validity and clinical utility," failing to note that absence of evidence was not evidence of absence, that, in fact, the decision amounted to letting the marketplace decide which diagnoses should stay and which should go.

Skodol also ventured an explanation for not simply choosing one of the established personality theories, with its validated concepts and measures, and instead cobbling together a model that, as the APA work group noted on the website, was still "pending empirical validation." "We knew we couldn't incorporate anybody's model in toto," he told me, "because the APA wasn't going to pay royalties" to any copyright holder.

Whatever the rationale, the proposal left Widiger hopping mad. "The empirical support is a farce," he wrote in an e-mail to his colleagues, the section "embarrassingly bad." It would become "the laughingstock of the DSM and psychiatry," he predicted. "It's a monumental mistake."

Widiger wasn't alone in being appalled. John Livesley went public with his charge that the proposal was "a disaster." He withdrew his name from the work group's journal article describing the changes and published his own dissenting opinion in March 2010, lamenting the proposal as a "lost opportunity" that "negates years of progress toward a scientific-based classification system." In April, Frances called the proposal a "cumbersome hodgepodge" whose dimensions were "the favorites of the few members of the work group who have personal research experience in this area." The comments submitted to the website during the spring ran strongly against the proposals. In September, a group of eight psychiatrists and psychologists, some of the biggest names in the business, ranging from the ancient psychoanalyst Otto Kernberg to the even more ancient father of cognitive-behavioral therapy, Aaron Beck, to the upstart political psychologist Drew Westen, put aside their differences to tell readers of the *American Journal of Psychiatry* that the proposal was "an unwieldy conglomeration" whose traits and facets "have not been investigated empirically," which meant that the model "no longer rests on the decades of research" that had been "the chief rationale" for making the change to a dimensional model in the first place.

In the fall of 2010, the task force staged what Skodol called an "intervention." "They hated the prototypes"—the descriptions of personality disorders that had replaced the criteria. "They reminded them of

DSM-II," he explained, and they weren't crazy about the rest of it, either. "You guys look like outliers," they told him, as they ordered the group back to the drawing board—this time with two "consultants" ("minders," one committee member called them) to assist in reformulating the proposals. In a series of weekly phone conferences, chaired not by Skodol but by one of the consultants, a new proposal was hammered out and a "simplified and streamlined" proposal was posted on the website in late June. Now there were five trait domains instead of six, and thirty-one facets instead of thirty-seven, and six types instead of five. The criteria for those types were back, reflecting the task force's mandate to, as Skodol put it, "make the section look more like the rest of them."

Skodol took his very public rebuke in stride. He understood his colleagues' protests. "I mean, if you had spent your career studying Dependent Personality Disorder"—one of the five slated for elimination—"then I can see why you would be upset." Entire data sets accumulated over years would have to be mapped onto new categories. In at least one case—Narcissistic Personality Disorder—the vehemence and volume of the public comments prevailed over the lack of empirical support, leading the committee to rescue it, against Skodol's wishes, from nosological oblivion. But, he told me, even if this was the "most political" of the decisions, "if you're going to welcome comments, it doesn't make sense not to respond to the comments."

Skodol seemed stung about just one aspect of the "politics." His group had taken seriously the mandate to switch to a dimensional system, but "the rest of the work groups didn't get it, and Darrel and David were never able to convince them that dimensionality was the way to go," he told me. "I don't think they had quite the clarity of vision that Bob Spitzer had when he did DSM-III. He had this vision, and he sold it until it was bought, and I don't know that Darrel and David ever did that."

Kupfer and Regier, in other words, had failed to do in DSM-5 what Frances (at least according to Widiger) had failed to do in DSM-IV: to ram through the changes that would decouple psychiatry from the categories that most of its leaders knew were fictional, that had once worked to restore the profession's reputation, but now threatened it. Maybe the problem was that Kupfer and Regier's "bottoms-up" approach registered with their foot soldiers as a lack of leadership, or perhaps the leap from categories to dimensions was so long, the stakes of missing so high, that Spitzer himself couldn't have sold it. Or maybe Freud was right. Maybe the trouble that surfaced in the personality disorders, the section of the DSM most indebted to the past, was only the latest symptom of a neurosis, of a dream that can't be fulfilled: to make psychiatry into just another specialized branch of medicine.

Chapter 17

I n September 2011, David Kupfer traveled across his home state to kick off "Categories and Controversies: The Ethical Dimensions of the DSM-5," a program at the Center for Bioethics at the University of Pennsylvania. He told the audience of about seventy-five how glad he was to be at the university that two of his children had attended and that housed many of his research partners. In these friendly confines, he seemed confident. "You don't have to pay attention," he said, "because I'm assured you have the slides, so if you wanted to wander around or take a nap . . ." He was casual and personal as he told us about his experience working on DSM-IV (which, he said, had left him with "no interest and no desire" to work on DSM-5, but he'd nonetheless been talked into taking the reins) and about the importance of innovating while still maintaining continuity with the past. In a nod to the day's topic, he gave assurances about the importance of public input and displayed the statistics from the public comments, which now totaled 10,751. He explained that DSM-5 would be a living document, although he still wasn't sure how or when or under what circumstances DSM-5.1 and further updates would be issued. And he ended with an announcement, delivered with mock seriousness. "We've decided on the color of the cover," he said. The slide showed the familiar DSM cover, only in purple instead of the DSM-IV-TR's gray. "It was a huge debate, but that's been settled," Kupfer said with a smile.

Kupfer acknowledged the DSM-5 troubles only obliquely, noting almost in passing that there were "individuals who will say from the outset that it's ridiculous to revise DSM-IV," a charge he breezed past with a brief reminder of the current book's shortcomings. But just as I was contemplating that nap, he turned to a subject that was, at least to me, new and startling.

"I want to tell you a little about the competition," he said, a group at Columbia, led by a "young psychiatrist" named Helena Hansen. "They're not a group that has anything to do with DSM-5," he continued. They had invited Kupfer to one of their meetings. "I didn't have to wear a vest to protect me," he joked, "and it was a great experience." Kupfer reported that Hansen and her team were proposing a "DSM receptor," a group "outside the usual suspects" that would "periodically convene" to monitor "the implications of DSM-5 on society" and "collaborate closely with the DSM task force" to reckon with the findings, and that Kupfer was planning to take them up on their offer.

"I call them my friendly gadflies," he said. He didn't add "as opposed to some other gadflies I know," but anyone who had been following the developments would get the point: the APA was taking concerns like Frances's seriously enough to appoint a committee of ombudsmen.

When I tracked her down, Helena Hansen wasn't at Columbia, but rather at New York University, where she was a professor of anthropology and psychiatry. She told me she was indeed part of a group looking into the social dimensions of psychiatric nosology. They had responded to the APA's call for public comment, had gotten some money from the Robert Wood Johnson Foundation to hold a meeting on the subject— the session Kupfer had attended—and sent out an article for review.

"There has been a continual struggle to recognize and incorporate socio-cultural considerations into the DSMs," she told me in an e-mail. "This has not been seen as mainstream to the project, which is focused on buying credibility for psychiatry through biological formulations."

She sure sounded as if she had the chops for the gadfly position. But there was a problem: my e-mail was the first she'd heard of Kupfer's plan.

"I am not sure what Kupfer meant by gadfly," she wrote.

I sent her my transcription of his talk.

"This is amazing!" she wrote. "Wow. Well, I am tickled that we are now a 'committee of experts.'"

Hansen seemed willing to do the job. But she wasn't exactly waiting by the phone for Kupfer to call and offer it to her. "We are just hoping the piece gets published," she told me.

Back in California, the unfriendly gadfly sent me a staccato message in mid-November that seemed more fit for a telegram than an e-mail. "Approaching endgame. This is turning out to be much worse than I anticipated. A truly shitty way to end a career."

Frances's dour dispatch contrasted sharply with the ebullient one he had sent just a few weeks before. "A random and geographically diverse pick-up team of previously unknown idealists joins forces to create a grassroots movement that saves DSM-5 from itself and spares the world an orgy of diagnosis and a worsening epidemic of prescription drug use." And that was just the subject line.

The man who had once portrayed himself as "pretty Spockean (as in *Star Trek*, not Benjamin)—too rational, old, and indifferent to take things personally"—was evidently having some mood swings.

Among the idealists who had buoyed him was psychologist David Elkins, head of one of the American Psychological Association's divisions. He had written an open letter to the APA, complaining about the DSM-5's lowered diagnostic thresholds, shaky evidence, carelessness with the public health, and, of particular concern to psychologists, its "reconceptualizations of mental disorder as primarily medical phenomena." Elkins posted the letter on a petitions website on October 25, and it had attracted nearly five thousand signatures by November 8. That was the day that the president of the American Counseling Association sent a letter on behalf of his 115,000 DSM-buying members to the president of the APA. It reiterated the petition's objections about the quality of the science behind DSM-5. It called for the book to acknowledge that "mental disorders may not have a biological component" (although it did not explain just how it would be possible to have a mental disorder that did not somehow involve the brain). And it urged the APA to make public the work of the scientific review committee it had appointed to review the proposed changes, as well as to allow an evaluation of "all evidence and data by an external, independent group of experts."

This was a "tipping point," Frances wrote me. It wasn't the first time he'd thought that. In February 2010, the tipping point was going to be his open letter to the APA board. At the end of that year, it was going to be my *Wired* article, which would "bring Darrel to see DSM-5 through the eyes of the world that lives outside the bunkers." In the summer of 2011, he thought it would be his blog detailing the scientific shortcomings of DSM-5. But this time, he thought, the APA—its trustees if not its DSM bureaucrats—would have to see how bad things were. It was one thing to dismiss his protests as the raving of a jealous ex-chairman clinging to his passing glory (and royalties) and quite another to ignore these two powerful groups of professionals—and customers—not to mention the two or three hundred people from around the world signing the petition every day.

Of course, the APA was still hearing from Frances. His fingerprints were all over the letters from the psychologists and counselors, and he continued to chide them in his blogs—BlackBerryed in from San Diego and Carmel, as well as from Italy and Israel and Turkey and wherever else he happened to be traveling (often presenting his PowerPoint on the impending disaster)—and in the interviews he was granting to journalists all over the world. And he was now, he told me, "rattling some cages" on a back channel to the APA trustees and officers, with whom he was "trying to negotiate a face-saving compromise." (I think he meant their faces.) Even as he repeated his claim about the unimportance of bosses ("The most useless person on the battlefield is Napoleon," he wrote), he was in the thick of the battle, more godfather than general, perhaps, but directing the war just the same.

And he was trying to direct me more than ever.

"Cast of fascinating and colorful characters who deserve recognition and will greatly enrich human interest in your story," read the subject line of a note introducing me to a former television news producer ("bright, active, and great contacts"), a "somewhat eccentric and fascinating British lady who knows all there is to know about social networking," and a "seasoned mental health consumer advocate." And these weren't even the same previously unknown idealists who, just a few weeks earlier, he had nominated as the "unsung heroes" of my book.

"This will likely be the most important interview you do for the book," he wrote, when I told him about an interview I'd scheduled with an APA trustee. He gave me some advice on how to "get him comfortable" with me and warned me that I shouldn't "spook him" by letting him know just how much contact he and I had had.

"Don't waste your best brains," he advised me, when he heard about another interview, whose subject, Frances thought, "was a nice enough guy but peripheral."

He was trying to help someone he believed to be an ally, I think. But as allies go, I was problematic. I had sent him a peace offering for the bullshit quote—a copy of *On Bullshit*—but it continued to rankle. "I was in Dubuque, Iowa, in the courtroom testifying . . . before a jury of upstanding cornfed godfearing people who got to discover [via] Greenberg just how foul mouthed was this defender of the constitution," he wrote. "Thanks again, Gary."

But it wasn't the prosecutors and juries he was most worried about. It was the real enemy, the antipsychiatrists, to whom "your brilliant opening" had given ammunition. He allowed that maybe I hadn't meant this outcome, but that just made matters worse. "It was my lips that sank this ship," he wrote, "but you know sin on this one too . . . You are not concerned enough to avoid giving them aid and comfort." Heedless of the consequences of my own words, I was encouraging patients to discontinue treatment.

"I am pretty light about most things in life, but this is not a joke and you still don't get it," he scolded. It was an unusually excoriating performance for someone who, true to his word, had previously favored teasing me—for instance, calling me "Paula Caplan in drag"—over yelling at me.

Of course, it's not as if Caplan or any other antipsychiatrists needed my help, not when Frances himself was delivering one blistering blog after another. The Citizens Commission on Human Rights, the agitprop wing of Scientology, was hanging on his every word and gleefully reprinting news articles about this "one-time pillar of the psychiatric establishment," as one report put it. Even the real Paula Caplan had reached out to congratulate him for his courage in an e-mail he forwarded to me under the subject line "Fate has an ironic sense of humor."

"Everything I say," he lamented, "is seized by the antipsychiatry fanatics and misused for their own unfortunate purposes."

The more his criticisms of DSM-5 were turned against his profession, the more he protested that he was Panza, not Quixote. Neither was he Saul, suddenly truth-struck on his way to Damascus and testifying to the new revelation, nor was he an apparatchik-turned-dissident denouncing his former comrades for their ideological excesses, nor was he a deposed emperor confessing to his own nakedness even as he exposed the new boss's. He was a loyal opponent, not an enemy of the state, and he wanted to make sure I understood that.

"Where you see intelligent conspiracy, I see dopey incompetence," he wrote. "In movie terms, you see APA and DSM-5 as *The Parallax View* meets *The Stepford Wives*. I see it as the Keystone Kops meets *The Gang That Couldn't Shoot Straight*."

"Dereification is just as dumb as reification," he told me. "A construct is just a construct—not to be worshiped and not to be denigrated." Psychiatry, he was saying, has to live in the tension between the desire for certainty about the nature of our suffering and the impossibility of understanding it (or ourselves) completely. A DSM that tries to end this tension by turning itself into a living document was bound to collapse into chaos; that was the cardinal error of the incompetent DSM-5 regime. But to criticize the nosological enterprise, and with it psychiatry itself because it can't achieve certainty was to erect a straw man and then burn it—and to endanger the good the profession could do. This, Frances told me, was the greater mistake. And he was sure I was making it.

"I like to think the best of you," he wrote. He wanted to think I was not so much against psychiatry in principle as "angrily disillusioned [that] there is no Santa Claus"—offended that it can't be as scientific as, say, physics. I was, he said, referring to James Joyce's *Ulysses*, an "upside-down Jesuit," demanding an explanation that religion never claimed to offer and then enthusiastically denouncing it for its failure to provide it.

If this was the case, then, like Kupfer and Regier, I was guilty only of incompetence. But there was another possibility. "The less charitable interpretation of your blind spot is that it fits your Caplanesque world-view"—that I was prejudiced against psychiatry, suspicious of its claim to dominion over our inner lives, and that its failure to live up to a trumped-up scientific standard, so baldly on display in the unfolding debacle, was only a convenient excuse for me to denounce it.

Which I suppose is true. Not that I am somehow determined to see psychiatry ridden out of the medical kingdom. Nor do I think all psychiatrists are drug-pushing Pharma dupes. But it hadn't been my idea to turn psychoanalysis into a branch of medicine in 1926. Neither had I had anything to do with the decision, made four decades ago, after the attempt to render the psyche as just another organ in the body had led to disaster, to save psychiatry by creating a DSM ripe for the reifying and then, when the categories became cumbersome or inadequate or just plain embarrassing, to blame others for taking them too seriously. Nor was it I who kept insisting, against all evidence, that the mind could be understood as the output of neurotransmitters, its suffering as chemical imbalances, and psychiatry as a Santa Claus doling out drugs from an ever-growing bag.

And here's where Frances had me dead to rights: in my worldview, for which I cannot blame Paula Caplan, there are more choices to explain events than Parallax or Keystone, conspiracy or coincidence. We are in the grip of history, I believe, and if its long arc does not bend in any foreordained direction, it is also not random. Which means that hamartia—the fatal, unrecognized flaw—is always tragedy waiting to happen and needs only the right story to be seen for what it is.

Frances might not agree with that. He's a literary man, but he also constantly warned me against reading meaning into the DSM. Still, our dispute wasn't only about the significance of the flaw, but about its nature as well, about what exactly it consisted of and where it was to be found. Since we'd met, he had been urging me to read *A Canticle for Leibowitz*, a novel by Walter Miller. At the end of November, I told him over the phone that I'd just finished the book, which turned out to be a pretty good piece of science fiction squarely in the postapocalyptic tradition. The title character, an electrical engineer named Isaac Leibowitz, has survived a twenty-sixth-century nuclear holocaust that has led to the Simplification, an era in which the elite and educated have been exterminated by the Simpletons, who have outlawed learning and destroyed books. But Leibowitz, along with a band of "bookleggers," has set out to preserve the world's scientific knowledge in a monastery library. (Leibowitz converted to Catholicism after the war.) That effort earns Leibowitz martyrdom and beatification, but his Memorabilia lives on, and by the thirty-eighth century, the knowledge contained in it has escaped the monastery, once again wreaking a holocaust, but not before a small group manages to blast off from Earth in a rocket ship, carrying, so we presume, the Leibowitzian Memorabilia and its destructive knowledge to another world.

"What's the ending mean?" he asked.

"That you have your choice between ignorance and survival or knowledge and death."

"And?"

"And what?"

He told me that Miller had been a tail gunner in World War II who had participated in the destruction of Montecassino, a Benedictine abbey in Italy. "He wrote the book as an expiation. He's writing about wise guys like you and me throwing hand grenades at traditions that we think are stupid. But those traditions have a value we might miss," he said. "It's the intellectuals who create the nuclear weapons. The dumb traditionalists turn out to have it right. A lot of false beliefs help people cope with life."

Frances's thin voice descended nearly into a growl. "So don't throw grenades unless you know what you are doing, Gary. Don't throw grenades. There are some traditions if you fuck with . . ." He trailed off. "You wouldn't want to tell a placebo responder he's on placebo."

The APA wasn't so happy with me, either.

Early in November, just about when Frances was admonishing me, I contacted its press office to clarify a point from my interview with Regier and to nail down the exact order of events that resulted in banishing the drug companies from its educational programs and from the stock portfolios of DSM contributors. I also asked if an APA official would comment on the psychologists' petition, now that it had amassed so many signatures. So far the press office had stayed silent, except to note that the petition was just one of the "thousands of comments" that had been heaved over its transom—all of which were "being reviewed by task force and work group members."

After a few days, I received this message from the APA's director of communications, Eve Herold.

> Dear Gary,
>
> We have received several requests from you for access to APA experts and positions on issues related to the DSM for the book you're writing. I wanted you to know that we will not be working with you on this project. Last year we gave you free access to several of our officers and DSM experts for the article you wrote for *Wired*. In spite of the fact that we went to considerable lengths to work with you, the article you produced was deeply negative and biased toward the APA. Because of this track record, we are not interested in working with you further as we have no reason to expect that we would be treated any more fairly in your book than we were in the *Wired* article.

I think she meant "biased against."

Glad as I was to be spared the APA's talking points, I didn't understand why it would preemptively surrender its opportunity to correct my errors or respond to its critics, who they had to know were talking to me. I also wondered how Herold was going to stop her "experts"—at least the ones who didn't work directly for her organization—from being in contact with me, which many of them had been doing all along, gladly and forthrightly. The confidentiality agreement hadn't stopped them. Would a communiqué from headquarters?

But mostly I was wondering if I would lose my job as a Collaborating Investigator in the field trials. I'd already put in eight hours or so, completing the Field Trials Human Subjects Protection Basic Training and mastering the Informed Consent Process, learning how to fill out the Patient Log, how to Register the Patient, how to log onto the Portal, how to Push the Data to the Clinician Database, looking over the REDCap Flowchart and Disorder Quick Reference Troubleshooting Guide, reading the sixty-page System Manual, and sitting through the ninety-minute Webinar. I'd taken the quizzes and practiced on the case vignettes, and finally, just a week before Herold's blow-off, I'd received an e-mail from the field trials team, informing me that I had completed the training and would soon be given access to the "LIVE database." Had I worked so hard and come so far, only to be cut from the team just as I was about to take the field?

I had my answer the next day in an e-mail from the field trials' operations manager. It wasn't a pink slip at all, but rather a congratulations on my having successfully completed the DSM-5 field trials training, and a new login and password for the field trials site.

It was astounding that the APA would forgo the opportunity to spin its story to me—not to mention so baldly display its Kremlin tactics, and in writing no less—and yet let me in for an unfiltered look at their prized field trials. Most likely, no one had figured out that the biased writer and the Collaborating Investigator were the same person (although I made no effort to conceal this fact, using the same contact information in both capacities). But another e-mail from the operations manager—a note that had come just a few hours after Herold's—suggested a different explanation. That message told me to disregard any e-mail I might have just gotten from her. As it happened, I hadn't received anything. But just in case I wanted an opportunity to disregard it, she attached the errant e-mail. It was a note from Kupfer and Regier, thanking me (for the third time) for participating in the field trials, but also urging me to complete the training, and letting me know that the task force had extended the deadline to do so. "We realize how challenging it is for practicing clinicians to find time to participate in research," they wrote, before reminding us about the CME credits and the free copy of the DSM-5, complete with our names listed in the back, that awaited us in May 2013.

It sounded as if they were having trouble getting those five thousand clinicians on board. Perhaps, like Michael First, who told me it was "hard to find a spare six hours to do it," they were just too busy, or maybe they thought a free book and their name in agate type were insufficient compensation for the task. Whatever the explanation, it appeared that I was among the very few. I may have been persona non grata in the communications department, but over at the research department, people like me were much in demand. Plague rat or not, they couldn't afford to toss me overboard.

Recruiting my first trial patient was easy enough. Lee and I were still in that phase of therapy in which we really liked each other—positive transference/countertransference, the Freudians would call it. She would not want to displease me—a good thing, as it turned out, when the test proved to take an hour and forty-five minutes to complete.

Not that Lee got nothing out of the deal. She did seem pretty thrilled to sit at my desk and use my computer. Back in the psychoanalytic days, surrendering my chair and my equipment would have been a meaning-rich event. What was it like for her to sit in my chair and use my computer? How did it feel to be asked for a favor by her therapist? That conversation is either silly or significant, depending on whether or not you believe that the secrets of who we are come into view most clearly in dreams and slips of the tongue and reactions to the unexpected, and deserve to be illuminated.

Lee and I did eventually talk about some of that. But those subjects hadn't been covered in my training as a Collaborating Investigator. Instead, I'd been drilled on the necessity of obtaining explicit informed consent, which meant acknowledging that "there may be no benefit for the patient from participating," and some risk—"that the patient may feel uncomfortable answering personal questions about thoughts and feelings." But, I was to assure the subject, those risks were minimal, and the patient could always "talk to the clinician about any concerns or upsetting feelings," and could bail at any time. I'd been warned to make sure she could not, while using my computer, gain access to confidential information. And, in the Webinar and the online training and the manual, I'd been given all the fine points of the software, how to save and retrieve and submit. Technical and legal considerations had replaced those hoary concerns about the actual meaning of the experience.

It's hard to imagine Lee was finding much meaning as she clicked on the Level 1 cross-cutting measures and the Level 2 measures for the Level 1 domains—mood, anxiety, sleep, and substance use—she'd flagged as troublesome, and answered the WHO Disability Assessment Schedule questions about "getting along with people" and "participation in society." Neither were we talking about what it meant for her to give me my chair and computer back, or watch me fumble through the next hour or so, opening the modules and going down the checklists and reading boldfaced alerts like this one:

> To make the diagnosis of Major Depressive Disorder, one has to rule out whether the major depressive episode is better accounted for by Schizoaffective Disorder and is superimposed on Schizophrenia, Schizophreniform Disorder, Delusional Disorder, or Psychotic Disorder Not Otherwise Specified. To do so you SHOULD inquire about history of schizoaffective disorder, schizophrenia, and/or any psychotic symptoms!!

I navigated the menus and proceeded through the forty-nine pages of mood disorders and the thirty-one pages of anxiety disorders, the eighteen pages of sleep-wake disorders, the sixty-three pages of substance use disorders (many pages of which could be skipped simply by deciding that I did not want to explore the possibility that Lee suffered from cannabis use disorder or circadian rhythm sleep disorder, but it wasn't entirely clear how I was supposed to know exactly which ones to skip; in all that training, I'd been left to my own devices to study up on the diagnoses themselves), and I concluded that she suffered from Major Depressive Disorder—Severe and Insomnia Disorder and Alcohol Use Disorder—in Full Remission, all the while feeling retroactive sympathy for Bill Narrow, who knew long before he put hand to mouse that Virginia Hamm was a hoarder just as much as I knew that Lee was a depressed insomniac with a drinking problem, but had to go through with the exercise anyway.

On the other hand, Narrow had a part in designing this 501-page monster and I didn't.

But what about when the fix wasn't in? What about someone I didn't really know? The second interview I was supposed to conduct was with a new patient, and Claudia fit the bill. She had shown up on a rainy night twenty minutes late for her first visit after three increasingly frenzied phone calls in which I assured her that her GPS was correct about how to get from where she was to my building and one more as she wandered the hallways looking for my office, which she did not find until, after another phone call, I went out to meet her. She was easy enough to spot, a tiny woman with a pixie haircut, frantically flitting from doorway to doorway like a lost Tinker Bell. When I found her, she pressed her hands together under her chin *Namaste*-style and bowed slightly, my credibility as guru evidently established simply by my knowing my way around my building. It was a gesture she repeated three or four times in the course of our visit, just after I'd made a comment. After she left, I tried but could not for the life of me recall what those comments might have been. It's possible my memory got lost in the jumble of details that poured out of her mouth at top speed (she suffered from what we therapists call *logorrhea*), but more likely, I hadn't said anything particularly insightful, being too busy absorbing her distress and confusion, her depression and anxiety and paranoia, her fragmented stories of her fraught love affairs with men and women, the way she flew from bed to bed like a hummingbird, alighting just long enough to sip some nectar, searching for the next flower before she was even finished with the last—the most recent being a man whom she had, after a flurry of texts and e-mails and aborted trysts, accompanied to a hotel room, only to find his girlfriend already installed, and she, for reasons she couldn't quite explain, but maybe it was the three martinis they drank, went ahead with his suggested sexual encounter with the girlfriend—and her troubles at her graphic design job, which she was afraid she was about to lose, or maybe she had lost already, she wasn't sure, but she was too afraid to ask her boss, with whom she had been having sex, but who was leaving the company and his replacement was gay, so he probably wasn't going to exchange job security for sex (not, she assured me, that this was what she'd been doing with the boss). Plus which she somehow had ended up with the boss's pet birds, three squawking cages full, who needed care and feeding beyond what she could give any longer, and what she really wanted to know from me was what to do about the birds.

Being with Claudia was like riding a raft through white water. I might be skeptical of the value of the DSM, but I was ready to try anything to channel these rapids into an orderly stream of information, a diagnosis that would grant me the ability to communicate efficiently about Claudia to at least one clinician—me. So I was glad to offer her the opportunity to participate in the study (and the free visit in return), and she, for reasons she never stated, but most likely at least in part because she didn't exactly know how to say no to men, was glad to consent.

The very next week, after one more visit, one more fruitless attempt to piece together some coherent story out of the fragments of her life, I surrendered my desk and computer to Claudia. Her finger hovered above the mouse frequently as she read over the items, sometimes out loud. She sighed and laughed and, a couple of times, had an extended conversation with the computer (only one side of which I could hear). Twice she came to a complete stop, staring at the screen for a minute or so without scrolling or clicking or reading, transfixed, I thought, by something else entirely. After forty-five minutes, she stood up, made her little bow, and returned to her chair.

I pushed the data. We had our work cut out for us. She'd scored high in all the cross-cutting domains except substance use, where she had a zero—a strange result, I thought, since so many of the escapades she had described in our first session were fueled by alcohol. I fumbled through the diagnostic interview a little less with her than I had with Lee. But then again, I had more time to plot my course through the criteria while Claudia pondered every question closely. She wasn't sure if she had "feelings of worthlessness or excessive and inappropriate guilt" or "excessive anxiety" or a "distinct period of abnormally and persistently elevated, expansive or irritable mood that lasted 4 consecutive days and was present most of the day nearly every day." She would give an answer and take it back and venture another, hovering over her response like a checkers player who never lifts his fingers from his piece, until I finally had to say, "Let's go on," and she let the last move stand.

Claudia was certain about some criteria. She did not drink too much. She was not confused about sex. And she did not have a "diminished ability to think or concentrate, or indecisiveness."

I don't think she was lying. I think she was, as we therapists say, in denial. And who could blame her? She was too mercurial for introspection, and even if she hadn't been, these weren't exactly the best conditions under which to reveal her frailties and flaws. I was, after all, still more or less unknown to her, our lack of intimacy at wild odds with my probing, no less so than it is in the gynecologist's office, only here there was no sheet to cover her, no nurse to hold her hand or distract her, and

I was not crouched where she couldn't see me, but looking right in her eyes as I asked questions made indecent by their detachment from anything real or live between us. Efflorescent inner life rendered as symptom by a stranger wielding the DSM's computerized language as if it were a speculum: who would not resist?

It had been a little more than an hour since Claudia had relinquished the computer, nearly two hours since we had started this dispiriting adventure. I decided to skip the substance use disorders despite my doubts about her answers and click right to the part I had originally thought might yield something useful, a way to organize my own thoughts in the face of her chaos: the personality disorders section.

At first, it looked straightforward enough. There was ample "evidence of impairments" in her "experience of self as unique with clear boundaries between self and others," in the stability of her self-image and her "ability to regulate [her] emotional experience." Yes, she had some problems with intimacy. But how much impairment? REDCap wanted to know. On a scale of zero to four, just how fucked up was Claudia?

Here I was given a choice. I could "proceed directly to rating" and pull a number out of the air, or I could get a "detailed description of levels." I went for the details, which turned out to be extensive, three pages of description about "identity" and "self-direction" and "empathy" and "intimacy." Was she a Level 2—"Excessive dependence on others for identity definition, with compromised boundary delineation"? Or did she have the "weak sense of autonomy/agency" and "poor or rigid boundary definition" of a Level 3? Or was her experience of autonomy/agency "virtually absent," and her boundaries "confused or lacking," which earned her a Level 4? Was her self-esteem "fragile" (Level 3) or merely "vulnerable" (2), or perhaps riddled with "significant distortions" and "confusions" (4)? Was her capacity for empathy "significantly compromised," "significantly limited," or "virtually absent"?

Was her desire for connection with others "desperate," "limited," or "largely based on meeting self-regulatory needs?"

I had no idea. And even if I had, or if I knew how to get this confused and confusing woman to parse it for me, there still loomed thirty pages or so to get through, box after box to check about her self and interpersonal functioning, her separation insecurity and depressivity, her negative affectivity and disinhibition, the types and facets and domains of her traits, hundreds of boxes, or so it seemed, before I could make my final diagnosis, and, with the authority vested in me as a Collaborating Investigator of the American Psychiatric Association, determine which of the constructs that deserve neither denigration nor worship, that aren't real but still can be measured from zero to four, that need to be taken seriously enough to warrant payment and maybe a round of medication but not so seriously that anyone would accuse them of existing, which fictive placeholder would join her height and blood pressure and her childhood illnesses and surgeries and all the other facts of her medical life. At which point I realized that no matter what diagnosis I settled on, I wouldn't so much have tamed her rapids as funneled them into the diagnostic turbines, raw material for the APA's profitable mills.

I was longing for the pre-DSM-III days when I could have read this paragraph:

> This behavior pattern is characterized by ineffectual responses to emotional, social, intellectual, and physical demands. While the patient seems neither physically nor mentally deficient, he does manifest inadaptability, ineptness, poor judgment, social instability, and lack of physical and emotional stamina.

I could have then written down this diagnosis, perhaps cruel but to the point: inadequate personality. Not that *ineffectual* and *deficient* are any easier to define, but at least the DSM-II wasn't asking me to rate them on a scale of zero to four. At least it didn't first claim that they were real enough to measure and then insist that they weren't real at all.

"I think we'll stop here," I said.

"How did I come out?" Claudia asked.

It was a totally reasonable question. She'd just invested more than two hours in this procedure. After this kind of grilling, anyone would wonder. And Claudia might have been hoping the same thing I was— that somehow this process would provide some kind of clarity about her.

"Oh, I won't know right away." It was only a partial lie. Overwhelmed by the data, I had already forgotten which diagnoses I'd reached, and now that I'd clicked Send, I couldn't go back and look. I wouldn't know until I opened the files into which I'd been downloading the forms as we went.

I wanted to ask her how this interview had been for her. I wanted to apologize to her for the inadequacy, the pointlessness, the sheer idiocy of the exercise, for the two hours I'd spent with her during which we had not only failed to get closer to each other or to an understanding of her troubles but actually, I worried, moved further away. It was nearly nine at night. I'd been in my office since eight that morning. So I thanked her for helping me out and scheduled her next appointment and said good night.

I never saw Claudia again. I don't know why. She just didn't show for her next appointment and never returned my phone calls. Maybe she decided therapy wasn't for her, or I wasn't the therapist she should see. Maybe she ran out of money. But I'll always think it had something to do with those two hours of flailing about in the fields of the DSM, that my failure to take the measure of her suffering had turned into her failure to measure up, that the futility of the field trial had made the whole therapeutic enterprise seem futile, that when the DSM's desiccated vocabulary, at least in the hands of a nonbeliever, proved no match for the immensity of her suffering, Claudia had lost that most precious thera-peutic commodity: confidence.

Just before Christmas, the APA sent out *Inside DSM-5 Field Trials: Your Voice in Action!*, a newsletter for us participants. "The journey into the future begins with a few small steps," it proclaimed. But apparently not enough of us were taking them. "We understand that these steps can be time consuming, or even a bit confusing," the article continued, "but we believe that the value of training and participating extends far beyond that of the field trials." It didn't say exactly what other benefit lay in store for us, but it did reassure us that the APA staff was standing by to help us achieve it.

Farther down the page was the reason the APA had had to resort to badgering us. Of the 5,000 clinicians who had signed up, only 1,000 had so far started training, only 195 had completed the training, and only 70 had enrolled any patients. The newsletter writers did their best to sound upbeat—"in fact, nearly 150 patients have joined the study," they wrote, leaving out the fact that the goal was 10,000—but anyone with a calen-dar could see the problem. More than a year after the sign-ups began, three months after Kupfer and Regier had sent out their plea for co-operation, and only two months before the data had to be in, the RCP trials had scarcely begun.

That look at the calendar revealed an even more disturbing problem. The APA had originally planned two sets of field trials—the first to re-veal the bugs, the second to make sure they'd been shaken out. The sec-ond phase was originally scheduled to end in February 2012. But even though the academic center field trials were progressing better than the clinician version—and by some accounts were largely finished, although no one would say—their findings still weren't in, and no release date had been given. Neither had the APA announced the inevitable result: that the second phase would have to be canceled if the DSM-5 was to be published on time. That news had just appeared when a new timeline was posted on the website.

Something else had shown up quietly on the website. The banner at the bottom of every page, which, as recently as July 2011, had proclaimed that the APA represented "38,000 physician leaders in mental health," had been changed. The organization now represented only 36,000 doctors. And at the end of 2011, the treasurer delivered grim news to the remaining members: Annual income from the drug industry, once $18 million, was now only $4 million. Meeting revenues were off by $1.6 million. Ad revenues had sunk to $6 million, off their high of $10 million. Membership dues were down by $500,000. Thanks to cuts in expenditures, the APA was still running a surplus of about $2.85 million, but, the treasurer reported, "this is due to a [$5.6 million] surplus for American Psychiatric Press," whose most profitable property was, as it had long been, the DSM. Without the DSM, in other words, the APA would have lost nearly $3 million.

These numbers only strengthened the concern among critics like Frances that in its haste to freshen its cash cow, the APA was trampling over science. That, of course, was impossible to prove, but one thing was clear: toward the end of 2011, the APA was patrolling its intellectual property lines more vigilantly than ever, as a woman in England found out the hard way. For a couple of years, Suzy Chapman, a patient advocate, had been running a blog called *Dsm5watch*. Chapman, a caregiver for a patient with chronic fatigue syndrome, was interested primarily in developments related to CFS, but her blog covered the entire revision process (as well as that of the International Classification of Diseases). Unlike the APA, which removed old criteria and timelines as it changed them, Chapman had preserved excerpts from earlier iterations of the DSM-5, and her website, which also collected news and opinion pieces about DSM, had thus become one of the largest and most reliable repositories of revision-related information on the Web.

This may or may not be why, on December 22, she received a letter from Cecilia Stoute, the licensing and permissions manager of the American Psychiatric Press. It wasn't a Christmas card.

"It has come to our attention," Stoute wrote, "that the website http://dsm5watch.wordpress.com/ is infringing upon the American Psychiatric Association's trademark DSM-5 (serial number 85161695) and is in violation of federal law by using it as a domain name." Chapman's "unauthorized actions," Stoute continued, "may subject you to contributory infringement liability including increased damages for willful infringement." To avoid that outcome, Chapman must "immediately cease and desist any and all use of the DSM-5 mark" and remove it from her domain name.

"I thought it was a hoax," Chapman told me—an impression reinforced by a second letter she received, this one instructing her to remove the DSM-5 mark from a second website, as well as a Facebook page and a Twitter account. But those domains didn't belong to her and never had. They were run by the psychologists who originated the petition. Those sites remained online despite the APA's copyright, as did Dsm5.com, Newdsm5.com, Dsm-5diagnosis.com, Dsm5band.com (INSANITY NEVER SOUNDED SO GOOD!), and even Dsm5sucks.com.

But no matter how outlandish the claim or how selective the action or how shaky the APA's legal grounds, and no matter how much the move reeked of intimidation, Chapman felt she had no choice but to comply. "I could not finance a legal wrangle with the APA," she told me, adding that she feared that her blog's host would remove her site at the first sign of trouble, wiping out years of work with a single keystroke. So she changed her blog name to *Dxrevisionwatch*. As she feared, the new URL caused her readership to plummet to nearly zero—but not for long. On January 3, Frances wrote about Chapman's travails in his *Psychology Today* blog. Within a couple of weeks, traffic to her website was double its pre-putsch levels.

That's probably not what the APA had in mind.

The incident left Chapman wondering about the APA. "What kind of organization slaps heavy legal threats on a member of the public just two days before Christmas, when it would be hard to get legal advice? What kind of organization is so lax that it issues cease-and-desist letters without having first established who owns the contested domains?"

The answer was obvious: an organization that was both intelligently conspiratorial *and* dopily incompetent. Or, as they might say in Hollywood, *The Gang That Couldn't Shoot Straight* meets *The Parallax View*.

Chapter 18

Speaking of conspiracies, Darrel Regier had a theory about Allen Frances's complaint that the DSM-5 would extend the reach of psychiatry into everyday life. "The idea of medicalizing normality," he told a reporter in late January, "comes from a perspective that there are no psychiatric disorders, and you need to avoid stigmatizing people by giving them one."

It's possible that Regier had joined the crowd who believed that the former most powerful psychiatrist in America had become a devout antipsychiatrist. Or maybe he had just misunderstood what Frances really meant. But it's also possible that Regier was getting desperate.

You couldn't exactly blame him. The middle of January 2012 was the start of a terrible month-long period for him, the APA, and the DSM-5.

The first storm blew in from offshore on January 19, when Fred Volkmar gave a talk to the Icelandic Medical Association. Volkmar and a couple of his Yale colleagues had dusted off the data from the DSM-IV field trials for childhood disorders and then applied the proposed DSM-5 criteria to the same subjects. They determined that only 44 percent of the subjects who had received a diagnosis in the original study would have made it onto the proposed autism spectrum. And only twelve of the forty-eight original Asperger's patients—the same cases that had unexpectedly strengthened the case for including Asperger's in the DSM-IV—would have qualified under the new regime.

Volkmar had presented much of this data before, at a November meeting of the American Academy of Child and Adolescent Psychiatry in Toronto, but he wasn't in any hurry to have it known by the general public. "I wasn't exactly hiding it," he told me. "But I am (or have been) friends with a number of people on the committee, and I knew that this would cause bad feeling." And, he added, "I knew that the powers that be would take no hostages on this one." So he didn't approach reporters with the incendiary news that three-quarters of Asperger's patients might soon be losing their diagnoses (or wouldn't be getting them in the first place).

But then Benedict Carey, the *New York Times* reporter on the psychiatry beat, happened to call Volkmar on the eve of his trip to Iceland, fishing for news on the autism front. Volkmar still didn't draw attention to the data reanalysis, but he did send Carey the slides from his upcoming presentation, and as soon as Carey saw the slide listing its results, he grasped their significance. His front-page story, "New Definition of Autism Will Exclude Many," appeared on January 19 and quickly rocketed around the world via newspaper, TV, and blog. The *Times* followed up the next day with a story about the possible impact of a reduction in diagnoses on children and their families.

When he heard the news, GRASP's Michael Carley was already rethinking his position in favor of the DSM-5 proposal—and not only because of Volkmar's research. He'd gotten hold of another soon-to-be-published article, this one from a group at Louisiana State University, that had concluded the new criteria would exclude 37 percent of the patients, most of them at the high-functioning end of the spectrum. He now found himself siding with his son.

"It was one thing to make a change that relabeled people," Carley told me, "and another to make a change that they knew would exclude so many."

The promises the APA had issued since announcing the proposals now seemed like mere "damage control," Carley told his members. "We think those who reassuringly tell us, 'No one will be left behind,' really mean, 'No one will be left behind who deserves a diagnosis under the DSM-5 criteria.'" He now urged GRASPers to take action: by signing a petition opposing the changes and by flooding the APA's phone lines with complaints. "Yes, they are telling you to e-mail instead," he acknowledged. "But we ask that you please instead be the articulate, impassioned, and peaceful nuisance that is needed in this debate, and not adhere to their instructions."

The APA scrambled its experts, but they couldn't seem to agree on their talking points. "We have to make sure not everybody who is a little odd gets a diagnosis of autism or Asperger's disorder," David Kupfer told *The New York Times*. Cathy Lord echoed this concern, telling the same reporter that her work group wanted to make sure "that autism was not used as a 'fallback diagnosis.'" But she also reassured readers that "the committee's own data shows very few who currently have a diagnosis would be dropped." She didn't say why, if the problem was so insignificant, the committee had gone to so much trouble to fix it.

Another work group member, Bryan King, tried a different approach. The question of overdiagnosis had never even been relevant to the proceedings, he claimed. "There has never been an agenda for us to restrict or limit the numbers of people diagnosed with autism," he told *Medscape Medical News*, an industry outlet. "We've only wanted to get the criteria right," he continued, as if a reduction of diagnoses was only a side effect of a drastic reduction in the number of possible symptom combinations that could result in a diagnosis. And even if a few people lost their official labels, they had nothing to fear: if one label disappears, he said, "then a different label will appear in its place. There will always be a way to capture the need for treatment."

King didn't say exactly what label was waiting in the wings for those fallback-diagnosed, a-little-odd kids who may or may not exist. Neither, apparently, did he realize he was giving up the game, acknowledging that *capturing* rather than *establishing* the need for treatment had become the purpose of diagnosis, nor did he consider how antipsychiatrists would treat that comment. After all, if every complaint that brings a person to a doctor demands a diagnosis, the next thing you know you'll have a wholesale imperial medicalization of normality.

King was clear on one thing: Volkmar had unduly scared the bejesus out of people, at least to judge by the calls to King's clinic, where the phones, he said, had been "ringing off the hook."

At APA headquarters, despite Carley's efforts, it wasn't the phones that were taking the brunt. It was Regier's e-mail in-box, which, he told a reporter, had been deluged with "10,000 plus e-mails" in the wake of the *New York Times* articles. Regier added that he would have liked to respond to Volkmar's numbers with his own, but he "was not willing to give detailed data . . . until [they] are subjected to peer review and are published." He didn't add "like some people I know," but the implication was clear: Volkmar wasn't playing fair, and Regier was once again the victim of his own scrupulousness. And in case he hadn't sufficiently questioned Volkmar's integrity, Regier threw another elbow, telling a reporter that Volkmar had a new book coming out about Asperger's—a book whose market might well disappear with the diagnosis.

"I hope this is not what he said," Volkmar responded, when the reporter passed along the comment.

"There is certainly a better way to phrase this," Regier wrote back (after complaining that he hadn't had much luck in "changing how journalists present a story"). "The point I was making is that Fred has a particular interest in Asperger's," he explained. That, evidently, was the best phrasing he could find.

Only five days after the autism story broke, a Carey-penned DSM piece once again made the front page of *The New York Times*. This time around, the hook was a *World Psychiatry* article by Jerry Wakefield and Michael First questioning the evidence on which the proposal to remove the bereavement exclusion was based. Their argument was a detailed refutation of the research that Sid Zisook and his colleagues had mustered in favor of their notion that there wasn't enough difference between bereavement-related depression and all other depression to warrant the exclusion.

"An estimated 8 to 10 million people lose a loved one every year, and something like a third to a half of them suffer depressive symptoms for up to a month afterward," Wakefield told Carey. "This would pathologize them for behavior previously thought to be normal." The article went on to detail the other DSM-5 proposals that threatened to raise the prevalence of mental disorders—Attenuated Psychosis Symptoms Syndrome, Binge Eating Disorder, Premenstrual Dysphoric Disorder. Carey quoted a psychiatrist who forecast a wider use of drugs as a result and let Frances issue yet another warning about the medicalizing of normality. Some experts were worried about the "corrosive effect" all this "politicking" might have on the revision process, Carey wrote, but others—including Steve Hyman and his successors at NIMH—thought it was mostly beside the point, which was why they were no longer interested in the DSM. "Nature does not respect psychiatric categories," Carey concluded, and added that while there might someday be a nosology that nature would respect, "until then, there . . . will be the diagnostic manual."

Carey gave Jay Scully an opportunity to defend the APA's position. Rather than address the questions raised by the article, however, Scully decided to blame the messengers. "We've got electronic media around the clock, and we've made drafts of the proposed changes public online, for one thing," he told Carey. "So anybody and everybody can comment on them, at any time, without any editors." It was a curious tactic, and one that didn't shed much light on the subject of diagnostic inflation, but then again, Scully couldn't respond to that worry with reassuring statistics about prevalence from the field trials—and not because, as Regier had implied, the detailed data awaited analysis or because professional decorum demanded reticence, but because there was no such data, and there would never be any.

Helena Kraemer, chief architect of the field trials, had said as much earlier in January. Writing in the *American Journal of Psychiatry*, she had "set out realistic expectations" for her project, starting with the "contentious issue" of prevalence. Rates were going to change, Kraemer warned. Some new criteria were going to pick up more mental disorder in the population, and some were going to exclude people who might previously have been included. The only way to avoid these outcomes would be "to require that any existing difference between true and DSM-IV prevalence be reproduced in DSM-5"—or, to put it another way, to rig the game to leave prevalence unchanged. "Thus," Kraemer concluded, "there are no specific expectations about the prevalence of disorders in DSM-5."

But who was expecting that diagnostic rates would remain unchanged? Surely not Wakefield and First and Frances, or any of the civilians worried about the reach of psychiatry. Like Kraemer, they fully expected prevalence to change; what worried them was the possibility this would lead to epidemiological chaos. But unlike Kraemer, they weren't in a position to find out, and, as she made clear in her very next sentence, she was not going to do that.

"The evaluations primarily address reliability," Kraemer wrote, as if it somehow followed that because prevalence rates were bound to change, they weren't worth looking into.*

She didn't explain further, so it is possible that this is not what she meant. Perhaps Regier had decided the problem that attracted him to the field—the Midtown Manhattan Study's wild prevalence rates—was

*The APA did eventually try to use the academic field trick to assess prevalence by comparing each subject's DSM-IV and DSM-5 diagnosis, and measuring whether the new criteria would create more cases of any particular disorder. But because the two diagnoses were made by two different raters, the results were of questionable value. It was, as one insider put it, a "half-assed way to determine prevalence."

suddenly unimportant, or Kupfer had decided to leave the question to his imaginary gadfly friends. Maybe Kraemer thought her readers would leap over the gap in logic and assume that the only reasonable thing to do was to abandon the subject of how many people would be declared mentally ill in favor of the question of whether psychiatrists could agree on which mental illnesses they had. (Of course, as she had announced the previous May and repeated in the *AJP* article, people should temper their expectations about that subject as well.) But whatever the reasoning, it was clear that the field trials hadn't been designed to address the issue. In fact, it seemed as if they'd been designed not to, as if the prevalence question needed to be avoided at all costs because the answers might be too disturbing, because they couldn't help but point to the fact that the diagnostic sands were still shifting, and thus undermine confidence in the APA.

Okay, maybe that's too much like *The Parallax View*. Certainly the APA's disorganized, off-the-point, whiny response was pretty Keystone Kops. And even the most sure-footed organization might well have been knocked to its knees by the rush of events.

Scully and his crew barely had time to draw breath before *The New York Times* struck again—this time with a pair of op-ed columns about Asperger's appearing on the same day, one by a psychiatrist who acknowledged that it was overdiagnosed (and looked forward to a time when "biological markers" would separate the sick from the weird), and the other by Benjamin Nugent, a writer whose psychologist mother, an expert in Asperger's, had diagnosed him with the disorder when he was a teenager, but who, after he "moved to New York City and . . . met some people who shared my obsessions," realized he wasn't sick at all.

Before the APA could accuse all these writers of believing that mental illnesses don't exist, or wonder if the Church of Scientology had bought *The New York Times*, the news that the DSM-5 would throw kids out into the diagnostic cold had spread to more than one hundred outlets in twelve countries. In Great Britain, a group of dissenting psychologists and psychiatrists called a press conference. "The proposals in DSM-5 are likely to shrink the pool of normality to a puddle," one of them said, and the sound bite made it into papers and blogs all over the world. *The Lancet*, perhaps the most venerable of all medical journals, ran, in a single issue, a report on research showing Attenuated Psychosis Risk Syndrome to be invalid, an editorial decrying the removal of the bereavement exclusion, and a moving essay by the Harvard medical anthropologist Arthur Kleinman about his grief after losing his wife of forty-six years. A year later, Kleinman wrote, "I still feel sadness at times and harbour the sense that a part of me is gone forever.... I am still caring for our memories. Is there anything wrong (or pathological) with that?" Even politicians were piling on. State legislators in Illinois and New York introduced bills proposing to make the DSM-IV definition of autism, Asperger's, and Pervasive Developmental Disorder the law of their lands, "even if," as the Illinois version put it, "subsequent changes to the diagnostic criteria are adopted by the American Psychiatric Association."

So it's no wonder the APA was on its heels and in disarray. Or at least that's my explanation for their surprisingly ineffectual response. When they weren't launching ad hominem attacks or whining that they were the misunderstood victims of their own good intentions, or repeating their long-stale talking points to reporters and in mostly ignored press releases, they were silent. They didn't bother responding, by letter or column, to the onslaught in *The New York Times*. They didn't answer Kleinman or *The Lancet* or hold a news conference of their own to counter the British renegades' arguments. They didn't expound on the philosophical and scientific conundrums posed by psychiatric diagnosis. They didn't argue that diagnostic uncertainty was the rule rather than the exception in medicine. They didn't warn people not to take the DSM too seriously. They didn't even make the obvious point that the two articles in the *Times*—one of which thrashed the APA for diagnosing too few people, the other for diagnosing too many—were at least an indication that it wasn't trying to fix the game either way. Perhaps the APA's leaders were shell-shocked, or tired, or simply lacked the intellectual horsepower to respond. Maybe they really believed, as David Kupfer told *MedPage Today*, that even though the deadline was rapidly approaching, "the door is still very much open" to changes. Or maybe they had figured out that when the DSM-5 came out in May 2013, none of these complaints, no matter how trenchant or eloquent, not Frances's or Wakefield's or First's, not *The New York Times'* or *The Lancet's*—not one of them would matter. Maybe they decided that since they had the ball—indeed, they owned the ball—they could just duck their heads and run out the clock.

There was one other DSM-related op-ed in *The New York Times* in late January. I wrote it. "You've got to feel sorry for the American Psychiatric Association," it began, "at least for a moment." I wasn't being entirely ironic. I did feel a little sorry for the APA. Not that the organization deserved my sympathy or needed my help, but there was something nearly pathetic about its inability to mount a spirited defense of its own work, about the fear that prevented it from telling us what all its members knew: that the disorders listed in the DSM were not real diseases, but, as my essay put it, "useful constructs that capture the ways people commonly suffer," that this is why the arguments were fraught and endless, and that it was foolish to think this task force would come up with anything better than previous task forces: provisional categories that would inevitably change with time. The APA couldn't, or wouldn't, say this—perhaps because it would turn into fodder for its enemies—so I said it for them. It seemed like the least I could do.

Plus I got to quote Herb Peyser: "We're like Cinderella's older stepsisters. We're trying to stick our fat feet into the delicate slipper so the prince can take us to the ball. But we ain't going to the ball right now." I thought this image captured the problem perfectly. I still do.

I did not receive a thank-you note from the APA's Office of Communications. That might be because I ended the essay by saying that even if it wasn't going to the ball anytime soon, once the DSM-5 came out, the APA would be laughing all the way to the bank. But I did get an e-mail from Frances, sent at six a.m. the day the article ran. In its entirety, it read:

From: Allen Frances
To: Gary Greenberg
Subject: As the scorpion told the frog

What do you expect, I am a scorpion.

Sent from my Verizon Wireless BlackBerry

I asked him to elaborate and got this back:

When you had an incredible platform to help contain DSM 5 damage, you couldn't contain your antipsychiatry quixotic instincts and instead had bigger fish to fry. This is unfortunate for a Panza like me (with much smaller ambitions like protecting kids from antipsychotics) because your broadside against psychiatry allows the DSM 5 crowd to simply shrug you off . . . So in tilting against windmills, you made yourself irrelevant to DSM 5.

I'm not sure where Frances got the idea that I wanted to be heard by the DSM-5 crowd. It was clear, however, why he saw my article as anti-psychiatry: because I had said out loud, while standing on that "incredible platform," that his profession's authority rested on nothing more than agreement among experts. Not that he denied this, but he was sure it should not be said so publicly, and it was making him wonder if he'd made a mistake by being so candid with me.

"I often ask myself why I am so good to you when I know you will stab psychiatry in the back," he had written earlier. He answered his own question. "It is the Prince Myshkin in me." But, as was often the case when Frances called himself an idiot, it seemed his real barb was directed elsewhere.

Frances's winter of discontent was lasting into spring. "The man is an absolute fool and an incorrigible tool," he wrote of one DSM-5 activist. The psychologists' petition was "dying as the feckless humanists fiddle." Paula Caplan had started her own petition, calling for a boycott of the DSM and for congressional hearings into the harmful effects of psychiatric diagnosis. Infighting among the groups opposing the APA was growing. "This is getting really disgusting," he wrote.

There were a couple of bright spots. Late in February, the Department of Health and Human Services confirmed that the ICD-10 would not be implemented until October 2014, meaning that the APA no longer needed to hurry the DSM to publication in 2013. In early March, a psychologist's blog post about the bereavement exclusion attracted 65,000 hits in four days—"a spontaneous revolt by the large community of the bereaved," Frances wrote in the *Psychiatric Times*—and his latest hope for a tipping point. And the APA handed him a rhetorical opportunity when it hired James Tyll, a former Pentagon flack, to handle its DSM communications, and he promptly told a *Time* reporter that Frances was a "'dangerous' man trying to undermine an earnest academic endeavor."

"Fresh from DoD," Frances riposted in *The Huffington Post*, "it may be difficult for the new spokesman to leave behind combat clichés. Who knows? I may have become a picture card in his deck of high-value targets."

But overall Frances's tone was darkening. "How can you possibly continue to fiddle?" he asked his former friends on the back channel. In an open letter he urged the board of trustees to keep the bereavement exclusion, get rid of Disruptive Mood Dysregulation Disorder and Attenuated Psychosis Symptoms Syndrome, and abandon Hebephilia "before more harm is done." Take these steps, he wrote, and they would prevent a further loss of "public and professional faith," reduce the likelihood of overdiagnosis and overmedication, and "allow me to throw my cursed BlackBerry into the ocean." And in case that wasn't enough to spur them to action, he added that "as the responsible leaders of the APA, you cannot avoid your fiduciary responsibility to regain control of the staff and to rein in a runaway DSM-5 process." Otherwise, he wrote, they risked "dramatically reduced DSM-5 sales, APA budget shortfalls, declining membership, and the potential loss of the DSM franchise."

After all his appeals to common sense and professional wisdom, to aristocratic humility and the spirit of moderation, Frances was apparently reduced to hoping that it was true what they say about capitalism: that money talks.

"Wonderful news," Frances blogged in late April. He had caught wind of some changes—that Attenuated Psychosis Symptoms Syndrome and Mixed Anxiety-Depression would be placed in the Appendix of the DSM-5, as would Internet Use Disorder, and that Hebephilia was not going to get its own diagnostic category (although it would probably be listed as a subtype of Pedophilia). Regier and Kupfer attributed these changes to data from the field trials, but to Frances, this meant that they had finally, and wisely, concluded that there was indeed such a thing as bad publicity.

"For the first time in its history," he wrote, "DSM-5 has shown some . . . capacity to correct itself." There were still many outstanding concerns (and just in case the APA had lost track, he listed twelve of them), but it seemed that "extensive criticism from experts . . . public outrage . . . negative press coverage," as well as the data, had paid off. Frances wasted no time in using this as a rallying point for his troops, urging them to exploit "this opening chink in the previously impervious DSM-5 armor" and "take this last opportunity to be heard."

More bad news was soon filtering out from the field trials, though, including a rumor that Major Depressive Disorder and Generalized Anxiety Disorder, longtime staples in the psychiatric pantry, had achieved extremely low reliability scores, an indication that those little tweaks, coupled with the poor design of the study, had made a huge difference, and this strengthened Frances's fears that the reliability numbers would be a "stain on psychiatry."

"Looks like I wasted my time," he wrote me. "Cassandra, not Cincinnatus."

Though it had relented on some of the diagnoses, the APA was showing no signs of changing its tactics. Indeed, it reprised one of its earliest moves. In mid-April, just a couple of weeks before the APA's annual meeting, members of the task force and work groups received a communiqué from Kupfer and Regier, reminding them that the confidentiality agreement to which Spitzer had objected (but which they had signed) had new implications now that studies were appearing in the academic press using the proposals they had generated.

"We encourage the wide dissemination of these important studies," the memo read, but lest anyone get it in their heads to go Volkmar on the APA, Kupfer and Regier wanted to "remind you that the content and work products that have been generated as part of your ongoing activities . . . is [sic] considered to be the property of the APA." This meant that "permission is required for its use," which in turn required that any outside publisher obtain a license from the APA to use its intellectual property. As for people who might have unwittingly violated the copyright agreement already, "please let us know immediately so that we can work out any copyright issues before publication."

So it wasn't just outsiders such as Suzy Chapman who needed to fear the copyright police. Nor was it only publication that might attract their notice. "We ask that you refrain from submitting any manuscripts . . . without first consulting the APA's American Psychiatric Publishing," Kupfer and Regier wrote. Simply circulating a paper was a no-no. "It is imperative that our publishing arm and attorney be made aware of any such instances," and also of any papers already under consideration. Indeed, it seemed, any attempt to use the material published on the DSM-5 website in any venue not approved by the APA would be considered a violation of a copyright that the lawyers were gearing up to enforce vigorously.

The APA had evidently figured out that money doesn't just talk. It can also prevent talking.

"What possible copyright excuse can there be?" Frances asked, when I told him about the memo.

"It is just too nutty," he wrote a week later. The memo, the "crazy low reliabilities," the fact that essential questions had not begun to be addressed, the way Kupfer and Regier were living inside an echo chamber and doing all they could to seal off the DSM from the outside world, the flagrant violation of the most basic academic and scientific freedoms—suddenly this wasn't just Keystone Kops antics anymore.

"I used to compare them to the Kremlin," he wrote. "But they are really North Korea and that is a whole lot more dangerous. Expect chaos."

Chapter 19

A little bit of chaos did break out at the APA's 2011 annual meeting in Philadelphia, in the form of a couple hundred Occupy the APA: Boycott Normal protesters, waving signs (DSM—MEDICALIZING THE SYMPTOMS OF LIFE) and chanting chants ("Hey, hey, APA! How many kids did you kill today?"). Kim Jong-un would probably have approved of the notices urging attendees to check the credentials of strangers approaching them with questions (because people "presenting themselves as journalists are not always who they say they are") and to refer the unbadged to the Office of Communications and Public Affairs; the Supreme Leader might even have given an extra food ration to the security guard who broke up a family photo session in the main lobby, citing an APA edict banning unauthorized picture taking.

But the Occupiers were corralled at one entrance to the sprawling convention center, and at least one unsanctioned (and officially persona non grata) journalist—that would be me—roamed the halls unmolested, asking questions of whomever he liked, and if the scene was a little more tense than in Honolulu, brotherly love reigned supreme over chaos and fascism most of the time. John Livesley's highly public resignation from the personality disorders work group, announced just the week before, didn't stop him from participating collegially in forums with the remaining members, and Andrew Skodol met the continuing, now nearly universal outcry against the personality disorders proposals with charm and equanimity. Michael First learned that despite his criticisms, the APA was probably going to renew his franchise on two DSM-related products—the Structured Clinical Interview for DSM Disorders and a handbook of differential diagnosis—and would ("after I sign my life away") provide him with advance copies so he could get to work. Darrel Regier and David Kupfer were all smiles and handshakes as they greeted colleagues before their first presentation about the DSM, held on the first morning of the meeting.

The session was just a warm-up, an opportunity for Kupfer and Regier to reiterate the shortcomings of the DSM-IV, to talk about paradigm shifts without quite saying whether or not the new book would constitute one, to once again list all the effort, time, and money that had gone into the revision. As he had in Hawaii, Lawson Wulsin, the APA's liaison to other medical specialties, gave his advice on psychiatry's ongoing struggle for respectability and money. "Mental illness has been promoted to constituting a respectable public health problem," he said. This meant that psychiatrists now had a huge opportunity, but only if they could "learn how to work outside their comfort zone, and how to get well paid for it." The key to this, he continued, was joining other medical specialties in "integrated care settings," where they could deliver "measurement-based care." The DSM-5, with its focus on dimensional measures, would be one of the tools psychiatrists could use to "do well and win at that game."

The afternoon symposium was the main event—the public announcement of the results of the field trials. Before the packed room could hear the numbers, however, Helena Kraemer once again described her methodology—and the problems with the DSM-III and DSM-IV that she had attempted to remedy. Since she'd presented it the previous year in Hawaii, her critique had become a full-on broadside against Spitzer and Frances. Their sample sizes were too small. They had created conditions that were too pristine. They had invited conflicts of interest, letting work groups design the field trials, allowing clinicians to choose subjects most likely to qualify for the diagnosis in question, taking too much of a hand in adapting the kappa statistic to the DSM-III, focusing too much on maintaining prevalence rates in DSM-IV. "There was a bias in those studies," she said. Spitzer and Frances had feathered their own nests, but no matter how good the results made their DSMs look, they were "badly inflated and that causes a problem now."

The resulting problem—unreasonable expectations of how reliable psychiatric diagnosis should (or could) be—had a solution. It was the downward adjustment she had first suggested at the previous annual meeting, the one where she announced that a kappa of .2 would be "acceptable."

"I regret that now," she said, but not because such a low number was unacceptable. What she actually meant was that a result of .2 "*might* be accepted." A very low kappa, she allowed, was a "point of worry," but by no means should it be automatically discarded. In fact, an overall reduction in reliability numbers would signify not that the criteria (or the tests) were faulty, but that the APA's researchers had succeeded in duplicating the messiness of the real world.

By that standard, the field trials were an unalloyed triumph. It was left to Regier to announce the results of the studies conducted at academic medical centers. He led with schizophrenia, which had achieved a kappa of .81 in DSM-III and .76 in DSM-IV, but in the DSM-5 came in at .46. Alcohol Use Disorder scored a .40, compared with .81 in DSM-III. Agreement on Oppositional-Defiant Disorder was .41, much lower than the .66 found in DSM-III and the .55 in DSM-IV. Some of the new disorders received relatively solid ratings—Hoarding Disorder notched a .59, Binge Eating Disorder a .56, and Disruptive Mood Dysregulation Disorder a .50. But others were dismal, like Mixed Anxiety-Depression, whose kappa of less than .01 was deemed "uninterpretable," as were kappas for four other disorders, including the once stalwart Obsessive-Compulsive Disorder. Results from the personality disorders trials were also confounding; Toronto's Centre for Addiction and Mental Health, one of Canada's leading psychiatric hospitals, managed a .75 reliability in identifying Borderline Personality Disorder, while clinicians at the august Menninger Clinic in Houston scored only a .34 using the same criteria. Some reworked disorders did fare better than did their predecessors—PTSD, at .67, was eight points higher than the DSM-IV trial and beat DSM-III by twelve; ADHD was also a few points better than it had been, although Regier had to acknowledge that "we're still going back and forth" on whether there would be eighteen or twenty-two criteria; the autism spectrum rang up a solid .69, although that was much lower than the .85 of the DSM-IV trial for autism.

But these high-ish numbers were the exceptions, and if the audience members had managed to recalibrate their expectations, perhaps by reminding themselves that in golf lower is also better, they were not able to suppress a murmur when Regier announced that the kappa for Major Depressive Disorder—whose criteria were, other than the removal of the bereavement exclusion, unchanged—was .32 and that Generalized Anxiety Disorder had scored a paltry .20.

Something had gone terribly wrong. Those two diagnoses were the Dodge Dart and Ford Falcon of the DSM, simple and reliable and ubiquitous, and if clinicians were unable to agree on who warranted them, there were only a few possible conclusions: that the DSM-III and DSM-IV had been unreliable from the beginning, that the DSM-5 was unreliable, or that the field trials were so deeply flawed that it would be impossible to say with any kind of certainty just how reliable the new book would be.

Darrel Regier is not a demonstrative man. But even so, he seemed strangely cool, as if he had pumped himself full of Valium before announcing results that were not merely bad but disastrous. Hadn't he promised all along that the field trials would bear out the revisions and staked his (and the APA's) reputation, as well as the fate of the DSM-5, on the results? And didn't the lower kappas and the discrepancies among sites signal a return to the dark days before DSM-III, when diagnoses depended more on where they were rendered and by whom than on what was wrong with the patient? Here he was, announcing a miserable failure, but if he grasped the extent of the debacle, nothing about his delivery showed it.

That might be because he had an explanation, one that seemed to satisfy him. "It's important to go back and look at where we were and where we've come," he told us. "We're in a different era of statistical sophistication now." Unlike Spitzer and Frances, "we gave [clinicians] a set of options and they had to choose," he explained. In that unsophisticated era, clinicians "didn't have other diagnoses to confuse them," which is why they got such high kappas. But the DSM-5's "state-of-the-art design" had ensured that they would be confused, and the dismal numbers were the proof of the DSM-5's validity.

The problem, in other words, was not in the numbers but in ourselves. We'd swallowed what Spitzer and Frances had dished out; their comfort food had fattened our expectations, and if the new numbers challenged our unschooled palates and proved a little hard to digest, they at least represented the way psychiatric diagnosis works in the real world. We were just too unsophisticated to understand that failure is success.

One failure couldn't be gussied up, no matter how hard Eve Mościcki, head researcher for the APA's Practice Research Network, tried. And try she did, as she presented the results of the Routine Clinical Practice trial, the one in which I had participated. She tried the Kraemer gambit, lowering the bar at the outset by explaining that "this is a first-time presentation" that would offer only "a flavor of the results." She tried Regierian obfuscation, telling us only how many patients had been enrolled, but not how many of the five thousand clinicians who signed up had actually completed the study. ("I don't have the exact numbers off the top of my head," she said during the Q&A, but she finally had to acknowledge that only 640 had submitted data on at least one patient.) She tried distraction, blaming the failure on bureaucratic delays and the unexpectedly long software training rather than on the study's design, its imposition of a near-impossible burden of conducting hours-long interviews using unfamiliar instruments whose clinical value was questionable and whose reimbursement value was zero. She tried the corporate mission-statement approach—reframing the "unique challenges" faced by the APA as "opportunities for innovative resolutions." She even went Hollywood, calling her talk "Trials, Tribulations, and Triumphs," as if it were an elevator pitch for a movie about a plucky heroine overcoming adversity.

If all her bobbing and weaving hadn't tipped us off to the extent of the fiasco, it became obvious about fifteen minutes into her talk when, after one last reminder that her study was about the feasibility and usefulness of the revisions and not their reliability, she finally flashed some data on the screen—a bar graph depicting how easy (or hard) clinicians found the new criteria to use.

"For ADHD, the majority of clinicians thought it was very easy or extremely easy," she said. The same was true, she went on, for autistic disorders, anxiety, and depression. This might have been a bright moment in an otherwise bleak afternoon but for one thing: according to the graph, while the narrowest majority (52 percent) had indeed given a thumbs-up to ADHD and anxiety disorders, the number who thought the autism and depression criteria and measures were very easy or extremely easy to use was below 50 percent. Mościcki didn't seem to notice this discrepancy between the story she was telling us and the data she was showing us. Perhaps she thought that since she was presenting only a flavor, she was free to add sweeteners to taste, or maybe she just didn't care what we thought, or figured that no one would point out the discrepancies, no matter how obvious, for the same reason that people are reluctant to mention that a coworker smells bad or has left his fly unzipped: because you really don't want to embarrass him.

And up to a point, she was right.

Mościcki switched from "ease of use" to "usefulness." She put up the slide about ADHD and autism diagnoses.

"It looks to me like . . . I want . . ." She trailed off and peered at the slide, which showed even more anemic results than the earlier one. It was as if she had never seen it before, although she may only have been calculating the odds of getting away with this forever. "It looks to me like almost a majority for ADHD thought the criteria were pretty useful, and for autism, clearly the majority thought the criteria . . ."

A man's voice rang out in the darkened room. "It's not a majority," he said. "Look, thirty-seven plus seven"—the "very" and "extremely useful" numbers—"doesn't equal fifty."

The interrupter, who turned out to be a blogger for *Scientific American*, didn't bother asking exactly what "pretty useful" was supposed to mean. He didn't ask Mościcki if she thought it was kosher to make up a diagnostic entity called *trauma*, which she acknowledged she had teased out of the anxiety disorders and which looked suspiciously like a category she had cooked up so she could parade its 62 percent favorable rating. He didn't point out the lunacy of spending all that time (including mine) and money to find out not whether the criteria or the cross-cutting measures were reliable or valid, but rather only whether clinicians liked the DSM-5, as if the APA were looking for Facebook friends. He didn't raise the question of selection bias, that is, whether or not the same factors that motivated the few volunteers who actually followed through also predisposed them to give the DSM a Like. He didn't have to do any of this. Nor did he have to deconstruct propaganda or slog through weedy statistics. He just did the simple math and came to the obvious conclusion.

"This is totally appalling," he said.

"It's okay, it's okay," Mościcki replied. It was not clear whom she meant to comfort. "This is a first look. If it's not a majority, it's a large number of them."

But her antagonist wasn't buying it.

"This is deceptive," he said, as he slung his backpack over his shoulder, spun on his heel, and stormed out.

Like the kid in the story about the emperor's clothes, he had managed to say out loud what everyone in the room, or at least those who could add, must have been thinking: that Mościcki had crossed the Frankfurt Line, the one between bullshit and lies.

The conference featured at least one glimmer of good news for nosologists. Regier mentioned it a couple of times in his various talks, but the honor of revealing it went to Charles O'Brien, a University of Pennsylvania psychiatrist and head of the DSM-5 work group for substance-related disorders.

Before O'Brien got down to the business at hand—his committee's proposals—he turned to the business of business. "People should understand that when they read things in the newspaper about Pharma influence, I don't believe it," he said, as he made the conflict-of-interest disclosure required of every speaker. "We stopped that a long time ago, even though in the past we might have had some consultancies." O'Brien didn't say exactly what they had stopped, but it clearly wasn't the consultancies. Indeed, he was still working for three drug companies. "Only two of them are actually producing drugs that you can prescribe or buy," he explained, and this work "is really socially important, because there are very few medications available and not many companies are working on this." The public fails to understand this, and psychiatry (or at least psychiatrists' income) is the victim of its ignorance.

This was a riff that could not help but ingratiate O'Brien with his audience. And he needed all the help he could get. He had to explain to his colleagues, many of them skeptical, why his group had eliminated the categories of *substance abuse* and *substance dependence*, which the DSM-IV had used to sort out the people who merely get in trouble with drugs from those who get addicted to them. In their place, the committee proposed the supercategory of *substance use disorders*, which, it said, occurred whenever there was a "problematic pattern" of substance use that led to "clinically significant impairment and distress." O'Brien's group, perhaps remembering that no one had yet defined clinical significance, had listed eleven further criteria. If an impaired patient met two of them, he or she had the disorder. So, for instance, if in a twelve-month period you "often" drink "larger amounts or over a longer period than intended," and experience "craving or strong desire or urge to use alcohol," you qualified for Alcohol Use Disorder. The few studies that had been done using the new diagnoses indicated that many people looked forward intensely to their next party and, when they got there, took that third martini or extra toke—enough, in fact, to cause some Australian researchers to forecast a DSM-5-related 60 percent increase in the prevalence of drug-related diagnoses.

O'Brien thought these warnings were balderdash, but he also thought the DSM-IV was balderdash. "I feel free to criticize DSM-IV," he said, because he'd been part of that revision, which he now characterized as "a bunch of wise men sitting around a table and asking what happens when people start using drugs."

"Although we thought we were wise, we were wrong," he said. "There is no evidence to support this idea of drug abuse."

Not that people don't use drugs to their own or others' detriment. But the problem isn't that sometimes the use causes collateral damage (abuse) or becomes habitual (dependence). The problem is "compulsive, out-of-control drug seeking." O'Brien would have preferred to call the reformulated disorder *addiction*, but "some people have a kind of allergy to the word," believing that it carries too much stigma. Avoiding the a-word is "useless," O'Brien said. "When you have the president talking about addiction to oil, the word has lost its pejorative tone," and besides, even if the president did mean it pejoratively, addiction is "what the average doctor is going to call it." But the chair was evidently out-voted, and the anodyne new name won the day.

Whatever its name, O'Brien had no doubt about the nature of the problem. "Addiction is a brain disease," he said. Of course, this was the tacit assumption of the DSM, not to mention of psychiatric nosology for the last hundred years: that what psychiatrists were treating were illnesses that originated in the brain, and that someday they would find out exactly where and how. That promise, O'Brien reminded the crowd, had gone unfulfilled. "Let's take depression or anger or any of the other things we diagnose," he said. "They're all subjective. You have to get hints from what the patient says and how they say it, but you have no test for it."

On the other hand, "we do have tests for craving," he said. "I think craving could become the first biomarker in psychiatry. I can show you where it is in the brain." And so he did, flashing a photo on the screen. "If you're an addict," he said, "you're noticing this person is booting right now." Actually, you didn't have to be an addict; the picture featured a tied-off arm, a blood-filled syringe stuck into a tracked-up vein. What would be different if you were an addict—at least it would if you had just been given a shot of carbon-11 raclopride, a radioactive marker, and a PET scanner had just detected its emissions—is the way your brain would light up upon beholding this image. "This is the caudate, this is the putamen," O'Brien said, pointing to the next slide, a chart of an addict's neural activity. "There's a complete correlation here between the subjective feeling of craving and the degree of inhibition of the binding of raclopride." Similarly, said O'Brien, show an alcoholic an image related to drinking, and you will notice "increased blood flow to the cingulate gyrus, the anterior cingulate, the insula, and the nucleus accumbens down here." In both cases, you're seeing disturbances in dopamine metabolism, "the reward system," as O'Brien put it. You're seeing addiction—not the experience, which can only be described in words

320   Gary Greenberg

and assayed subjectively, but the thing itself—caught when it thought no one was looking, naked and unmistakable.

Of course, there was a catch. "The clinician would have to have a brain-imaging machine," said O'Brien. "But these are getting to be very common," he added. He didn't have to explain to this crowd what that really meant: that devices like brain scanners could be huge profit centers, a way to go outside their comfort zone and get well paid for it, as Lawson Wulsin would put it, to win at the game by delivering the measurement-based care that insurers crave.

It's too bad the doctors' brains weren't being scanned as they gazed upon the evidence that their most fevered cravings were on the verge of fulfillment, that after a century of wandering in the biomedical desert, one psychiatrist was ready to lead them home.

O'Brien ended his talk by pointing out that it's not just boozers and cokeheads whose addiction (and, presumably, recovery) can be verified by the magic machines. "We've listed gambling with the use disorders and we've put Internet Use Disorder in the Appendix," O'Brien said. He'd saved it to the end, but this news was hardly an afterthought. By poaching what the DSM-IV had called Pathological Gambling from the disorders of impulse control work group, his committee had pulled off a coup. It had made official what once was only folk wisdom: that we could be addicted to behaviors as well as to drugs. We could be workaholics and shopaholics, sex addicts and love addicts, hooked on cyberporn and jonesing for carbs. (Indeed, the first question O'Brien fielded was from the head of the Food Addiction Institute, who demanded to know why food addiction hadn't been included.) Any strong desire could be put under surveillance and diagnosed with dead certainty, and any behavior with the telltale signs, anything that set that circuitry in motion, could be called a disease.

The brain scanner, O'Brien said, "tells us directly what's going on." And that's the beauty part: no need to take your hints from what junkies or boozers say or how they say it. Indeed, there's no need to talk (or listen) to them at all. Neither is there any reason to pay attention to those English professors and other amateurs who, emboldened by the DSM's simple language, might kvetch that it might not be such a good idea to pathologize desire in a country where people line up at midnight to buy the newest iPhone, where greed is a virtue and the pursuit of wealth a spectator sport, where an entire economy depends on an endless cycle of craving and not-quite-satisfaction. When the DSM is finally full of words like *nucleus accumbens* and *putamen*, these critics will be out of business.

And so will the rest of us. Because if the brain scanners fulfill their promise, psychiatrists will finally be able to cut out the middleman entirely, and with him the subjectivity that was once psychiatry's bread and butter, but which, especially when it comes to diagnosis, has become its bane. After all, who needs dimensional assessment forms, let alone the stunted conversations that allow clinicians to fill them in, when you have raclopride?

While Regier was presenting the results of the field trials, the 159 voting members of the APA Assembly were taking up a question of great importance to him. Roger Peele, the assembly's representative to the DSM-5 task force, had proposed an action paper that called for all the dimensional measures Regier had proposed—the cross-cutting assessments, the severity scales, and the personality disorder ratings—to be placed in Section 3, the task force's new name for the Appendix, where they would await "further study."

"I wanted to avoid a repeat of Axis V," Peele told me, referring to the DSM-IV scale that asks a clinician to rate a patient's overall functioning from 1 to 100. Once that measure had been instituted, Peele remembered, "insurance companies used it as a basis to deny service." The result was predictable—"One of the first things you were told when you joined a hospital staff was, 'Doctor, all Axis V's on this ward are a forty or less'"—and regrettable.

"It makes a farce of psychiatry," he said.

And it wasn't just the insurance companies whose demands turned psychiatry into a game of Diagnosing for Dollars. A public sector psychiatrist, Peele knew that bureaucracies like his were number-crazy. If the DSM offered measures, then clinicians were sure to be compelled to use them, and their workload would increase—a problem obscured by the Facebook approach to evaluating the measures. "The 'liking' of severity scales . . . by clinicians volunteering to be part of the DSM-5 field trials is not necessarily representative of the vast majority of American clinicians who did not volunteer to be part of such trials despite many opportunities to do so," he wrote in the resolution.

Perhaps the burden of the dimensions would have been worthwhile, and the method of evaluating them unimportant, had they had any scientific integrity. But "most, if not all, are not based on science," Peele told me—and that was assuming you could even find out what they were. "Some of them are so immature that if you go to the website, they aren't even shown." And indeed, even at this late date, a click on the tab for many proposed measures returned the message that "recommendations . . . are forthcoming. We encourage you to check our Web site regularly for updates."

The day before the assembly meeting, Regier had had a chance to defend himself to a committee with the power to endorse the resolution to the full body. He spoke longer than anyone else at the meeting, but nothing he said swayed the committee, which recommended the passage of the resolution; and the very next day the assembly voted unanimously to send the dimensional measures, which Regier had once promised as the key to springing the APA from its epistemic prison, to the elephant burial ground.

As he had in Hawaii, Michael First spent the beginning days of the meeting hanging out with this year's gathering of the Association for the Advancement of Philosophy and Psychiatry. It wasn't quite so captivating this time around. "Too much name-dropping of philosophers whose work I am not familiar with," he told me, "so the arguments are too hard to follow."

Still, First knew enough about philosophy and its significance to the DSM to have once put his name on a paper urging the task force to appoint a DSM-5 work group that would take up "conceptual issues" such as the definition of mental disorder. "Conceptual questions are not minor 'side issues' to be dealt with in improvised ways," the group wrote. "Conceptual clarification is a critical partner to good scientific work . . . [and] advances the scientific rigor of our work." The paper was published in 2008. The task force never responded.

Four years later, and too late for them to have any impact, the philosophers were given a chance to philosophize at one of the annual meeting's official symposia—"Philosophical and Pragmatic Problems for DSM-5." But, as they had in Hawaii, they remained mostly on the fringes, this time at a Crowne Plaza a few blocks from the convention center, where the elevator actually stopped at the floor of the meeting room. Everyone attending had heard David Kupfer assert that the DSM was all but completed, and the panels on ideology and the role of science in medicine and other chewy issues seemed more like pathologists' probes at a postmortem than clarifications contributed by critical partners.

First was the discussant for the symposium, which the APA had scheduled for the same time slot as the field-trial session. He had asked me to report the results to him. He shook his head as I read them off.

"Point twenty for GAD?" he asked. "Really?"

He ventured an explanation. The new criteria required a clinician to determine if the patient's anxiety led him or her to avoid activities "with possible negative outcomes" or to procrastinate "due to worries" or to "repeatedly [seek] reassurance." These, First thought, were vague notions, poorly written and untested; it was no surprise that clinicians could not agree on them.

This much, he acknowledged, was speculation. But that was his point: he had to speculate, and so would the people who had to figure out what to do with the DSM-5, because the field trials had not been designed to find out what had gone wrong, nor was there time for a second round to see if the problem, whatever it was, had been fixed. There was only one possible solution, First said: to go back to the DSM-IV definition.

I thought I might have glimpsed, for the first time, some Firstian schadenfreude, but he sounded more disappointed than gloating, like a professor explaining a concept to hardheaded students for the umpteenth time. He told me he was beginning to give up hope that the APA would listen to him, that indeed he was already looking beyond the publication of DSM-5. As the problems of the new book became clear, he thought the APA might draft him back into service, giving him a chance once again to do what he'd been born to do. After the conference, I suggested that if the DSM-5 turned out as he feared it might, he was likely to have his work cut out for him. "Yes," he said, "but I do like a challenge."

Susan Swedo, chief of the Pediatrics and Developmental Neuroscience Branch at NIMH, started her talk on the second day by announcing she'd changed her title from the original "Neurodevelopmental Disorders, Including Autism Spectrum Disorder, Intellectual Developmental Disorder and Learning Disorder" to "Making National Headlines." And it wasn't because the new title was catchier.

"I felt if I just addressed what is being said about our criteria versus what they actually say," she explained, "maybe you'd come away with a better idea of what we are doing."

As much as she might have wanted to deliver the straight skinny to her colleagues, Swedo also wanted to settle some scores.

"The most glaring [headline] was in *The New York Times*," she said. It had reported that Volkmar's data had been "presented at a major medical meeting." Swedo took a beat. "That major medical meeting turned out to be the winter meeting of the Icelandic Medical Association."

The crowd tittered, and Regier laughed into his microphone.

"Thank you for laughing," Swedo said. "Because there are about 250,000 people in Iceland, which means there are maybe half a dozen child psychiatrists in the country."

If there were any Icelandic patriots in the crowd to defend their homeland (or just to tell Swedo that Iceland's population is about 320,000), they kept silent. Reporter Ben Carey was definitely not present, so he couldn't point out that his article didn't call the Iceland conference a "major medical meeting." And Fred Volkmar was back in New Haven, so he wasn't able to remind Swedo that he had first presented his data in fall 2011, at the American Academy of Adolescent and Child Psychiatry's annual conference, which is about as major as a meeting gets, and one at which she was also on the program.

Darrel Regier was there, and he had to listen as Swedo described her field-trial results as "superb," then, as if remembering the kerfuffle over the meaning of kappa, corrected herself. "I'm sorry. Not superb. Very good. Superb only compared with the rest of DSM." Regier wasn't laughing anymore, but he didn't object out loud to the slight, either. He was, after all, a veteran of scorched-earth campaigns; he must have known Swedo wasn't taking prisoners, that it was best to stay out of her way.

It's too bad no one was in attendance from the Asperger's Association of New England, the group to which Nomi Kaim belongs. It would have been interesting to hear the organization's response when Swedo, after complaining about all the people who had blown up her e-mail in-box after Carey and Volkmar had unnecessarily struck "fear in their hearts" and dismissing Volkmar's study as "comparing apples to Apple computers" (but without refuting his data), explained why she thought it was safe to ignore their objections. "Most of the individuals who belong to the AANE call themselves Aspies," she said, "but that may need to be a new diagnosis introduced in future editions of the DSM, because Aspies don't actually have Asperger's Disorder, much less Autism Spectrum Disorders."

In the Q&A, I asked Swedo how she knew this.

"By my interactions with them," she said. "We have been petitioned by so-called Aspies and literally they are writing to us and saying I am an Aspie . . . and they describe what, if they had seen a psychiatrist, might have been called Obsessive-Compulsive Personality Disorder."

"So based on your interaction, you can conclude that people who call themselves Aspies don't have Asperger's?" I asked. Was she really diagnosing people whom she knew only through their letters of complaint? Did she maybe want to qualify this or elaborate on her earlier comment that Aspies were simply "Norwegian bachelor farmers, just a little awkward . . . but we would consider them to have a normal variation"? Did she mean to confirm in a public forum the worst fears of people with Asperger's and their families: that the APA, convinced that they had made it on to the sick rolls illegitimately, was determined to kick them off?

Swedo backpedaled a little, allowing that some of the AANE members might indeed have Asperger's, but still, she insisted, "there is an element of folks . . . who do not meet the criteria for DSM-IV." Whatever they had, and they may well have had something (after all, they were harassing her), "it just didn't have the same flavor as Asperger's."

Not that it really mattered, as Swedo's answer to another questioner indicated. By now, she was sitting next to Regier and other panel members at a table, and the man wanted to hear from any or all of them what role the availability of services had played in the revision. Swedo took the mic. She told him a story about the field-trial clinician who had sent her a note saying, "My patient did not meet criteria for autism, but I know he has it, so I gave him the diagnosis anyway."

This would have been the perfect time for Swedo to dress down her correspondent with the same withering sarcasm she'd used on Volkmar and Carey. After all, wasn't this a perfect illustration of all that was wrong with the DSM-IV—that it had turned clinicians' instincts, leavened by sympathy, into a diagnostic epidemic? Hadn't the purpose of DSM-5 been to put an end to this kind of discretion and revoke the benefits of diagnosis from all those undeserving bachelor farmers?

Apparently not.

"I think this is actually quite appropriate," Swedo said. "If the clinician's gut feeling is that the patient has the disorder, it's appropriate for them to get [the diagnosis], to give them the services, the treatment, whatever needs to happen."

Swedo paused briefly. But if she was weighing the implications of suggesting that doctors ignore the new criteria the APA had just spent $25 million to fashion, if she was reconsidering what her comments meant for her profession's scientific credibility or for the reputation of the man sitting right next to her, if she was even aware that she had just admitted that the whole enterprise was a confidence game, a way to give doctors plausible scientific cover even as they continued to diagnose and medicate their patients based on their gut feelings, their whims and fancies and judgments, it wasn't evident when she resumed her answer.

"So politically it's gotten a little messy," she said, "but scientifically and clinically I think we remain committed to the idea that the purpose of the DSM is to provide clinicians with a road map. We're not driving the car."

And the map doesn't really matter, because even if clinicians load the DSM into their GPS units, they're going to take the routes their gut tells them are best. And if a doctor decides to head for uncharted territory, to lead his colleagues into the land where irritable children suffer Bipolar Disorder, or where attraction to thirteen-year-olds is Hebephilia, or a slave's thirst for freedom is a symptom of drapetomania, if he thinks his MD plates entitle him to take his patients off-road or the wrong way down a one-way street or, for that matter, over a cliff, well, that's not the APA's fault.

Within two hours of the release of the field-trial data, Allen Frances had written a new blog post: "Newsflash from APA Meeting: DSM-5 Has Flunked Its Reliability Test."

"The DSM-5 has managed to fail in ways that go beyond my poor imagination," he wrote. "Reliability this low . . . gravely undermines the credibility of DSM-5," and the result would be a "book no one can trust." The field trials thus signaled a "DSM-5 emergency"—an imminent loss of the authority that the DSM-III had earned and the DSM-IV had preserved—and the only way to "salvage this deplorable mess" was to reinstate the second round of field trials, which, of course, would mean delaying publication.

Speaking of deplorable messes, the blog (which appeared on the *Psychology Today* website) contained a table of the results with misaligned columns, indecipherable abbreviations, and unintelligible figures. It looked as if it had been assembled hastily on a BlackBerry, which it had—but not Frances's. I'd sent the list to him while Bill Narrow was droning on about something or other, and he'd copied and pasted it with my clumsy thumbwork intact.

Partly I did it because I was bored. And partly I did it for the same reason that your cat drops a beheaded mouse on your doorstep: to express gratitude for your care and feeding, and, maybe, to curry further favor. Although sometimes you have to wonder if Snowball is trying to make a point by leaving a bleeding carcass for you to find first thing in the morning—to remind you, perhaps, that while you may have an electric can opener, in the tooth-and-claw world she still has an advantage. Cats are sly and complicated creatures.

I wish I could say that I was too, and that I had somehow tricked Frances into revealing one of psychiatry's dark little secrets when he wrote:

> The great value to the field of DSM-III was that it established reliability and preserved the credibility of psychiatry at a time when it was becoming irrelevant because it seemed that psychiatrists could not agree on a diagnosis. Everyone knew that the reliability achieved in DSM field testing far exceeds what is possible in clinical practice, but DSM-III took the major step of proving that reliability could be achieved at all.

But I'm not that clever. And Frances doesn't need to be tricked into saying this, nor would he agree that it has ever been a secret. In his world, the DSM was never more than a book of useful constructs validated in idealized settings, and this is not a problem because the point was never to establish the truth about mental disorders. But Frances had a questionable conviction as well: that he could trash the DSM-5 without trashing his profession.

"The controversy stirred by my critique of DSM-5 is a terrible moment in the history of psychiatry," he told me the month after the annual meeting. "This is the worst thing to happen to the field's credibility since Rosenhan—and psychiatry is a field that especially requires credibility to be effective. I know I have done grave harm."

Frances reasoned that the damage to misdiagnosed and overdiagnosed patients was a graver harm than undermining psychiatry's credibility with the truth. It was the kind of calculation Cincinnatus might have made, hoping to hasten his return to the farm. Frances had gambled that the fragile edifice Spitzer had erected and he had reinforced would withstand the weight of the truth, that one of the guardians of the noble lie could reveal it and yet somehow preserve the authority the lie had purchased. And even as he fended off more antipsychiatrists drafting him unwillingly into their cause and more attorneys eager to use his own criticisms to undermine his (and his profession's) credibility, he continued to be certain he'd made the right choice.

It's possible he was compelled by unconscious inner necessity to blurt out the truth, or that contrition or self-loathing or that old Freudian notion, the *death instinct*—the inbuilt yearning for the chaos that the lies of civilization, noble and otherwise, hold at bay—drove him. He would say that what he did was much simpler than that, that it grew from an easy calculus, nearly bureaucratic in its plainness: that the only chance to preserve the DSM's hard-won authority was to stop the APA from going ahead with the worst of its ideas—especially those, like removing the bereavement exclusion, that would badly cashier the reputation of his beloved profession. He would also say that it doesn't require vast sophistication to grasp the reality: that a language by which two doctors can agree on a name for a patient's subjective suffering is a signal achievement no matter how contrived, and worth preserving despite its many flaws.

In this, he may have overestimated the value of that language. He may also have overestimated the tolerance of Americans for bullshit. But above all, Allen Frances may have overestimated himself.

Chapter 20

O r maybe it was just me he overestimated.

In October 2012, I join Frances and Manning in a hotel room near Harvard Medical School, where Frances is scheduled to address a bioethics seminar. A documentarian working on a film about the DSM is setting up her equipment. She has finally caught up with Frances after a four-month chase. He has decided that she should interview the two of us together. It's not entirely clear to me if she is on board with that idea. Since June, Frances has mostly been quiet about the DSM. He is still blogging for *The Huffington Post* and *Psychology Today* and the *Psychiatric Times*, where he has weighed in on gun control and the presidential election and offered "to stop being an amateur columnist" if David Brooks would "stop being an amateur psychologist." But the DSM has never been far from his mind, and as soon as the lights are on and the camera is running, he is back to it and drawing me into his explanation of all that has gone wrong with the DSM-5. I may be an upside-down Jesuit and he a world-weary rationalist, but for the moment, we're just a couple of friends on the inside of the same joke. The filmmaker seems entertained, although it's possible she is simply egging us on in hopes of capturing some outrageous Francesism on film. But he's become more careful. In fact, he tells the camera, he's learned his lesson, the one about how impertinent remarks might, in the wrong hands, turn his attacks on DSM-5 into attacks on psychiatry.

The director describes an Internet video she has seen, put out, she says, by Scientology's Citizens Commission on Human Rights, in which the narrator somberly intones that even the head of the DSM-IV thinks psychiatry is bullshit. Frances looks over at me, vindicated.

The thing I don't understand, he tells me (and I'm working from memory here; I didn't tape our meeting), is that you think the words in the DSM are capable of great harm. So why aren't you worried about the harm your words can do?

The question makes me think of the infamous line with which Janet Malcolm opened her book *The Journalist and the Murderer.* "Every journalist who is not too stupid or too full of himself to notice what is going on knows that what he does is morally indefensible." Malcolm was writing about the way Joe McGinniss had seduced and betrayed Jeffrey MacDonald, promising exoneration and then penning indictment. But Frances is accusing me of more than luring him into candor with assurances that my criticism of psychiatric diagnosis was tempered by a recognition of its uses, and then using him as a cudgel in my own crusade against psychiatry. Indeed, he has always insisted he doesn't care about his own image, and while that may be a little too much protest, it's not hard to believe that his worries are genuine, and that my real betrayal is using his comment to harm the people who need to have confidence in their doctors (and keep taking their drugs) to get better. If the discrepancy between opportunity and knowledge remains under wraps, it seems, that's not bullshit. That's wisely deploying the placebo effect. That's medicine.

The camera is rolling, or whatever it is that digital cameras do. I'm pinned and wriggling, scrambling for some way to explain why I don't seem to care about what happens when people glimpse what's behind the curtain. It isn't the first time a psychiatrist has warned me that criticizing the profession would lead to dire consequences. It's the profession's stock response to anyone who attacks it, and I have a stock rebuttal: that I am sure more people have been hurt by the DSM, or at least by the treatments that follow diagnosis, than by anything I ever wrote. Yet it seems inadequate to the moment. I say some words, but they don't really make sense, and they surely don't answer his question. Frances sits back in his chair.

He has the right to his satisfaction. It is true that I didn't give a moment's thought to the question of whether reporting Frances's comment (along with a lot of evidence that he is right) would hurt anyone. I always figure people are better off with the truth, which is probably why I went into both the therapy and the journalism businesses—and why I get angry when one of those professions hides its own uncomfortable truths. But as much as I like the way that sounds, maybe I'm just too full of myself to see that I'm using Frances and the patients, that they have become character and audience, and that I'm using truth as well, not as a virtue but as a narrative device, as the MacGuffin for exposing humbuggery and chronicling comeuppance, and that to undermine the already shaky foundations of a profession that offers the last and only hope for some patients—that has succeeded, at least in some cases, at quelling their hallucinations, modulating their mood swings, allaying their anxiety, and restoring them to some semblance of normal functioning—and to bring low the confidence man at the expense of his potentially satisfied customers is simply indefensible.

But then again, so is psychiatry, at least when it comes to the DSM. And not because the DSM-5 was botched or because the profession is a cabal of Pharma collaborators, although it harbors its fair share of both incompetents and conspirators, but because even at its best, even in the view of honest and eloquent men like Steve Hyman and Allen Frances, psychiatric diagnosis is fiction sold to the public as fact. And not the Supreme Fiction that Wallace Stevens says begins "by perceiving the idea / Of this invention, this invented world," but a fallen fiction whose authors, if they are to hold on to their power, must insist that they have gathered together the scattered particulars of our suffering and sorted them according to their natural formations, even as they harbor the knowledge that they have done no such thing. That knowledge can be locked up, like Leibowitz's Memorabilia in its monastery, but it will always escape when the DSM is opened for revision and doctors once again argue over matters that their science cannot settle.

Later that day, Frances is once again called upon to defend psychiatry against his own charges. In an elegant wood-paneled room at Harvard, just after he has told a group made up mostly of doctors why expert consensus—the method that has yielded the DSM—is both necessary and dangerous to public health, Arnold Relman, the eighty-nine-year-old former editor of *The New England Journal of Medicine*, professor emeritus at Harvard, and a longtime critic of for-profit health care, suggests that this tension is worse in psychiatry than in other specialties because psychiatric experts lack biological findings that can anchor diagnosis in something beyond the symptom. Where is psychiatry's pneumococcus, Relman seems to be asking. Frances has fielded this question before, and he has a ready answer: that diagnostic uncertainty and lack of treatment specificity haunt all of medicine.

It's a version of the argument Steve Mirin and Darrel Regier once made to the editors of *The Washington Post*, and it was not entirely wrong. There are plenty of illnesses that are described purely in terms of their symptoms—chronic headache, for example, or idiopathic neuropathy—and devastating diseases, such as multiple sclerosis and cancer, that seem unlikely to have a single form caused by a single pathogen like pneumococcus. And while it is true that those diseases are often diagnosed by lab studies, if only to rule out other known causes of their symptoms, psychiatry is still not so different from other specialties in this sense.

But even if medical nosology, taken in the aggregate, is as fictive as psychiatric nosology, even if many of its diagnoses are merely descriptions of the problem in a medical language, still it would have its pneumococcus and its polio and its diabetes, not to mention its heart diseases and bone fractures, its blood counts and biopsies and X-rays, its antibiotics and vaccines, its cobalt-chromium stents and titanium joints, its brain surgeries and organ transplants. Even if its unknowns far surpass its knowns, medicine undeniably has its slam dunks. Even when they are found by accident, as they often are, and even when they seem miraculous, as they often do, these are not miracles or mere serendipities, but the discovery of the natural laws that govern our suffering. Medicine's sure knowledge of those laws saves our lives and earns doctors our deference.

This is precisely what psychiatry lacks. Without a single mental disorder that meets the scientific demands of the day, let alone enough of them to make the DSM more than an invented world, and with its claim to "real medicine" still mostly aspirational, it cannot make good on its assertion that psychological suffering is best understood as medical illness. So it must guard its position jealously. Lacking confidence in itself, psychiatry must work ever harder to command ours. This is what unites the APA, with its circle-the-wagons paranoia, its deceptions and duplicity and tortured language, and Allen Frances, with his invocations of Leibowitz and his warnings about patients gone wild. He and Darrel Regier may be bitter opponents, but they both have the fear that comes with knowing the fragility of the edifice they share.

The APA had at least one opportunity for a slam dunk in the DSM-5. In an article published in *The American Journal of Psychiatry*, an international group of seventeen prominent men—including clinicians, psychoanalytically minded personality theorists, historians of medicine, biological psychiatrists, critics of biological psychiatry, and Bob Spitzer—urged the

DSM Task Force to include in the DSM-5 a disorder they called *melancholia*. "Melancholia," they wrote, is "a syndrome with a long history and distinctly specific psychopathological features." Melancholia is Winston Churchill's black dog, Andrew Solomon's noonday demon (an image he borrowed from Isaiah), William Styron's darkness visible—a form of depression noted by doctors since Hippocrates and characterized by an unshakable despondency and sense of guilt that arises from nowhere, responds to nothing, and dissipates for no apparent reason.

The authors drew on thirty years of research to describe five clinical characteristics by which melancholia could be distinguished from other kinds of depression. Among those characteristics were biological findings that set the melancholics apart, notably *hypercortisolemia* and disturbances in *sleep architecture*. A sleep study could show whether or not patients had the reduced deep sleep and increased REM time characteristic of melancholia. And a dexamethasone suppression test (DST)—in which patients were given a synthetic steroid to see if it suppressed the activity of their own hormonal system—could determine whether their cortisol, a stress hormone, was in overdrive. Patients who meet the criteria for melancholia are much more likely than other depressed people to show this abnormality. They are also much more likely than other depressives to respond to two treatments: tricyclic antidepressants (drugs discovered in the late 1950s and in wide use before the Prozac era) and electroconvulsive therapy (ECT), better known as shock treatment, and they show less response to both placebos and cognitive-behavioral therapy. Melancholia, the proponents concluded, was a "distinct, identifiable, and specifically treatable affective syndrome." It might even be, although they didn't say this, a type of depression that actually was the result of a real chemical imbalance, a disorder onto which our biochemistry could be mapped.

The proposal included plenty of standard scientific evidence—clinical and lab studies, case histories, literature reviews—and, with its tie to cortisol, melancholia seemed to fit in with emerging theories about depression and stress. So you would think that the APA would have leaped at the opportunity to finally prove to dismissive doctors in other specialties and to a skeptical public that, at least in this one case, psychiatrists were real doctors treating real diseases that could be discerned with real tests and treated with real cures.

But you would be wrong. Melancholia not only failed to gain inclusion, it was not even given much consideration. Only five days after he had received the group's proposal, in October 2008, mood disorders work group member William Coryell was already telling Max Fink, one of melancholia's main proponents, that the odds were very long. The main obstacle was exactly what Fink and his colleagues thought was one of the great strengths of the proposal: the biological tests, especially the DST. "I believe the inclusion of a biological measure would be very hard to sell to the mood group," Coryell wrote Fink—and not because the test was unreliable. "I agree there is more data to support using the DST for melancholia than for using any other measure for any other diagnosis," he conceded. Even so, the DST would be "very hard to sell since it would be ... the only biological test for any diagnosis being considered." Coryell didn't finish the thought, but the implication was obvious: a test for melancholia would make the lack of biological measures elsewhere in the DSM that much more glaring. It was a success that would only highlight the APA's failures. (Coryell declined to comment.)

Sixteen months later, when the APA posted its first draft of the DSM-5, Coryell was proven correct. Melancholia didn't even show up in the mood disorders section; it had merited only a single line in a section of "conditions proposed by others"—a category it shared with Parental Alienation Syndrome and Male-to-Eunuch Gender Identity Disorder, among others.

"I [am] flabbergasted that our suggestion ... has been excluded from consideration," Fink wrote to Coryell. "Carving out a well-defined type of mood disorder, one that carries with it the promise of homogeneous samples and optimized treatment outcomes, is a small step in the development of the classification, but it is one that has been extracted from Nature grudgingly, and deserves greater attention and consideration within . . . DSM-5."

"I believe you and your colleagues are fundamentally correct," Coryell replied. But, he added, his belief had "not been shared by any of the other work group members," so there was "no point in pursuing it further." Coryell ventured a new explanation for the outcome: that the proposal would "entail a fundamental change in the boundaries" of a diagnosis (MDD) that was "among the most enduring and stable" of the DSM's categories. "Evidence for such a sweeping modification would need to be quite extensive and compelling."

But an ambiguous research record hadn't stopped the work group from gerrymandering the bereavement exclusion out of MDD, nor was it stopping other work groups from considering destabilizing changes like the removal of Asperger's or the introduction of entirely new diagnoses like DMDD. On the other hand, those diagnoses had one advantage over melancholia: they didn't threaten to introduce a biological measure into the DSM and make the rest of the book look bad in the bargain. Offered a key to one of the cells of its epistemic prison, the APA had decided that the cost of freedom was too high.

In June 2012, the APA posted a change to the permissions policy on its DSM-5 website. "The APA owns all products generated by the Work Groups developing DSM-5," it declared. This included, they asserted, not only proposed criteria, but also the discussions that led to the work groups' decisions. To those who wondered how this squared with the insistence that this was the most transparent DSM ever, the APA issued a reassurance: "Requests will be considered for permission to describe the criteria and development process in narrative form." The organization wasn't trying to erase history, only to control it.

There was no explanation of this change. It was hard not to think that it had something to do with my having shown up at the annual meeting and peppered the presenters with questions, from which the APA's communications experts could only conclude that their embargo had not stopped me from writing my book.

On the other hand, the new policy also came shortly after Allen Frances put his scathing description of the development process on the op-ed page of *The New York Times*. The APA, he charged, was guilty of "arrogance, secretiveness, passive governance and administrative disorganization." It had failed to rein in its experts, who had in turn (and predictably) manufactured new disorders, heedless of the fact that "new diagnoses in psychiatry can be far more dangerous than new drugs." And now he had come to a reluctant conclusion—that the APA "is no longer capable of being sole fiduciary of a task that has become so consequential to public health and public policy," and that it should be stripped of the diagnostic franchise.

Frances acknowledged that there was no obvious immediate successor, but he suggested the Department of Health and Human Services, the Institute of Medicine (a section of the National Academy of Sciences), or even the World Health Organization. He mentioned one obvious contender, the National Institute of Mental Health, only to dismiss it as "too research-oriented and insensitive to the vicissitudes of clinical practice." Since sponsoring the planning conferences at the beginning of the DSM-5 effort, the NIMH had indeed remained on the sidelines—not because nosology was out of its bailiwick, but because the institute had lost faith in the DSM. "Our resources are more likely to be invested in a program to transform diagnosis by 2020," NIMH director Thomas Insel told me, "rather than modifying the current paradigm."

The NIMH is placing its bets for a new paradigm on a program it calls the Research Domain Criteria (RDoC), a name that recalls the Research Diagnostic Criteria, the Washington University initiative that led to the transformation of diagnosis in the DSM-III. Just as Spitzer and his colleagues had been confronted with widespread dissatisfaction with the diagnostic system among psychiatrists, so too had Insel heard the discontent among his peers on his frequent trips to hospitals and universities around the country.

What Insel heard "over and over again" on his tour was that psychiatrists were tired of being trapped by the DSM. "We are so embedded in this structure," he told me. He and his colleagues had spent so much time diagnosing mental disorders that "we actually believe they are real. But there's no reality. These are just constructs. There's no reality to schizophrenia or depression." Indeed, Insel said, "we might have to stop using terms like *depression* and *schizophrenia*, because they are getting in our way, confusing things." Thirty years after Spitzer burned down the DSM-II and built the DSM-III in its ashes, psychiatry might once again have to "just sort of start over."

Spitzer's error, at least according to Bruce Cuthbert, the NIMH psychologist in charge of RDoC, was not that he tried to cram psychological suffering into faux medical categories, but that he continued to think of suffering as a function of the mind. "So many of our disorders historically have been conceived of as disorders of mind," Cuthbert says. This leaves scientists in an impossible position. "As scientists we have to measure things," he says. "What else can we do?"

But the attempt to measure the mind has led to nothing but dead ends like the old, now discredited theories about depression and serotonin. "There was going to be a one-to-one map between our putative mind diseases and biology," says Cuthbert. "Whoops! It wasn't that simple."

The way to start over, according to Cuthbert and Insel, is to forget about the mind and look directly to the brain for understanding our suffering. We shouldn't take the fact that people have been describing disorders of the mind such as melancholia for more than two thousand years or schizophrenia for more than a century as evidence that those diseases exist and then try to find them in the brain, Cuthbert said.

Instead we should ask, "What does the brain do? What did it evolve to do? And we know that now."

What we know now, Cuthbert explained, is that "there are very specific circuits in the brain that perform somewhat specific things." Previous attempts to map the brain onto disorders of the mind failed not only because they were looking for mind disorders, but also because they had the brain's role in psychopathology wrong. The trouble didn't originate in individual brain structures like the hippocampus or frontal cortex. Neither was it in droughts and floods of neurotransmitters. Rather, it was to be found in circuits of neurons, the pulsating networks that experience builds in the brain, each their own little ecosystem in the vast electrochemical jungle between our ears. Understanding circuits, or even knowing that they existed, wasn't even possible a generation ago, but now, thanks to MRI, PET, and other brain-scanning technologies, "we know there are circuits for fear," Cuthbert said. "We know there are circuits that guide us to approach things that are desirable and to go get them, like the food that we need for nourishment. We know there are circuits for memory. So we know something about the organization of these circuits now, and we have an idea that these circuits are involved in lots of different disorders."

Cuthbert doesn't expect neural circuits to map onto the DSM disorders any better than neurotransmitter metabolism has. But then again, this may not matter. If, for instance, researchers can trace the neurocircuitry of the startle response, figure out all the electrochemical events that make an animal blink and hunch and shrink away from a sudden noise, then they will be on their way to understanding the anxiety found in many DSM disorders. The arousal itself having been elucidated, it will no longer be merely a scattered particular waiting to be gathered under the correct diagnosis. Indeed, fictive placeholders will no longer be necessary. They will be replaced by the natural formations that the brain scanners have detected as the sources of this particular kind of suffering.

Cuthbert pointed to a chart titled "Draft Research Domain

Criteria Matrix." Its rows list the five natural formations the NIMH is interested in: negative valence systems, including threat, fear of loss, and frustration; positive valence systems, including motivation, learning, and habit; cognitive systems (attention, perception, and memory); systems for social processes (facial expression identification, imitation, attachment/separation fear); and arousal/regulatory processes (stress regulation). Its columns are eight units of analysis—such as genes, molecules, and cells—which the NIMH would like researchers to use to investigate the domains. So, for instance, a scientist interested in working memory (a cognitive system) might want to look into the dorsolateral prefrontal cortex, while a researcher in the negative valence domain could propose a study about the *hypothalamic-pituitary axis* or the *bed nucleus of the stria terminalis* or *corticotrophin-releasing factor*. Ultimately, so Cuthbert and Insel hope, the matrix will be filled in with knowledge about these domains, and the neural substrates of the distress of people with attachment/separation fear or difficulties in regulating stress will be elucidated, pinpointed, and presumably targeted for treatment, without any need for recourse to putative mind diseases.

Cuthbert was not clear about whether it is the mind that is putative or only its diseases, although the fact that most of this research is going to take place on animals is a clue to the relative place of the human mind in this scheme. And, indeed, it is hard to see how the idea that human consciousness is something more than the sum of its parts—an idea that, however muted, still lingers in the notion that a state of mind such as depression can be something real, something that surpasses and unites its scattered particulars—can survive an effort such as RDoC. Not that the program signals the death knell of the self (and not that psychiatry, for all its influence, could slay the idea of human agency that has developed over the last five thousand years or so), but it does seem to signal the profession's intent to complete its abandonment of the mind as the location and source of our suffering, an effort that began in earnest when Spitzer kicked psychoanalysis out of the DSM and that might end as it turns to circuits and systems whose primary virtue is that they can be measured. It seems to signal a future in which diagnosticians will let the brain talk in its own language of inputs and outputs, of ganglia and dendrites, of myelin sheaths and afferents; tell its owner what it is saying; and then provide treatments that are no longer targeted at mythical chemical imbalances or fictive disorders but at the faulty circuits that are causing distress.

At the APA meeting in Honolulu, Insel laid out his vision of that future. He showed an animation illustrating the differences in brain development between children with ADHD and normal kids, differences that he said originated very early in life. "We call this attention deficit/hyperactivity disorder," he said, but "think about it for a moment. Attention, that's cognition; hyperactivity, that's behavior; so this is a cognitive-behavioral disorder. That's the way we define it, the way we characterize it, the way we study it, the way we treat it." He looked over at the PowerPoint screen, where the two kinds of brains were still projected. "This to me looks like a disorder of cortical maturation. Imagine if we took everyone with myocardial infarction and said they had a chest-pain problem. Yes, these kids do have attention deficit, they do have hyperactivity, that is part of it, but if you don't begin to think about ADHD as a disorder of cortical maturation, you'll never ask the key questions . . . Maybe we could use this as the target to develop treatments instead of always thinking about the observable symptoms."

The same is true of schizophrenia, Insel continued, and presumably of other psychiatric disorders. "Behavior is a late manifestation of brain disorders, so if mental disorders are brain disorders and we've only allowed ourselves to define them based on manifest symptoms and signs, we're talking about getting into this game in the ninth inning. And in medicine we don't do so well when we get into the game very late."

Psychiatrists, not to mention their patients, can't afford to wait until people actually suffer to intervene—and, if RDoC is successful at laying bare the neural and genetic substrates of our suffering, they won't have to. They will be able to render a diagnosis before there is even trouble, based on what they can see in the brain.

And since the brain is nothing but electricity and meat, since, that is, it is real, brain-based diagnosis will also be real, not reified real but really real, and psychiatric nosology will finally put paid to the century-old promissory note—not by finally connecting signs and symptoms to biology and chemistry, but by getting out of the mind business and placing all the money on the brain. In the system the RDoC envisions, there will be no more reminders to clinicians not to think of diagnoses as actual diseases, no more worries that the DSM is taken too seriously, no more whining about epistemic prisons, no more fights over symptom counts or disorder names, no more exclusion criteria, no more doomed attempts to ride the royal road of descriptive psychiatry to the kingdom of anatomical pathology, no more unworkable definitions of mental illness, and, above all, no more bullshit.

On the other hand, maybe not. In 2020, or whenever RDoC comes to fruition, after the animals have been startled or frustrated or taught a new maze and had their brains duly mashed and assayed, after the matrix has been filled in, Insel and Cuthbert or their successors will still have to name those circuits and then define all those words. They will have to say exactly what those measurements of neurons in the stria terminalis or cortisol in the spinal fluid are measuring. And then they will have to do what Kraepelin and Salmon and Spitzer and Frances and First and Regier and every other would-be psychiatric nosologist has had to do: figure out what *fear of loss* is and where it leaves off and *attachment/separation fear* sets in, and how much of each is pathological and when and whether to say that the measured symptoms add up to an illness. They will once again be faced with the fact that there is very little that is important about us that can be defined in such a way as to measure it, and that numbers and words may be incommensurable vocabularies, two irreconcilable languages in which to understand us.

The mind may well be an illusion, something the brain does to entertain us while it goes on about its business, whatever that business is, but it's a gorgeous illusion and very convincing. I'll bet you think you are in there reading this, just as I am sure I am in here writing it, and when you are doing that, or when you are anxious or depressed, I'll bet you are pretty sure it's because of something other than some crossed-up brain circuits. The mind is also a resilient illusion. The idea that we are agents, that our brains serve us just as our other organs do—in this case providing us with the means to author our lives—and that this is in some sense what it means to be human, has survived all sorts of assaults, and it may survive this one as well.

But then again, popes and dictators and philosopher kings have never had so many drugs at their disposal or a huge scientific-looking book claiming to list the natural varieties of our suffering. Nor have they been able to hold out the tantalizing possibility of elucidating the brain's role in consciousness, of finding us in its hundred billion or so neurons, its five hundred trillion synapses, its ten-to-the-millionth-power possible connections. Neither have they presided over a populace quite so eager to turn over their (and their children's) troubles to their brains and to the doctors who claim to know how to understand them, or quite so willing to gobble down mind-altering medications whose mechanisms of action and long-term effects are as unknown as their capacity to blunt feeling is known. So conditions might be ripe for a neuroscience-inflected psychiatry to usher in a new understanding of ourselves as the people of the brain and for us, with the help and encouragement of our doctors and the drug companies, to become the kind of selves who believe in and benefit from that understanding, and for whom the RDoC's matrix is the troubleshooting manual.

Not that an assault on human agency is what psychiatrists like Insel are after. Despite the creepy *Minority Report* overtones of his idea that we can be mentally ill (and ready for treatment) *before* we actually do anything, it's impossible to spend an hour or so with him and Cuthbert or, for that matter, with any of the doctors with whom I have spent so much time over the last couple of years and think that they are motivated by anything other than a wish to relieve suffering. Their purpose in cataloging our troubles is surely not to turn us into Shrink McNuggets. But they are in the grips of forces bigger than they are, bigger than any of us. It's not their fault that medicine is a service industry, that diseases are market opportunities, and that a book of them is worth its weight in gold.

After my visit with Frances in Boston, I e-mailed to ask him to name a diagnostic category that in his view made the strongest case for psychiatric diagnosis.

"Why do you hate psychiatrists so much? Is it because I pinched your cheek?" he wrote back.

I persisted. I wanted to hear about a slam dunk, the psychiatric equivalent of strep or diabetes, a single diagnosis that indicated a single pathology and a single treatment. But I would have settled for less, just one solid example of the value of a diagnostic system.

"Really silly questions," he replied. "Your bias is showing."

Frances did offer a defense. Not for the first time, he told me that "psychiatry done badly can be very harmful, psychiatry done well within its proper competence can be noble. The trick is to develop a healing relationship, to care for the person not just the disorder, to diagnose and treat cautiously, and to see the healthy part of the person not just the sick." All of which is inarguable, if a little hazy, but it doesn't really answer the question of why pulling off that trick requires a thousand-page catalog of disorders that are not real—other than to inspire confidence among bureaucrats, and among people who are comforted when a doctor names their suffering. Nor does it explain how exactly that book can keep psychiatry within its "proper competence." Neither does it acknowledge Freud's warning that medical education is the worst possible training for people who take on the troubles of the psyche, a warning issued long before the medical-industrial complex turned suffering into a commodity and psychiatry into a profession in which clinician communication must be efficient and the "healing relationship" must be established in ten-minute medication management visits.

"It isn't bias to be skeptical," I wrote. "And it's not antipsychiatry to question psychiatry. And it's not silly, in the context of a book about diagnosis, to ask how nosology relates to the practice of psychiatry." I gave Frances a hypothetical case, a psychotic person he has diagnosed with Bipolar Disorder. "How does that diagnosis help him to proceed?" I asked. It was the question former APA president Paul Fink once answered by saying, "I got paid."

"Like to help," Frances answered. "But the question makes no sense to me. Suggest you read a textbook of psychiatry."

At $80.99, *Kaplan & Sadock's Concise Textbook of Clinical Psychiatry* seems like a real bargain, compared with the $410.99 *Kaplan & Sadock's Comprehensive Textbook of Psychiatry*. At 700 pages, it isn't exactly concise, but it is a lot shorter than the 4,884-page full-size version, not to mention 200 pages shorter than the DSM-IV. So maybe Benjamin and Virginia Sadock, authors of the *Concise Textbook*, are just trying to save space, but when they tell students that "DSM-IV-TR attempts to describe the manifestations of the mental disorders," they don't mention that there's no reality to those mental disorders or warn students of the dangers of reification.

They do, however, tell the young doctors that it is a "major challenge" to separate the bipolars from the depressives, and they discuss the "difficulty of distinguishing a manic episode from schizophrenia." They explain that "depressive symptoms are present in almost all psychiatric disorders," that "every sign or symptom seen in schizophrenia occurs in other psychiatric and neurological disorders," and that "the distinction between generalized anxiety disorder and normal anxiety is emphasized by the use of the words 'excessive' and 'difficult to control.'" But, the book reassures the students, these difficulties can be overcome through careful clinical observation. Even if the categories don't exist, in other words, people can nonetheless be sorted into them.

"Once a diagnosis has been established," Sadock and Sadock write, "a pharmacological treatment strategy can be formulated." That may involve psychosocial treatment, but as just about any psychiatrist will tell you, the days in which psychiatrists underwent psychoanalysis as part of their training are long gone, as are the days in which psychiatrists routinely practiced talk therapy, so that treatment is most likely not going to be provided by them. When it comes to the technique that remains their sole bailiwick—pharmacotherapy—"no one drug is predictably effective." For bipolar patients, the doctor has at her disposal lithium, anticonvulsants such as Depakote, tranquilizers such as Ativan, and antipsychotics such as Haldol and Zyprexa. "Often," advise Sadock and Sadock, "it is necessary to try several so-called 'mood stabilizers' before an optimal treatment is found."

Even when the diagnosis is established, the treatment is still uncertain. And there is a good reason for this. According to Sadock and Sadock, "the objective of pharmacologic treatment is symptom remission." Bipolar isn't the only case. There is no specific treatment for any of the disorders Sadock and Sadock present, and many drugs are used for many conditions: antidepressants to treat obsessions, antipsychotics to treat depression, mood stabilizers to treat anxiety, and so on. Psychiatrists, in other words, are not treating the disorders they diagnose.

The categories, after all, aren't natural formations; symptoms, the scattered particulars, are all they have to go on and all they can treat.

Which doesn't mean they shouldn't treat them. "Not everyone needs to see a psychiatrist for the treatment of a mental disorder," Frances told me. "But if the problem is moderate to severe, persistent, and impairing, medication is likely to be needed. In my view, this should mostly be provided by psychiatrists, not primary care doctors who are usually out of their depth." He is surely right about this. Psychiatrists do indeed have a wealth of experience in treating people's distress with drugs. No clinician can deny the value of that knowledge, the way that people in the throes of a manic episode or a psychotic break or a disabling depression can be helped by drug therapy. Nor can anyone deny that this uncertainty about diagnosis and treatment is exactly what makes the expertise of the psychiatrist essential.

But you don't have to hate psychiatrists to point out that their expertise is mostly empirical and their treatments potentiated at least as much by hope as by chemistry. Or, to put it another way, that psychiatry, much more than other medical specialties, is still deeply in the debt of ancient medicine. The Platonic ideal of a world of suffering carved up into its natural formations remains exactly that—an ideal, one that psychiatric nosology can't yet approach. And you also don't have to hate psychiatrists to think that this gap, the distance between what the profession claims and what it actually knows, between its opportunity and its knowledge, is vast, and that even as the jury remains out on the legitimacy of psychiatry's claim to understand mental suffering, more and more people are taking daily doses of drugs whose mechanisms are poorly understood and whose long-term consequences, on the body and on the body politic, are uncertain. You don't have to hate psychiatrists to think that the ever-expanding DSM is not a book that can help psychiatrists stay within their competence, that indeed it encourages them to do the opposite. You don't have to hate psychiatrists to think that a book that dresses up symptoms as diseases that are not real and then claims to have named and described the true varieties of our suffering is all clothes and no emperor. And you don't have to hate psychiatrists to think we—patients, doctors, therapists, all of us—might be better off without it.

Or maybe the APA *was* trying to erase history. In early November 2012, the draft of the DSM-5 disappeared from the DSM-5 website, removed, according to a note on the home page, "to avoid confusion or use of outdated categories and definitions." It wasn't enough to threaten legal action against people who might want to use the draft criteria as part of a research project or, I don't know, a book about the development of the DSM-5. It is, of course, possible that the APA really feared that a paper using outdated criteria would slip by a peer reviewer or that a doctor would render a diagnosis based on discarded definitions. But it is also possible that the APA hit the delete button for the same reason Soviet apparatchiks airbrushed old photos: to prevent embarrassment.

The move was so arrogant, and so unnecessary, and so heedless of the public trust the APA holds—in short, it was so incompetent that it made me wonder if Frances had been right all along: that the trouble with the DSM-5 was purely bureaucratic, that if it turns into the disaster he has predicted, it will not be because the APA has found itself perfectly situated to exploit the capitalist imperative to turn all need into markets and thus to manufacture need by the carload. Neither will it be because a diagnostic empire built on air must at some point come crashing down, as if some tragic principle were at work, ensuring that hubris inevitably meets justice. Nor will it be because the attempt to catalog our suffering is doomed to be a fool's errand, that our troubles will always outdistance our attempts to take their measure. It will be because the Keystone Kops bungled the job. Only naiveté or animus toward psychiatry or a writer's fervent wish for drama could make someone read more into the unfolding events than incompetence, to see the DSM-5 as anything other than one more step in the long, random walk of human folly.

But there is a reason insiders trot out the one-bad-apple defense when disasters occur. It distracts from the more disturbing truth—in this case, that a profession that has been struggling to establish its credentials for more than a century, that has lurched from crisis to crisis, always for the same reason, always because it cannot make good on its claim to be treating diseases as other doctors do—that such a profession has something rotten at its foundation: its have-it-both-ways, real-until-it-isn't diagnostic manual.

You don't have to be a hater to think that the DSM, no matter how often it is revised or how competently, will never manage to pour the old wine of human suffering into the new skin of scientific medicine. And you don't have to resort to biblical analogies to show that the Bible of psychiatry is failing to do what it is presumably intended to do, and what would bolster the argument for bringing our mental suffering under the medical gaze: to improve psychiatric treatment. You don't even have to be an upside-down Jesuit or a Leibowitz unwittingly sowing the seeds of destruction. You could be Tom Insel, who is neither an antipsychiatrist nor a Jesuit of any spatial orientation, who is, in fact, America's psychiatrist in chief.

"Whatever we've been doing for five decades," he told me, "it ain't working. And when I look at the numbers—the number of suicides, number of disabilities, mortality data—it's abysmal, and it's not getting any better. All of the ways in which we've approached these illnesses, and with a lot of people working very hard, the outcomes we've got to point to are pretty bleak"—especially, he added, compared with the "extraordinary" progress in other fields, such as the 70 percent drop in mortality from cardiovascular disease since he went to medical school or the steep reductions in deaths from auto accidents and homicides. "There are some people for whom some of what we do is enormously helpful," he said. But even so, "we don't know which treatments are working for which people." And this litany of failure, he said, "gets us back to your interest in nosology. Maybe we just need to rethink this whole approach."

That's what Pliny Earle said in 1886, and what Thomas Salmon said in 1917, and George Raines in 1951, and Robert Spitzer in 1978, and Steve Hyman in 2000: that without a working nosology, psychiatry is a failure, that the current nosology (whatever it is) is sadly lacking, that the profession needs a new paradigm. You don't have to be an antipsychiatrist to wonder if incompetence can possibly explain all that futility, or if a profession that, despite its repeated failures, continues to "cherish expectations with regard to some mode of infallibly discovering the heart of man," as Melville once put it, deserves our confidence. You only have to know what Tom Insel knows and is honest enough to say out loud.

Insel may be right that a deeper foray into the thickets of the brain will yield what psychiatry has long sought: a taxonomy of disorders validated by biochemical findings. And Frances may also be correct that in the meantime mythical disorders are better than no disorders at all, that without them patients won't listen to their doctors or get the benefits of having a name for their pain. But no one knows what would happen if psychiatrists simply let themselves out of their epistemic prison by no longer pretending to know what they can't know. No one knows what would happen if they simply told you that they don't know what illness (if any) is causing your anxiety or depression or agitation, and then, if they thought it was warranted, told you there are drugs that might help (although they don't really know why or at what cost to the brain, or whether you will be able to stop taking them if you want to; nor can they guarantee that you—or your child—won't become obese or diabetic or die early), and offer you a prescription.

There are undoubtedly patients who would balk. Depressed people might be less willing to surrender their orgasms to Prozac if they don't think they are correcting a biochemical imbalance called Major Depressive Disorder. Psychotic patients might object to a lifetime of taking drugs that blunt their emotions, cloud their cognition, make them gain weight, and shorten their life span if they don't think they are being treated for Schizophrenia. Parents might hesitate to ply their kids with stimulants and antipsychotics if they believe that they are merely calming them down rather than treating their ADHD or BD (or, once the DSM-5 goes into effect, their DMDD). After all, this is a country whose pharmacological Calvinism has led to a four-decade-long war on drugs used merely to change the way we feel, and that harbors disdain—especially when it comes to our mental lives—for treating symptoms rather than underlying causes.

But other people would surely be willing to take the gamble. Indeed, they already are. Seventy-two percent of the prescriptions for antidepressants in the United States are written for patients who are not given a psychiatric diagnosis of any kind, who suffer from troubles ranging from tiredness and headaches to "abnormal sensations" and "nonspecific pain." It's impossible to know exactly how the prescribing doctors sold their patients on the idea of using the drugs, and while it's likely that at least some doctors told patients they had depression but then didn't write that down in the chart, it's also easy to imagine a conversation in which the doctor confesses her uncertainty about diagnosis, but suggests that other patients with similar symptoms have benefited from the drug and encourages the patient to give it a try.

Of course, this is exactly the kind of problem that Frances thinks arises when nonpsychiatric physicians (family doctors and other primary care providers account for 80 percent of those prescriptions) go beyond their proper competence. He may be right about this, but that doesn't necessarily mean specialists are more restrained in their prescribing habits, nor is whatever advantage they might have over their nonpsychiatrist colleagues the result of being better at figuring out which of the nonreal mental disorders listed in the DSM their patients have. Rather, it is more likely to come from their greater experience in treating symptoms, in making the artful judgment of which potion is likely to help which patient. If this—the ability to match symptom with drug—were the only claim that psychiatry made, if psychiatrists stopped pretending that they know the proper names for our suffering, then perhaps the profession could finally free itself from the prison it has built.

Of course, a psychiatry that gave up a common scientific language, and the perquisites it garners, might also not have a DSM, or at least not one that looks anything like the DSM we have now. But by no longer insisting that it is just like the rest of medicine, and by renouncing its noble lies about the scientific status of psychiatric diagnosis, the profession might become a more honest one than it is now. Given that psychiatrists demand honesty from their patients, honesty is perhaps the least we should ask of them. It might even build our confidence. (And theirs: with less to defend itself about, psychiatry, or at least the APA, might have less need for secrecy and paranoia, and less need to diagnose all its opponents with Antipsychiatry Disorder.)

But there is no doubt that an honest psychiatry would be a smaller profession. It would have fewer patients, more modest claims about what it treats, less clout with insurers, and reduced authority to turn our troubles into medical problems simply by adding the word *disorder* to their description. It would, in other words, be more likely to stay within its proper competence. Its restraint would depend not on the modesty of aristocrats, who have proven themselves to be unreliable in that respect, and not on government regulation, which, even if it were possible, has recently fallen into disrepute, and not on the discovery of the boundary between mental health and mental illness, which will always prove elusive, but on that much more modern and effective arbiter, the one master to whom we all seem to submit: the marketplace.

Speaking of marketplaces, an honest psychiatry would not be such a good thing for my profession, at least not if it meant the end of the DSM as we know it. We talk therapists have arguably been the book's prime beneficiaries. While psychiatrists are treating the floridly psychotic, the raving manic, the suicidal and the catatonic and the delirious, we, by and large, get to minister to the walking wounded. Thanks to Bob Spitzer's expansive approach to the DSM, we can casually jot down "Generalized Anxiety Disorder" or "Adjustment Disorder" and talk (on the insurance tab) with our patients about the meaning of life, while right down the hall psychiatrists are making momentous decisions about whether a man who thinks his bones have been sucked out of him is bipolar or schizophrenic and which drugs to prescribe. While they have to take the DSM at least a little seriously, we can pretend it doesn't exist, give it the cynical bureaucrat's shrug, denounce it even as we cash those insurance company checks. And when it comes time to revise it or explain it or defend it, and its flaws are once again open to scrutiny, it's the psychiatrists who take the heat.

Not that I feel particularly sorry for them, but it is clear that for us nonpsychiatrist clinicians, the stakes are purely monetary. Without those codes and the access they give us to insurance companies' compensation schemes, the unfettered marketplace will decide how much we are worth. Weekly visits with me right now cost the equivalent of a monthly payment on a car. I try to adjust my charges according to what a person can afford to drive. But while for some people that's a BMW, for others it isn't even a badly used Kia, and I have no doubt that shorn of their DSM-enabled insurance subsidy, fewer people could pay me anything at all. So I would make less money. In this, I am like workers everywhere in America, although at least for now my job can't be offshored.

An honest psychiatry might also lead the way to a new understanding of illness. The idea that disease is suffering caused by an identifiable pathogen that can be targeted and killed by medicine's magic bullets is a historical accident, one that originated at the height of the Industrial Revolution and that springs as much from commerce as from science. It has been an extraordinarily beneficial idea, but like all inventions, it has its drawbacks—notably that it has encouraged us to think that all our troubles will ultimately yield to the microscope and the pill.

"The future belongs to illness," Peter Sedgwick wrote in the early 1970s. "We are just going to get more and more diseases, since our expectations of health are going to become more sophisticated and expansive." Thanks to a DSM that has kept pace with those expectations, that future is here. It has arrived in a capitalist age, which means that we have placed our well-being in the not-so-invisible hands of a medical-industrial complex whose proprietors have a stake in reducing suffering to biochemistry. It has spawned a psychiatry that can't help giving us more and more diseases, at least not if it wants to meet the economic, if not the scientific, demands of the day.

Still, the problem with psychiatry may not be that it lags behind the other medical specialties, with their magic bullets and the science by which they identify the targets. Rather, it may be a harbinger of a time when the low-hanging fruit has been picked, when the inadequacies of modern medicine to the complexity of our suffering—physical and mental alike—have become manifest, and when the folly of encouraging us to give up the ghost for the machine is unmistakable.

Because there is one definition of mental disorder that is not bullshit. Mental disorder, like all disease, is suffering that a society devotes resources to relieving. The line between sickness and health, mental and physical, is not biological but social and economic. It is the line between the distress for which we will provide sympathy and money and access to treatment, and the distress for which we will not. For the past 150 years, we have relied on doctors to decide who gets those resources, and they in turn have furnished us with diseases that, they assure us, are not figments of their imaginations, but real entities that reside in tissues and cells and molecules, that can be observed and measured, and, if all goes well, treated. Psychiatry has tried its best to stake its claim to this bonanza, perhaps nowhere so ardently as in its attempt to fashion its book of woe, but it has not worked. This may be because the psychiatrists in question, or their technologies, have not been up to the job. It may be because that line can't be drawn without deciding how a human life is supposed to go, how it ought to feel, and what it is for—questions for which science, no matter how robust, is no match. It may be because the arc of history bends toward justice, and biochemistry may not be the fairest basis on which to determine whose suffering deserves recognition. But it may also be because the human mind, even in its troubles, perhaps especially in them, has so far resisted this attempt to turn its discontents into a catalog of suffering. And for this we should be glad.

Afterword

The careful reader will by now have detected the odor of a certain barnyard effluent suffusing this book. My opportunity to publish at the same time as the DSM-5 exceeds my knowledge of what is actually in the new manual. Indeed, it is very likely that you know more about its specifics as you read this than I do as I write in early January 2013. But I do know a little about the final product.

For this, I can thank the APA. Not that they decided to talk directly to me, but they did use the trustees' rubber-stamping of the final draft at the beginning of December 2012 as an occasion to release some details—among them, the price of the new book, $199. As expected, Hoarding Disorder and Disruptive Mood Dysregulation Disorder were in, Asperger's was out, and Attenuated Psychosis Symptoms Syndrome was in the Appendix, now officially renamed Section 3, where it would be joined by all the dimensional measures and the "trait-specific methodology" proposal for personality disorders. (Those diagnoses would revert largely to their DSM-IV versions.) Section 3 would also include "the names of individuals involved in *DSM-5*'s development." I'm looking forward to finding out if my name is among them.

The summary left unanswered some important questions. For instance, while it said that Asperger's would be "integrated" into the autistic spectrum, it did not spell out exactly how, or whether the APA would retain ownership of the name or relinquish it to all those Aspies in search of an identity. Neither did it illuminate a persistent rumor: that currently diagnosed Asperger's patients would be "grandfathered," keeping the diagnosis even if the disorder was eliminated. It mentioned that the bereavement exclusion had been replaced by "several notes within the text delineating the differences between grief and depression," but did not elaborate except to say that the change "reflects the recognition that bereavement is a severe psychosocial stressor that can precipitate a major depressive episode beginning soon after the loss of a loved one." What a clinician, astute or otherwise, was supposed to do with that recognition was not made clear.

The press release did offer some reassurances to a skeptical public. "We have sought to be very conservative in our approach to revising DSM-5," David Kupfer said. "Our work has been aimed at more accurately defining mental disorders that have a real impact on people's lives, not expanding the scope of psychiatry." And Jay Scully reminded reporters that the process had been "as open and independent as possible. The level of transparency we have strived for is not seen in any other area of medicine." An e-mail sent by Kupfer and Regier to task force and work group members in advance of the press release elaborated on just how open and independent that was. "We do ask that you focus your interviews on the disorder and refrain from talking about the criteria or text," it read. They apparently didn't want anyone to spoil the surprise.

The trustees' vote triggered a spate of news coverage, some of it summarizing the APA's summary, some of it opining for or against, and at least one article—in *The Washington Post*—repeating charges of corruption in the process, this time by reporting on the study that Sid Zisook, architect of the bereavement policy, once ran proving that Wellbutrin was effective in the bereaved. The APA responded with a press release under David Kupfer's byline, reiterating all that the task force had done to eliminate conflicts of interest and assuring the public that "DSM-5 includes material to make sure that it is understood that sadness, grief, and bereavement are not things that have a time limitation to them or go away within two or three months." What it meant that psychiatrists had to be told this, or what they would do now that they had been informed, Kupfer did not say.

Two weeks after the vote, psychiatric diagnosis was back on the front pages, this time when a young man armed with a semiautomatic weapon slaughtered twenty children at an elementary school in Connecticut. Dilip Jeste, the APA president, told Congress that the tragedy, which occurred "at the very time [that] federal and state funding for critical mental health services is under siege," was a reminder that, because mentally ill people in treatment are "considerably less likely to commit violent acts" than those who are untreated, Congress should "act to protect federal funding for mental health . . . research and services." Three days later, however, after the National Rifle Association's Wayne LaPierre told the nation that no matter how many rounds they can fire in an instant, guns don't kill people, "lunatics" kill people, and suggested that the solution to the problem was a registry of mentally ill people whose diagnoses would presumably lose them their Second Amendment rights, Jeste took a different approach. Not only was LaPierre's language "offensive," he said in a news release, but "only four to five percent of violent crimes are committed by people with mental illness," and that "only a small percentage" of the 25 percent of Americans who will come down with a mental disorder in any given year "will ever commit violent crimes." Gun violence, in other words, was not an indication of mental illness unless there was money to be made.

Al Frances responded to the trustees' vote with what he promised would be his last blog on the subject. "The saddest day in my 45-year career," he wrote, and urged clinicians to "ignore its ten worst changes," which he enumerated. "Apparently they deleted a few irrelevant things and approved all the junk that was left," he e-mailed.

Ten days later, Frances broke his promise, telling readers that the APA had "one last act to save DSM 5 before the curtain drops," and warning that unless the organization used the remaining time to fix the outstanding problems (and add a black-box warning about the dangers of overdiagnosis), the new manual would be "a financial as well as a clinical, scientific, and artistic flop." He repeated this warning in a series of e-mails to the APA's leaders, in which he promised to shut up if they heeded his advice. They did not take him up on his offer.

The APA wasn't the only organization ignoring Frances. In the wake of the trustees' approval, many proposals to boycott the DSM-5 sprang up—a dozen, by his account. He urged comity. "Any new boycott must unify the diverse opposition," he wrote, "not further fragment what is already a very fragmented field." But the groups did not coalesce into a single movement, nor did the antipsychiatrists among the dissidents heed his call to stop using his name ("without permission," he pointed out) to support their cause. Frances was left to explain once again that his attack on his profession's foundational text was not an attack on the profession itself.

For his part, Michael First was back on the inside. In late November, I asked him about a rumor I'd been hearing all fall: that the APA had called him to duty to help finalize the manual. "I can confirm it's true," he e-mailed, "but I really cannot say anything else. Sorry." He wasn't going to jeopardize his ability to do once again what he'd been born to do. An insider, who also wouldn't go on the record, made it clear that his role was limited: reviewing criteria for consistency, editing them for clarity, and making sure the book could be used by clinicians.

First was willing to give me his overall appraisal of the outcome. "The good news about the DSM-5 is also the bad news," he e-mailed. "While many little things have changed for the better, and clinicians will find the transition relatively easy to make, the fundamental problems with the descriptive approach remain." It still explains little, offers scant treatment guidelines, and "relies on categories that facilitate clinician communication but have no firm basis in reality. So I think it's an improvement," he concluded, "but it's also an acknowledgment that psychiatry, especially in its understanding of mental illness, is still in its infancy." Whether the profession can grow up remains to be seen.

Acknowledgments

At *Wired*, where this book got its start (and its title): Bill Wasik and Bess Kalb.

At Blue Rider Press: Aileen Boyle, Anna Jardine, Phoebe Pickering, David Rosenthal, and the inestimable Sarah Hochman.

For crack agentry: Jim Rutman.

For reading and comment on parts of the manuscript: Barney Carroll, Bill Musgrave, and Stuart Vyse.

For reading and comment on the entire manuscript: Rand Cooper, Gideon Lewis-Kraus, and Michelle Orange.

For interviews that no doubt turned out to be more than they bargained for, not to mention all those follow-up e-mails: Bill Bernet, Michael Carley, Gabrielle Carlson, Will Carpenter, Jane Costello, Bruce Cuthbert, Max Fink, Paul Fink, Steve Hyman, Tom Insel, Nomi Kaim, Ronald Kessler, David Kupfer, John Livesley, Catherine Lord, Steve Mirin, Bill Narrow, Roger Peele, Harold Pincus, Darrel Regier, Jay Scully, David Shaffer, Andrew Skodol, Bob Spitzer, Fred Volkmar, Jerry Wakefield, Barbara Wiechmann, Tom Widiger, and Sid Zisook.

For research materials and editorial assistance: Paula Caplan, Beth Card, Bart Laws, Ned Shorter, Steve Silberman, Katherine Sticklor, and Ken Kendler.

For careful proofreading: Ruth Greenberg.

For honesty, patience, and generosity: Michael First.

For honesty, patience, generosity, and hospitality, sometimes against their better judgment: Allen Frances and Donna "Peach" Manning.

And, as always, for bringing out my best and putting up with my worst, and for her blue eyes: Susan Marie Powers.

Notes

Chapter 1

2   *"In noticing a disease"*: Cartwright, "Diseases and Peculiarities of the Negro Race," Part 1, 332.

1   *"the disease causing Negroes"*: Ibid., 331.

1   *Two classes of persons*: Ibid., 332.

2   *"whipping the devil"*: Ibid.

2   *"submissive knee-bender"*: Ibid.

2   *"northern hornbooks in Medicine"*: Cartwright, "Diseases and Peculiarities of the Negro Race," Part 2, 506.

2   *"demonstrated, by dissection"*: Ibid., 505.

2   *"the membranes, tendons, and aponeuroses"*: Ibid., 506.

3   *dyaesthesia aethiopica*: Cartwright, "Diseases and Peculiarities," Part 1, 333.

4   *"the learned Dr. Cartwright"*: Olmsted, *Journeys and Explorations*, 122.

4   *"the nervous erythism"*: S. B. Hunt, "Dr. Cartwright on 'Drapetomania,'" 441–42.

5   *They underwent countless therapies*: For an account of the treatment of homosexuals, see LeVay, *Queer Science*, chapter 4.

5   *11 percent of the U.S. adult population*: Centers for Disease Control, "NCHS Data Brief, October 19, 2011," http://www.cdc.gov/nchs/data/databriefs/db76.htm.

5   *you got tired of feeling numb*: For side effects of antidepressants, see Glenmullen, *Prozac Backlash*.

5   *placebo effect*: Kirsch, *The Emperor's New Drugs*.

5   *this chemical imbalance does not, as far as doctors know*: Greenberg, *Manufacturing Depression*.

5   *more than seventy combinations of symptoms*: See DSM-IV-TR, 356. There are nine symptoms of depression, but patients need have only five in any combination to earn the diagnosis.

7   *"another [of] the ten thousand"*: Cartwright, "Diseases and Peculiarities," Part 1, 336.

10   *"Love is a madness"*: Plato, *Phaedrus*, 265e.

12   *Before John Snow*: The best account of this famous story is probably Steven Johnson's *The Ghost Map*.

12   *Louis Pasteur and Robert Koch*: Ullmann, "Pasteur–Koch."

14   *"blessed rage to order"*: Stevens, "The Idea of Order at Key West," *The Palm at the End of the Mind*.

page

14   *Adam and Eve:* Genesis 2:19–21.

15   *"loose, baggy monster":* Henry James, *The Tragic Muse*, 4.

16   *"insomnia, flushing, drowsiness":* Beard, *American Nervousness*, 7–8.

17   *"As long as I live":* Gay, *Freud*, 491.

17   *"It burdens [a doctor]":* Freud, *The Question of Lay Analysis*, 95.

17   *"the mental sciences":* Ibid., 88–90.

18   *"the patient's ambivalent feeling":* American Psychiatric Association, DSM-I, 34.

19   *a psychologist showed:* Ash, "The Reliability of Psychiatric Diagnoses."

19   *By 1962, despite various attempts:* Summarized in Beck, "Reliability of Psychiatric Diagnoses."

19   *doctors in Great Britain:* Sandifer et al., "Psychiatric Diagnosis." See also Kendell et al., "Diagnostic Criteria of American and British Psychiatrists."

19   *Erving Goffman and Michel Foucault:* See Goffman, *Asylums*, and Foucault, *Madness and Civilization*.

20   *The DSM instructs users:* American Psychiatric Association, DSM-IV-TR, xxxi–xxxii.

22   *"perhaps the most powerful psychiatrist in America":* Daniel Goleman, "Scientist at Work," *The New York Times*, April 19, 1994.

23   *"Here's the problem":* Allen Frances interview, August 16, 2010.

23   *the lead of the* Wired *article:* Gary Greenberg, "The Book of Woe: Inside the Battle to Define Mental Illness," *Wired*, December 2010, 126–36.

24   *"Bullshit is unavoidable":* Frankfurt, *On Bullshit*, 63.

24   *"neither on the side of the true":* Ibid., 56.

Chapter 2

26   *"The present classification of mental diseases is chaotic":* Salmon et al., "Report of the Committee on Statistics," 256.

27   *"It cannot be supposed":* Jarvis, *Relation of Education to Insanity*, 4–5.

27   *"Within the last fifty years":* Ibid., 6.

27   *"In an uneducated community":* Ibid., 8.

28   *"From all this survey":* Ibid., 11.

28   *"In the present state of our knowledge":* Grob, "Origins of DSM-I," 231. Emphasis in original.

28   *"had become marginal":* Shorter, *History of Psychiatry*, 144.

29   *"Pathological anatomy":* Kraepelin, *Lectures*, 27.

29   *"poetic interpretation":* Kraepelin, "Manifestations of Insanity," 512.

30   *he took a Kraepelinian approach:* Salmon, "Report of the Committee on Statistics," 256–59.

30   *the association issued the Statistical Manual:* Grob, "Origins of DSM-I," 426.

31   *its last edition ran to seventy-one pages:* American Psychiatric Association, *Statistical Manual for the Use of Hospitals*.

31   *a membership of only 2,295 doctors:* Grob, "Origins of DSM-I," 427.

31   *"Our experiences with therapy":* Quoted in Grob, "Origins of DSM-I," 428.

31   *Psychoanalysis proved easy enough to adapt:* For a detailed account of this shift, see Zaretsky, *Secrets of the Soul*, especially chapters 10 and 11.

32   *only 10 percent of their cases:* American Psychiatric Association, DSM-I, vi.

32   *"At least three nomenclatures":* Ibid., vii.

33   *"stepchild of [the] Federal Government":* DSM-I, x.

page
33   *Anxiety Reaction:* DSM-I, 32.

33   *Depressive Reaction:* DSM-I, 33.

34   *"disorders of psychogenic origin":* DSM-I, 24.

34   *"Instead of putting so much emphasis":* Menninger, *The Vital Balance,* 325.

34   *"Man in transaction with his universe":* Quoted in Wilson, "DSM-III and the Transformation of American Psychiatry," 401.

34   *it had become a professional backwater:* Wilson, "DSM-III," 403.

35   *"compared to other types of services":* Quoted ibid.

35   *The war over the homosexuality diagnosis:* For a full account, see Bayer, *Homosexuality and American Psychiatry.*

35   *Ego-Dystonic Homosexuality:* DSM-III, 281–82.

36   *"If groups of people march":* Bayer, *Homosexuality and American Psychiatry,* 141.

36   *"Referenda on matters of science":* Ibid., 153.

36   *"Psychiatry was regarded as bogus":* Robert Spitzer interview, August 27, 2010.

38   *"I was uncomfortable with not knowing":* Spiegel, "The Dictionary of Disorder."

38   *By 1972, the group had described:* Feighner et al., "Diagnostic Criteria for Use in Psychiatric Research."

38   *Research Diagnostic Criteria:* Spitzer et al., "Research Diagnostic Criteria: Rationale and Reliability."

39   *A. One or more distinct periods:* Ibid., 776.

40   *the nosology would inexorably gain substance:* Ibid., 781–82.

40   *"The use of operational criteria":* Ibid., 781.

42   *a conclusion he published in the* Archives of Sexual Behavior: Spitzer, "Can Some Gay Men and Lesbians Change Their Sexual Orientation?"

42   *a letter to the* Archives: Spitzer, "Spitzer Reassesses His 2003 Study of Reparative Therapy."

Chapter 3

44   *"In the morning, everyone would be screaming ideas":* Allen Frances telephone interview, November 23, 2011.

45   *people who "employ self-sacrificing and self-defeating behavior":* Siever and Klar, "A Review of DSM-III Criteria for the Personality Disorders," 304.

45   *"dumb idea":* Allen Frances e-mail, November 27, 2011.

46   *"The fact that we had a descriptive system only revealed":* Allen Frances interview, August 16, 2010.

47   *"loving the pet, even if it is a mutt":* Allen Frances e-mail, September 3, 2010.

48   *"seemed a bit like stamp collecting":* Hyman, "The Diagnosis of Mental Disorders: The Problem of Reification," 157.

48   *"The tendency [is] always strong":* James Mill, *Analysis of the Phenomena of the Human Mind,* 5. The quotation is from a footnote appended to a later edition of Mill's 1829 book by his son John Stuart Mill.

48   *"It became a source of real worry":* Ibid.

50   *"I realized that it got me nowhere":* Steven Hyman e-mail, October 5, 2012.

51   *the* Post *had twice come out against parity:* "The Mental Health Amendment," *The Washington Post,* April 28, 1996; and " 'Parity' in Health Insurance," *The Washington Post,* December 4, 2001.

page

51   *They "asked questions"*: "Changes Put APA on Right Track to Face Future," *Psychiatric News*, October 4, 2002.

52   *They'd asked twenty thousand people*: The questionnaire is available in Robins and Regier, *Psychiatric Disorders in America*, 401–26.

52   *The ECA's findings*: Ibid., 333.

52   *And the sick among us were really sick*: Ibid., 357.

52   *only 19 percent*: Ibid., 361.

55   *the paper came out in favor of parity*: "Equity for Mental Illness," *The Washington Post*, September 9, 2002.

56   *the Midtown Manhattan Study*: Srole et al., *Mental Health in the Metropolis*, vol. 1.

57   *"designed for classifying full-blown pathology"*: Ibid., 134.

57   *So rather than ask . . . they asked about*: Ibid., 388–91.

58   *a six-point classification*: Ibid., 134–38.

58   *"mental illness and mental health [differed]"*: Ibid., 135.

58   *the actual number is 81.5 percent*: Ibid., 138.

59   *It was more than double the rate of mental illness*: Ibid., 141–43.

59   *he cited the 23 percent figure accurately*: Regier et al., "The De Facto U.S. Mental Health Services System," 687.

59   *about 15 percent of Americans were mentally ill*: Ibid., 692–93.

Chapter 4

61   *"the mind is a set of operations"*: Kandel, "The New Science of Mind," 69.

61   *"all mental disorders"*: Ibid., 71.

61   *"We can think of mental disorders"*: Insel, "Rethinking Mental Illness," 2011 American Psychiatric Association annual meeting, Honolulu, May 14, 2011.

62   *"neurologizing tautologies"*: Meyer, "The Aims and Meaning of Psychiatric Diagnosis," 165.

62   *"driving the Devil out"*: Shorter and Healy, *Shock Therapy*, 30.

63   *it was hard to argue with the biological psychiatrists*: For a history of these discoveries, see Greenberg, *Manufacturing Depression*, chapters 7, 8; Healy, *The Creation of Psychopharmacology*, and Shorter, *History of Psychiatry*.

63   *depression, he announced, must be the result*: Schildkraut, "The Catecholamine Hypothesis of Affective Disorders."

64   *"The gold standard was the DSM criteria"*: Steven Hyman e-mail, October 5, 2012.

65   *"to the point that they are considered"*: Kupfer, First, and Regier, *Research Agenda for DSM-V*, xix.

65   *"yet unknown"*: Ibid.

66   *"In a way, I was born to do the DSM"*: Michael First interview, April 25, 2011.

71   *"I have a patient"*: Paul Fink interview, September 2, 2010.

72   *"There is no assumption"*: DSM-IV-TR, xxxi.

73   *"The purpose of DSM-III"*: DSM-III, 12.

73   *"consensus of current formulations"*: DSM-III-R, xxix.

73   *black-box warning*: http://www.fda.gov/downloads/Drugs/DrugSafety/Informationby DrugClass/UCM161641.pdf.

Chapter 5

page

76   *"When I heard about them"*: Allen Frances interview, July 7, 2011.

77   *Biederman thought he detected in these children*: Biederman, "Resolved: Mania Is Mistaken for ADHD."

77   *a small literature reporting a few cases of "hyperactive children"*: Ibid., 1091.

78   *"the essential feature of Bipolar Disorder"*: DSM-IV-TR, 382.

78   *"a distinct period of abnormally and persistently elevated"*: DSM-IV-TR, 362.

78   *Manic episodes have seven Criterion B symptoms*: Ibid.

79   *So Biederman set out to prove*: Wozniak et al., "Mania-Like Symptoms." See also Biederman, "Pediatric Bipolar Disorder Coming of Age."

79   *One in five of those patients*: Wozniak et al., "Mania-Like Symptoms," 873.

79   *Biederman's announcement provoked*: See, for instance, Klein, Pine, and Klein, "Resolved: Mania Is Mistaken for ADHD," and McClellan, "Commentary: Treatment Guidelines for Child and Adolescent Bipolar Disorder."

80   *"smallpox vaccine was ridiculed"*: Biederman, "Resolved," 1098.

81   *"disorders with bipolar features"*: DSM-IV-TR, 400.

82   *"thoughtful clinical investigators"*: Papolos and Papolos, *The Bipolar Child*, 32.

82   *"latest research findings" would recognize the symptoms*: Ibid., 55–59.

82   *"You have bipolar disorder"*: Anglada, *Brandon and the Bipolar Bear*, 16.

82   *"can't do their job right"*: Ibid., 17.

82   *Brandon most likely inherited it*: Ibid., 20.

82   *"Young and Bipolar"*: "Young and Bipolar," *Time*, August 19, 2002.

82   *6.67 percent of office visits*: Moreno et al., "National Trends in the Outpatient Diagnosis and Treatment of Bipolar Disorder in Youth."

83   *"The label may or may not reflect reality"*: Benedict Carey, "Bipolar Disorder Cases Rise Sharply in U.S. Children," *The New York Times*, September 3, 2007.

84   *there is "some medicine that could help"*: Anglada, *Brandon and the Bipolar Bear*, 21.

84   *rebranding atypical antipsychotics*: The APA had a hand in this effort. See Hales et al., *What Your Patients Need to Know About Psychiatric Medications*, 183–85.

84   *devastating side effects*: See, for example, Üçok and Gaebel, "Side Effects of Atypical Antipsychotics: A Brief Overview."

84   *twelve-to-twenty-year decrease in life expectancy*: See Whitaker, *Anatomy of an Epidemic*, 175–77.

84   *studies indicating that children's symptoms improved*: For a summary, see Kowatch et al., "Treatment Guidelines for Children and Adolescents with Bipolar Disorder."

84   *prevalence of BD among children*: Moreno et al., "National Trends."

84   *antipsychotic use in children and adolescents*: "Antipsychotic Drug Use Among Kids Soars," Associated Press, May 3, 2006.

85   *Gardiner Harris reported*: Gardiner Harris, "Proof Is Scant on Psychiatric Drug Mix for Young," *The New York Times*, November 23, 2006.

85   *stories such as that of Rebecca Riley*: David Abel, "Hull Parents Arrested in Girl's Poisoning Death," *The Boston Globe*, February 6, 2007.

85   *"In psychiatry Mr. Grassley has found"*: Benedict Carey and Gardiner Harris, "Psychiatric Group Faces Scrutiny over Drug Industry Ties," *The New York Times*, July 12, 2008.

86   *what Grassley found when he investigated Joseph Biederman*: Gardiner Harris and Benedict Carey, "Researchers Fail to Reveal Full Drug Pay," *The New York Times*, June 8, 2008.

page
86   *"move forward the commercial goals"*: Gardiner Harris, "Research Center Tied to Drug Company," *The New York Times*, November 25, 2008.

86   *"will support the safety and effectiveness of risperidone"*: Gardiner Harris, "Drug Maker Told Studies Would Aid It," *The New York Times*, March 20, 2009.

87   *this exchange, which followed his testimony*: Ibid.

87   *"I have never seen someone so angry"*: Harris, "Research Center Tied to Drug Company."

87   *"violated certain requirements"*: Liz Kowalczyk, "Harvard Doctors Punished Over Pay," *The Boston Globe*, July 2, 2011.

87   *Grassley wasn't stopping with Biederman*: Gardiner Harris, "Top Psychiatrist Didn't Report Drug Makers' Pay," *The New York Times*, October 3, 2008.

88   *He revealed that Frederick Goodwin*: Gardiner Harris, "Radio Host Has Drug Company Ties," *The New York Times*, November 21, 2008.

88   *a drug that has been "generic for decades"*: Statement of Frederick K. Goodwin, M.D., http://drgoodwin.com/index.php?page=nyt.

88   *Alan Schatzberg owned nearly $5 million in stock*: Harris, "Top Psychiatrist."

88   *"I have come to understand"*: Senator Grassley's letter is available at http://www.finance.senate.gov/newsroom/ranking/release/?id=56860a96-5fba-4fb9-9207-849e796998ad.

88   *nearly one-third of the organization's $62.5 million annual revenue*: Carey and Harris, "Psychiatric Group Faces Scrutiny over Drug Industry Ties."

89   *As the* Times *had reported earlier*: Benedict Carey, "Study Finds a Link of Drug Makers to Psychiatrists," *The New York Times*, April 20, 2006.

89   *the report of a team led by psychologist Lisa Cosgrove*: Cosgrove et al., "Financial Ties Between DSM-IV Panel Members and the Pharmaceutical Industry," 154–60.

89   *"Pharmaceutical companies have a vested interest"*: Ibid., 159.

89   *Restless legs syndrome*: GlaxoSmithKline, press release, June 10, 2003, www.gsk.com/press_archive/press2003/press_06102003.htm.

89   *"With every new revelation"*: Carey and Harris, "Psychiatric Group Faces Scrutiny."

91   *the $4 million or so the industry kicked down every year*: See APA Treasurer's Report, May 2012. Available at https://docs.google.com/file/d/0BzWdENl1wkVSYk5aXzRZelFYUjA/edit?pli=1. This report contains APA financial reports from 2005 to 2011.

91   *"my board thought that through"*: James Scully interview, September 13, 2010.

92   *it took nearly two years*: Regier et al., *The Conceptual Evolution of DSM-5*, xxv.

92   *"All the people at the top"*: Michael First interview, April 25, 2011.

92   *"a new diagnostic paradigm must be developed"*: Kenneth S. Kendler et al., "Guidelines for Making Changes to DSM-V," http://www.dsm5.org/ProgressReports/Documents/Guidelines-for-Making-Changes-to-DSM_1.pdf.

Chapter 6

93   *"I was bored stiff"*: Allen Frances e-mail, October 7, 2011.

93   *"Psychiatric classification"*: Allen Frances e-mail, October 11, 2011.

93   *"Perhaps not surprisingly, the diagnosis"*: Allen Frances e-mail, October 7, 2011.

94   *"confidentiality in the development"*: See Hannah Decker, "A Moment of Crisis in American Psychiatry," *h-madness* (blog), April 27, 2010, http://historypsychiatry.com/2010/04/27/a-moment-of-crisis-in-the-history-of-american-psychiatry/.

page
94 *the APA had insisted:* On its acceptance form, available at http://www.dsm5.org/about/Documents/DSM%20Member%20Acceptance%20Form.pdf.

94 *"We are rethinking":* "DSM-V Development Will Be Complex and Open Process," *Psychiatric News,* June 6, 2008.

94 *"I was dumbfounded":* Robert Spitzer e-mail, September 24, 2010.

95 *"I found out how transparent" . . . "I didn't know whether":* Robert Spitzer, "DSM-V: Open and Transparent?" *Psychiatric News,* July 18, 2008.

95 *"I told him I completely agreed":* Allen Frances interview, August 15, 2010.

95 *new diagnosis to be called Psychosis Risk Syndrome:* For a full description, see Carpenter, "Anticipating DSM-V: Should Psychosis Risk Become a Diagnostic Class?" and Woods et al., "Validity of the Prodromal Risk Syndrome for First Psychosis."

96 *a conversion rate of 25 to 30 percent:* See Cornblatt and Correll, "A New Diagnostic Entity in DSM-5?"

96 *"I had not been closely following":* Allen Frances interview, August 16, 2010.

97 *Carpenter explained to Pincus:* William Carpenter interview, September 10, 2010.

98 *"I still think it's a crazy idea":* Harold Pincus interview, December 9, 2011.

99 *pseudoneurotic schizophrenia:* Allen Frances telephone interview, November 23, 2011.

99 *"more kids getting unneeded antipsychotics":* Allen Frances interview, August 16, 2010.

Chapter 7

100 *"People are going to write dissertations":* James Scully interview, September 13, 2010.

100 *Zucker was known for research:* See Zucker and Bradley, *Gender Identity Disorder and Psychosexual Problems in Children and Adolescents.*

101 *a fetish Blanchard called* autogynephilia: Blanchard, "The Concept of Autogynephilia and the Typology of Male Gender Dysphoria."

101 *"out of step":* National Gay and Lesbian Task Force, "Task Force Questions Critical Appointments to APA's Committee on Sexual and Gender Identity Disorders," news release, May 18, 2008. http://www.thetaskforce.org/press/releases/PR_052808.

101 *"thorough and balanced":* American Psychiatric Association, "APA Statement on GID and the DSM-V," news release, May 23, 2008, http://www.dsm5.org/Newsroom/Documents/APAStatementonGIDandTheDSMV.pdf.

102 *"the DSM is a diagnostic manual":* Ibid.

103 *an immediate rejoinder:* Nada Stotland et al., "DSM-V: Open and Transparent? A Response," *Psychiatric News,* July 18, 2008.

104 *Regier wanted to know:* Darrel Regier, William Narrow, and David Kupfer interview, September 14, 2010.

104 *"I'm not on the task force":* Sidney Zisook interview, September 10, 2010.

105 *"We have enemies":* Stotland, "Presidential Address," 1102.

105 *"psychiatry is a pseudo-science":* Tom Cruise, interview by Matt Lauer, *Today,* June 25, 2005, http://msnbc.msn.com/id/8343367/site/todayshow/ns/today-entertainment/t/im-passionate-about-life/.

105 *"Michael First shamed me into it":* Allen Frances e-mail, December 18, 2011.

107 *"Setting the Record Straight":* Alan Schatzberg et al., "Setting the Record Straight," *Psychiatric Times,* July 1, 2008.

108 *"Soaring ambition is another matter":* William Carpenter, "Criticism vs Fact," *Psychiatric Times,* July 7, 2008.

page
109   *"letting nostalgia and passion"*: Alarcon, "DSM-5—The We Know Better/Holier Than Thou Crusade," *Psychiatric Times*, July 14, 2008.

109   *"You must understand"*: Allen Frances, letter to APA board of trustees, July 6, 2009. http://www.scribd.com/doc/17172432/Letter-to-APA-Board-of-Trustees-July-7-2009-From-Allen-Frances-and-Robert-Spitzer.

110   *The APA's financial picture*: APA's Treasurer Report, 2012.

110   *"In reality, clinicians in the United States"*: Michael First interview, August 24, 2010.

110   *the ICD . . . is available for download*: You can browse it yourself at http://apps.who .int/classifications/icd10/browse/2010/en.

112   *an unsettling if unsurprising discovery*: Clayton et al., "The Bereavement of the Widowed."

112   *"a full depressive syndrome"*: DSM-III, 333.

113   *The bereavement exclusion*: DSM-III-R, 223.

114   *he tried to define* disease: Spitzer and Endicott, "Medical and Mental Disorder: Proposed Definition and Criteria," in *Critical Issues in Psychiatric Diagnosis*.

114   *"present concepts that have influenced the decision"*: DSM-III, 6.

115   Mental disorder, *he argued*: Spitzer and Endicott, "Medical and Mental Disorder," 30.

115   *"These guys have some chutzpah"*: Kirk and Kutchins, *The Selling of DSM*, 113.

115   *"In DSM-III each of the mental disorders"*: DSM-III, 5–6.

116   *"The syndrome or pattern"*: DSM-III-R, xxii.

116   *DSM-IV devoted seven of its 886 pages*: DSM-IV, 843–49.

Chapter 8

118   *"psychiatric classification is necessarily"*: Frances, "DSM in Philosophyland: Curiouser and Curiouser."

118   *"recurrent and persistent thoughts"*: DSM-IV-TR, 462–63.

119   *"A diagnosis is a call to action"*: Frances, "DSM in Philosophyland."

120   *"I just wanted them to learn"*: Allen Frances e-mail, January 6, 2012.

120   *"One of the reasons"*: Robins and Guze, "Establishment of Diagnostic Validity in Psychiatric Illness," 983.

121   *They concluded that* T. pallidum: For a comprehensive history of the discovery of syphilis and its significance to modern medicine, see Quétel, *History of Syphilis*. See also Greenberg, *Manufacturing Depression*, 52–60.

121   *a five-step process toward validity*: Robins and Guze, "Establishment of Diagnostic Validity," 983–84.

122   *"validity tests . . . have not lived up"*: "Time for a Change?" *Psychiatric News*, August 21, 2009.

122   *Kenneth Kendler added another validator*: Kendler, "The Nosologic Validity of Paranoia."

122   *"the [diagnostic] categories"*: Kendler, "An Historical Framework for Psychiatric Nosology," 1939.

122   *"to consider our major diagnostic categories"*: Ibid.

123   *"critics of psychiatric diagnoses"*: Ibid.

124   *"A historic and scientific process"*: Ibid.

124   *"It sounded about right"*: Kendler et al., "The Development of the Feighner Criteria," 136.

page
124 *"wonderful property of iteration"*: Kendler, "An Historical Framework," 1940.

124 *"assure ourselves"*: Ibid.

124 "wobbly *iterations*": Ibid. Emphasis in original.

124 *"asymptotes to a stable and accurate"*: Ibid., 1939.

125 *paleontologist Stephen Jay Gould*: See Gould, *Wonderful Life*.

125 *"We follow the tape forward"*: Kendler, "An Historical Framework," 1938.

127 *"The 'disastrous result'"*: "APA Disputes Critics of DSM-V," *Psychiatric News*, August 21, 2009.

127 *"attempt to address"* ... *"The single most important precondition"*: Regier et al., "Conceptual Development of DSM-V," 649.

128 *"establish better syndrome boundaries"*: Darrel Regier e-mail, October 5, 2010.

128 *Some diagnoses, such as depression*: DSM-IV-TR, 413.

128 *Global Assessment of Functioning*: DSM-IV-TR, 32–34.

128 *National Institutes of Health had created PROMIS*: See www.nihpromis.org.

129 *"bottoms-up approach"*: Regier et al., "Conceptual Development," 648.

129 *"If they really want to do dimensional assessment"*: Michael First interview, September 28, 2010.

129 *"We don't expect the DSM-5"*: Darrel Regier e-mail, October 11, 2010.

129 *Diagnostic criteria "are intended"*: Regier et al., "Conceptual Development," 648–49.

Chapter 9

130 *"Advice to DSM V"*: Allen Frances, "Advice to DSM V . . . Change Deadlines and Text, Keep Criteria Stable," *Psychiatric Times* (blog), August 26, 2009, www.psychiatrictimes.com/display/article/10168/1444663.

130 *in the field trials the new criteria identified 15 percent more*: Lahey et al., "DSM-IV Field Trials for ADHD," 1682.

131 *the actual increase was 28 percent*: Akinbami et al., "Attention Deficit Hyperactivity Disorder Among Children," 2.

131 *"everything was on the table"*: Allen Frances, "Alert to the Research Community," *Psychiatric Times*, January 7, 2010.

131 *"over the cliff"*: Frances, "Advice to DSM-V."

132 *"I take more blame for DSM-IV"*: Allen Frances interview, August 16, 2010.

133 *"some of us have gotten"*: Shirley Wang, "Psychiatrists Bash Back at Critics of Diagnostic Manual Revision," *Wall Street Journal Health Blog*, January 8, 2009, blogs.wsj.com/health/2009//01/08/psychiatrists-bash-back-at-critics-of-diagnostic-manual-revision.

133 *"The development process has been so public"*: Alan Schatzberg, "Some Thoughts on DSM-V," *Psychiatric News*, August 21, 2009.

133 *"I'm too small a fish"*: Jane Costello e-mail, August 1, 2010.

133 *"I cannot in good conscience"*: Jane Costello resignation letter, available at http://www.scribd.com/doc/17162466/Jane-Costello-Resignation-Letter-from-DSMV-Task-Force-to-Danny-Pine-March-27-2009.

134 *the response came from Darrel Regier*: Regier supplied me with the letter via e-mail, November 11, 2010.

136 *"Since we considered"*: Darrel Regier e-mail, November 11, 2010.

page
136   *"When there is smoke"*: Carolyn Robinowitz interview, October 4, 2010.

137   *the APA issued a press release*: American Psychiatric Association, "DSM-5 Publication Date Moved to May 2013," news release, December 10, 2009, http:// www.dsm5.org/Newsroom/Documents/09-65%20DSM%20Timeline.pdf.

138   *"long vetting process"*: Beth Casteel e-mail, November 11, 2010.

138   *"I'm going to be quite critical"*: Allen Frances, "DSM-V in Severe Distress: Is a Happy Ending Possible?" January 15, 2010, http://columbiapsychiatry.org/videos/ dsm-v-severe-distress-happy-ending-still-possible.

140   *The APA posted a full draft*: Although it has since been taken down, the draft is available at http://web.archive.org/web/20100402094501/http://www.dsm5.org/ ProposedRevisions/Pages/Default.aspx.

141   *"Anything you put in that book"*: Benedict Carey, "Revising Book on Disorders of the Mind," *The New York Times*, February 10, 2010.

142   *"The 19 Worst Suggestions for DSM5"*: Allen Frances, "Opening Pandora's Box: The 19 Worst Suggestions for DSM5," *Psychiatric Times*, February 11, 2010, www .psychiatrictimes.com/print/article/10168/1522341?printable=true.

Chapter 10

143   *another letter to the trustees*: Frances, "To the Membership of the APA," *Psychiatric Times*, June 2, 2010, http://www.psychiatrictimes.com/dsm-5/content/article/10168/ 1565491.

143   *"I was of age in the '60s"*: Allen Frances e-mail, January 23, 2012.

144   *"I never yell"*: Ibid.

144   *"nice irony"*: Ibid.

145   *"This was the stupidest idea in the world"*: Allen Frances telephone interview, November 23, 2011.

145   *"After the third or fourth"*: Herb Peyser interview, January 23, 2012.

145   *Freud once said*: See Freud, *The Joke and Its Relation to the Unconscious*.

146   *"orderly and democratic process"*: David Shaffer interview, December 8, 2011.

146   *"David probably misinterpreted"*: Allen Frances e-mail, January 23, 2012.

149   *"that children with the broad phenotype"*: Leibenluft et al., "Defining Clinical Phenotypes of Juvenile Mania," 436.

149   *"claim to define a new diagnosis"*: Leibenluft, "Severe Mood Dysregulation," 131.

149   *"Justification for Temper Dysregulation Disorder with Dysphoria"*: "Justification for Temper Dysregulation Disorder," http://www.dsm5.org/Proposed%20Revision%20 Attachments/Justification%20for%20Temper%20Dysregulation%20Disorder% 20with%20Dysphoria.pdf.

151   *it announced a new "naming convention"*: American Psychiatric Association, "APA Modifies DSM Naming Convention to Reflect Publication Changes," news release, March 9, 2010.

153   *"distinctly unmedical"*: Schatzberg, "Presidential Address," 1163.

153   *"Some of the attacks"*: Ibid.

153   *New Orleans had "risen as the Phoenix"*: Ibid., 1162.

154   *"the negative attacks on industry"*: Ibid., 1164.

154   *"There are a number of new drugs"*: Ibid.

Chapter 11

page

155   *"Turning bereavement into major depression"*: Allen Frances, "Good Grief,"
      The New York Times, August 14, 2010.

156   *"Sure, there's a reality out there"*: Allen Frances interview, August 16, 2010.

156   *"The full truth"*: Allen Frances e-mail, February 2, 2012.

157   *"Like most medical specialties"*: Allen Frances interview, July 7, 2011.

158   *"stigmatization [and] inappropriate care"*: Wakefield et al., "Extending the
      Bereavement Exclusion," 433.

159   *"ignore the many other kinds"*: Ibid., 434.

160   *"define every undesirable consequence"*: Horwitz and Wakefield, *The Loss of Sadness*,
      220–21.

160   *"Psychiatry has made immense strides"*: Ibid., 225.

160   *"There are few signs"*: Ibid., 212.

161   *"It just doesn't make any sense to me whatsoever"*: Sidney Zisook interview,
      September 10, 2010.

161   *Zisook did some data mining of his own*: Zisook and Kendler, "Is Bereavement-Related
      Depression Different Than Non-Bereavement-Related Depression?"

162   *"provides some support"*: Ibid., 791.

162   *"Because work toward the DSM-V"*: Zisook et al., "Validity of the Bereavement Exclu-
      sion," 102.

162   *"validity of the bereavement exclusion"*: Ibid., 104.

162   *"Why should bereavement be singled out"*: Ibid., 105.

163   *"Idiotic"*: Jerome Wakefield e-mail, January 31, 2012.

163   *a study showing that GSK's Wellbutrin*: Zisook et al., "Buproprion Sustained Relief for
      Bereavement."

165   *"The DSM-IV position is not logically defensible"*: Kendler, "Grief Exclusion," http://
      www.dsm5.org/about/Documents/grief%20exclusion_Kendler.pdf.

165   *"that sadness in response to loss"*: Wakefield et al., "Extending the Bereavement Exclu-
      sion," 439.

Chapter 12

168   *"the best we can do"*: See Allen Frances, "The Most Important Psychiatrist of Our
      Time," *Psychiatric Times*, December 22, 2010.

170   *"Moving forward"*: Regier, "Diagnostic Threshold Considerations for
      DSM-5," 293.

170   *"the clinical judgment of a psychiatrist"*: Ibid., 285.

170   *the National Comorbidity Survey*: Kessler et al., "Lifetime and 12-Month Prevalence
      of DSM-III-R Psychiatric Disorders in the United States."

171   *"We had much greater confidence"*: Ibid., 286.

172   *Regier's team began to dig them out*: Narrow et al., "Revised Prevalence Estimates of
      Mental Disorders in the United States."

172   *"To put it mildly"*: Regier, "Diagnostic Threshold Considerations," 288.

172   *Wakefield and Spitzer pointed out*: Wakefield and Spitzer, "Lowered Estimates—but of
      What?"

page

172 *"What is striking about this debate"*: Regier, "Diagnostic Threshold Considerations," 289.

172 *"to define the problem out of existence"*: Kessler et al., "Mild Disorders Should Not Be Eliminated from the DSM-V," 1.121.

173 *"In response to this scientific critique"*: Regier, "Diagnostic Threshold Considerations," 289.

173 *"I wasn't aware that he had interpreted"*: Ronald Kessler e-mail, February 9, 2012.

173 *"Certainly some of the loudest concerns"*: Regier, "Diagnostic Threshold Considerations," 290.

174 *Just look at the history of "progress"*: Ibid.

174 *"It may be of interest"*: Ibid., 292–93.

175 *"Since the broad definition"*: Ibid., 293.

175 *"DSM-IV has a label for everyone you might want to treat"*: Roger Peele interview, November 4, 2011.

178 *his $600,000-per-year salary:* That is as of 2010, according to the APA's tax return, available at http://www.guidestar.org/FinDocuments/2010/130/433/2010-130433740-077883c7-9.pdf.

178 *"The spirit of moderation"*: Montesquieu, *The Spirit of Laws*, 49.

179 *"They [the dimensional measures] will continue to evolve"*: Darrel Regier e-mail, September 29, 2010.

Chapter 13

182 *more than eight thousand comments:* Joan Arehart-Treichel, "DSM-5 Work Groups Assess Thousands of Comments," *Psychiatric News*, August 20, 2010.

182 *"developed a strong sense of uniqueness and belonging"*: Bernstein, "DSM-5: Year Ahead and Year in Review," *Psychiatric News*, August 20, 2010.

184 *"I fought to get myself comfortable in high school"*: Nomi Kaim interview, June 16, 2011.

187 *"It was a total add-on"*: Fred Volkmar interview, March 1, 2012.

187 *The disorder was first described by an Austrian pediatrician:* See Wing, "Asperger's Syndrome: A Clinical Account," and Lyons and Fitzgerald, "Asperger and Kanner, the Two Pioneers."

187 *"an especially intimate relationship"*: Wing, "Asperger's Syndrome," 117–18.

188 *"pervasive lack of responsiveness"*: DSM-III, 89.

189 *"the syndromes are more alike than unalike"*: Wing, "Asperger's Syndrome," 121.

189 *"the term is helpful"*: Ibid., 124.

190 *Of the nearly one thousand subjects:* Volkmar et al., "Field Trial for Autistic Disorder in DSM-IV."

191 *"The Little Professor Syndrome"*: Lawrence Osborne, "The Little Professor Syndrome," *The New York Times Magazine*, June 18, 2000.

192 *"Some things made sense"*: Michael Carley and CC interview, October 13, 2011.

192 *"I . . . have yet to stand successfully"*: Carley, *Asperger's from the Inside Out*, 4.

194 *"At GRASP we envision a world"*: http://grasp.org/page/mission-statement.

197 *She ballparked it:* Wing, "Asperger's Syndrome," 119–20.

197 *Eric Fombonne, an epidemiologist working in England, reviewed:* Fombonne, "The Epidemiology of Autism: A Review."

197 *"secular increase"*: Ibid., 777.

page

198 *a rate of 34 per 10,000*: Yeargin-Alsopp, "Prevalence of Autism in a U.S. Metropolitan Area," 53.

198 *these results were "an underestimate"*: Ibid., 81.

198 *As of 2002, the CDC reported*: All CDC figures can be found in Autism and Developmental Disabilities Monitoring Network, "Prevalence of Autism Spectrum Disorders," available at http://www.cdc.gov/ncbddd/autism/documents/ADDM-2012-Community-Report.pdf.

198 *"opening Pandora's Box"*: Wing, "Reflections on Opening Pandora's Box."

198 *a prevalence rate in a city in Korea*: Kim et al., "Prevalence of Autism Spectrum Disorders," 907.

198 *blitzed the media*: "New Study Reveals Autism Prevalence in South Korea," Autism Speaks, news release, May 9, 2011.

198 *"the need for improved and wider autism screening"*: "Top Ten Autism Research Achievements of 2011," Autism Speaks, news release, December 20, 2011, http://www.autismspeaks.org/about-us/press-releases/top-10-autism-research-achievements-2011.

199 *"a stigmatizing hereditary disorder"*: Kim et al., "Prevalence of Autism," 910.

200 *"Lower rates in 9- and 10-year-olds"*: Yeargin-Alsopp, "Prevalence of Autism in a U.S. Metropolitan Area," 53.

200 *"Diagnosis of ASDs"*: Charman, "The Highs and Lows of Counting Autism," 874.

201 *"canaries [who] sensed before anyone else"*: Lethem, *The Ecstasy of Influence*, 73.

202 *"premature to add Asperger's"*: Michael First e-mail, March 20, 2012.

202 *"We probably were premature"*: Allen Frances e-mail, February 20, 2012.

202 *"It involves a use of treatment resources"*: Amy Harmon, "A Specialists' Debate on Autism Has Many Worried Observers," *The New York Times*, January 20. 2012.

203 *"The goal was not to change prevalence"*: Catherine Lord interview, March 29, 2012.

203 *most important factor in determining which diagnosis*: Lord et al., "A Multisite Study of the Clinical Diagnosis of Different Autism Spectrum Disorders," 309–11.

Chapter 14

206 *"People say, 'What's in a name?'"*: Dilip Jeste, "State of Classification of Neurocognitive Disorders," American Psychiatric Association annual meeting, May 17, 2011.

207 *"Attire is 'aloha business/casual'"*: http://web.archive.org/web/20110523195007/http://www.psych.org/annualmeeting.

208 *"invent[ing] out of thin air"*: Thomas Widiger, "The DSM-5 Personality Disorder Dimensional Model," American Psychiatric Association annual meeting, May 15, 2011.

209 *"I do sense a reactionary element"*: David Shaffer, "State of the Science on Diagnostic Classification: Implications for DSM-5," American Psychiatric Association annual meeting, May 17, 2011.

210 *"Allen and I have a big disagreement"*: Michael First interview, March 2, 2012.

212 *First stuck to small ball*: Michael First, "The Future of Psychiatric Nosology," Association for the Advancement of Philosophy and Psychiatry annual meeting, May 15, 2011.

213 *Kupfer and Regier demonstrate*: David J. Kupfer and Darrel A. Regier, "Diagnostic Assessment in DSM-5: Approaches and Examples," American Psychiatric Association annual meeting, May 16, 2011.

214 *"That's why we are doing a field test"*: Darrel Regier interview, September 14, 2010.

page
214   *"two rigorous study designs"*: American Psychiatric Association, "APA Announces Start of Field Trials for DSM-5," press release, October 5, 2010.
215   *"I'm surprised"*: Darrel Regier e-mail, October 6, 2010.
225   *"People's expectations of what reliability should be"*: Kraemer, "DSM-5 Field Trials," American Psychiatric Association annual meeting, May 17, 2011.
226   Spitzer *"could have employed"*: Kirk and Kutchins, *The Selling of DSM*, 61–62.
229   *"We'd better get smart about measuring"*: Lawson Wulsin, "DSM-5 Research and Development," American Psychiatric Association annual meeting, May 16, 2011.

Chapter 15

230   *"You have to understand"*: Allen Frances interview, July 9, 2011.
231   *"If it seems like this is coming"*: Allen Frances interview, August 16, 2010.
232   *"My narcissism couldn't survive the teenage insight"*: Allen Frances e-mail, April 22, 2010.
233   *"over a period of at least 6 months"* . . . *"The fantasies, sexual urges"*: DSM-IV, 528.
233   *"the symptom criteria alone"*: First and Frances, "Issues for DSM-V," 1240.
233   *"While we have been preoccupied"*: Linda Bowles, "Kinder Gentler Pedophilia," WorldNetDaily, http://www.wnd.com/1999/05/228/.
234   *"acknowledge the 'APA's clear opposition'"*: Linda Bowles, "Pedophilia: Good News Bad News," WorldNetDaily, http://www.wnd.com/1999/06/231/.
234   if someone *"has acted on these urges"*: DSM-IV-TR, 572.
235   *"Fewer than half of child molesters"*: Michael First e-mail, April 22, 2012.
237   *"too polemical"*: Kutchins and Kirk, *Making Us Crazy*, 164–65.
237   *"a tendency to feel inordinately threatened"*: Pantony and Caplan, "Delusional Dominating Personality Disorder," 127–30.
237   *"I really wasn't sure"*: Kutchins and Kirk, *Making Us Crazy*, 171.
238   *"It is disruptive to constantly tinker"*: Ibid., 172.
238   *Caplan did give Frances a shout-out*: Paula Caplan, "DSM-5 Heads' Comments Reveal Lack of Compassion and of Respect for Science," *When Johnny and Jane Come Marching Home* (blog), http://whenjohnnyandjanecomemarching.weebly.com/1/post/2011/05/dsm-5-heads-new-comments-reveal-lack-of-compassion-and-of-respect-for-science.html.
238   *On the appointed day*: This account is from Caplan, "Letter from DSM-5 Task Force Head Leaves Major Concerns Unanswered," *Science Isn't Golden* (blog), http://www.psychologytoday.com/blog/science-isnt-golden/201106/letter-dsm-5-task-force-head-leaves-major-concerns-unanswered-part-1. The public relations firm that arranged the conference call declined to comment.
239   *"the continued and continuous medicalisation"*: British Psychological Society, "Response to the American Psychiatric Association: DSM-5 Development," http://apps.bps.org.uk/_publicationfiles/consultation-responses/DSM-5%202011%20-%20BPS%20response.pdf.
240   *Regier made clear in his official response*: See "Society's Critical Response to DSM-5," *The Psychologist News*, July 13, 2011, http://www.thepsychologist.org.uk/blog/blog-post.cfm?threadid=2102&catid=48.
241   *"previous failures"*: Melville, *The Confidence-Man*, 77.
242   *"stranger entering"*: Ibid.

page

243   *"general resistance or indifference"*: Blanchard et al., "Pedophilia, Hebephilia, and the DSM-V," 336.

243   *"discriminable erotic age-preference"*: Ibid., 335.

243   *"Your neighbors' 7-year-old girl"*: Blanchard et al., "IQ, Handedness, and Pedophilia in Adult Male Patients," 292.

244   *"to minimize his embarrassment"*: Blanchard et al., "Pedophilia, Hebephilia, and the DSM-V," 339.

245   *"hebephilia exists"*: Ibid., 347–48.

Chapter 16

248   *"We are . . . test piloting"*: APA Research e-mail, July 8, 2011.

249   *"The most common reason"*: Now found at http://www.findthatpdf.com/search-80840213-hPDF/download-documents-ft-20note-20for-20web-20site.pdf.htm.

249   *"We have learned"*: Eve Mościcki e-mail, September 9, 2011.

249   *"Thanks for your candid note"*: Ibid.

250   *another note from Kupfer and Regier*: APA Research e-mail, September 20, 2011.

250   *DSM-5 proposal for Generalized Anxiety Disorder*: This once appeared at www.dsm5.org/ProposedRevisions1.2011/Pages/proposedrevision5478.html?rid=167.

251   *the old one*: DSM-IV-TR, 476.

261   *"A Personality Disorder is an enduring pattern"*: DSM-IV-TR, 685.

261   *"ensures that consideration will be given"*: DSM-IV-TR, 28.

262   *"I think this is the best way"*: Allen Frances e-mail, May 1, 2012.

263   *"I have never really been a doctor"*: Gay, *Freud*, 681.

263   *"They have the lowest reliability"*: Allen Frances e-mail, May 12, 2012. See Frances, "The DSM-III Personality Disorders Section: A Commentary."

263   *The kappas were .56 to .65*: Spitzer et al., "DSM-III Field Trials: I. Initial Interrater Diagnostic Reliability."

263   *"the personality disorders are not at all clearly distinct"*: Frances, "The DSM-III Personality Disorders Section," 1050.

263   *"Rather than being diagnosed"*: Ibid., 1051.

264   *"committed dimensionalist"*: Allen Frances e-mail, May 17, 2012.

264   *"I believe I was chosen"*: Thomas Widiger e-mail, May 21, 2012.

265   *"under active investigation"*: DSM-IV, 633–34.

265   *a paper, published just before DSM-IV*: Frances, "Dimensional Diagnosis of Personality Disorders—Not Whether but When and Which."

265   *"It might be more consistent"*: First et al., "Personality Disorders and Relational Disorders," 130.

267   *"uniform classification of general personality functioning"*: Ibid., 131.

267   *"That is why I pushed"*: Michael First e-mail, May 15, 2012.

267   *Regier, he said, had asked him*: Thomas Widiger e-mail, May 21, 2012.

267   *According to Widiger's distillation*: See Widiger and Simonsen, "Alternative Dimensional Models of Personality Disorder."

267   *"basic science research"*: Ibid., 123.

268   *"The devil, of course"*: Ibid., 126.

268   *"Nobody on the work group"*: Thomas Widiger e-mail, May 21, 2012.

page
268   *"a sense of self-identity"*: For the original proposal, see http://web.archive.org/web/
      20100323205756/http://www.dsm5.org/ProposedRevisions/Pages/Personality
      andPersonalityDisorders.aspx.
269   *insufficient "empirical evidence"*: Skodol, "Personality Disorder Types Proposed for
      DSM-5," 138.
270   *"We knew we couldn't incorporate"*: Andrew Skodol interview, May 24, 2012.
270   *"embarrassingly bad"*: Thomas Widiger e-mail, September 23, 2010.
270   *"lost opportunity" that "negates years of progress"*: Livesley, "Confusion and
      Incoherence in the Classification of Personality Disorder," 307.
270   *"cumbersome hodgepodge"*: Frances, "The DSM-5 Personality Disorders," *DSM-5 in
      Distress* (blog), http://www.psychologytoday.com/blog/dsm5-in-distress/201004/
      the-dsm5-personality-disorders-great-intentions-unusable-result.
270   *"an unwieldy conglomeration"*: Shedler et al., "Personality Disorders in DSM-5,"
      1027.

Chapter 17

274   *"There has been a continual struggle"*: Helena Hansen, e-mail, September 27, 2011.
275   *"This is amazing!"*: Helena Hansen e-mail, September 28, 2011.
275   *"Approaching endgame"*: Allen Frances e-mail, November 14, 2011.
275   *"A random and geographically diverse"*: Allen Frances e-mail, October 31, 2011.
275   *"pretty Spockean"*: Allen Frances e-mail, September 21, 2010.
275   *an open letter to the APA:* Available at http://www.ipetitions.com/petition/dsm5/.
276   *a letter on behalf of his 115,000:* Available at http://www.counseling.org/Resources/
      pdfs/ACA_DSM-5_letter_11-11.pdf.
276   *"bring Darrel to see DSM-5"*: Allen Frances e-mail, August 28, 2010.
277   *"trying to negotiate"*: Allen Frances e-mail, November 15, 2011.
277   *"Cast of fascinating and colorful characters"*: Ibid.
277   *"This will likely be the most important"*: Allen Frances e-mail, October 25, 2011.
277   *"Don't waste your best brains"*: Ibid.
277   *"I was in Dubuque"*: Allen Frances e-mail, November 4, 2011.
278   *"your brilliant opening"*: Allen Frances e-mail, October 16, 2011.
278   *"Paula Caplan in drag"*: Allen Frances e-mail, January 5, 2012.
278   *"one-time pillar of the psychiatric establishment"*: Rob Waters, "Therapists Revolt
      Against Psychiatry's Bible," http://www.salon.com/2011/12/27/therapists_revolt_
      against_psychiatrys_bible/.
278   *"Fate has an ironic sense of humor"*: Allen Frances e-mail, July 14, 2011.
278   *"Everything I say"*: Allen Frances e-mail, October 16, 2011.
279   *"Where you see intelligent conspiracy"*: Allen Frances e-mail, September 18, 2011.
279   *"Dereification is just as dumb"*: Allen Frances e-mail, January 15, 2012.
279   *"I like to think the best of you"*: Allen Frances e-mail, January 5, 2012.
281   *"What's the ending mean?"*: Allen Frances telephone interview, November 23, 2011.
282   *I received this message:* Eve Herold e-mail, November 7, 2011.
283   *"We realize how challenging it is"*: Lisa Countis e-mail, November 7, 2011.
290   *"This behavior pattern"*: DSM-I, 35.
292   *"The journey into the future"*: The newsletter is available at http://api.ning.com/files/
      AbciMXSvxet4NaqPJajU41T2kvOhgvc3JLSZdblrTDlfSyH4b2tKRiorse
      SDWZFCrifi7jgzHZyn7S5TvwzCpddFjQN—kLt/DSM5.fieldtrials.pdf.

page

293 *the treasurer delivered grim news:* http://www.ncpsychiatry.org/APA/APA%20
Assembly%20ReportNov2011.pdf.

293 *running a blog called Dsm5watch:* It can now be found at dxrevisionwatch.com.

294 *"It has come to our attention":* Cecilia Stoute e-mail to Suzy Chapman, December 22,
2011.

294 *"I thought it was a hoax":* Suzy Chapman e-mail, June 11, 2012.

294 *"I could not finance a legal wrangle":* Suzy Chapman e-mail, February 27, 2012.

Chapter 18

296 *"The idea of medicalizing normality":* Elizabeth Lopatto, "Psychiatric Group Push
to Redefine Mental Illness Sparks Revolt," *Bloomberg Businessweek,* January 27,
2012.

297 *"I wasn't exactly hiding it":* Fred Volkmar e-mail, June 26, 2012.

297 *"It was one thing to make a change":* Michael Carley e-mail, June 28, 2012.

298 *"damage control":* http://grasp.org/profiles/blogs/very-important-dsm-5-update.

298 *"We have to make sure":* Amy Harmon, "A Specialists' Debate on Autism Has Many
Worried Observers," *The New York Times,* January 20, 2012.

298 *"There has never been an agenda":* Debra Brauser, "Concern over Changes to Autism
Criteria Unfounded," *Medscape Medical News,* January 25, 2012.

299 *"10,000 plus e-mails":* This exchange, not reported in the press, is available at http://
grasp.org/profiles/blogs/dsm-5-update-a-poor-poor-descent-into-pettiness.

299 *a Carey-penned DSM piece:* Benedict Carey, "Grief Could Join List of Disorders,"
The New York Times, January 24, 2012.

300 *a World Psychiatry article by Michael First and Jerry Wakefield:* Wakefield and First,
"Validity of the Bereavement Exclusion to Major Depression: Does the Empirical
Evidence Support the Proposal to Eliminate the Exclusion in DSM-5?"

301 *"set out realistic expectations":* Kraemer et al., "DSM-5: How Reliable Is Reliable
Enough?," 13.

302 *a pair of op-ed columns:* Paul Steinberg, "Asperger's History of Overdiagnosis,"
and Benjamin Nugent, "I Had Asperger Syndrome, Briefly," *The New York Times,*
January 31, 2012.

303 *"The proposals in DSM-5":* See "Psychologists Fear US Manual Will Widen Mental
Illness Diagnosis," *The Guardian,* February 9, 2012.

303 The Lancet . . . *in a single issue, a report:* See http://www.thelancet.com/journals/
lancet/issue/vol379no9816/PIIS0140-6736%2812%29X6007-0.

303 *"I still feel sadness":* Kleinman, "Culture, Bereavement, and Psychiatry," 608.

303 *"even if," as the Illinois version put it:* Public Act 097-0972 available at http://www.ilga
.gov/legislation/publicacts/fulltext.asp?Name=097-0972.

304 *"the door is still very much open":* John Gever, "DSM-5 Critics Pump Up the Volume,"
MedPage Today, February 29, 2012.

304 *"You've got to feel sorry":* Gary Greenberg, "Not Diseases, but Categories of Suffering,"
The New York Times, January 29, 2012.

307 *"Wonderful news":* "Wonderful News: DSM 5 Finally Begins Its Belated and Necessary Retreat," *Psychology Today* (blog), May 2, 2012. http://www.psychologytoday.
com/blog/dsm5-in-distress/201205/wonderful-news-dsm-5-finally-begins-its-
belated-and-necessary-retreat.

308 *"stain on psychiatry"* . . . *"Cassandra":* Allen Frances e-mail, April 29, 2012.

page

308   *"We encourage the wide dissemination"*: Roger Peele provided the memo via e-mail, April 29, 2012.

309   *"What possible copyright excuse"*: Allen Frances e-mail, April 23, 2012.

309   *"It is just too nutty"* . . . *"I used to compare"*: Allen Frances e-mail, April 30, 2012.

Chapter 19

318   *a DSM-5-related 60 percent increase*: Mewton et al., "An Evaluation of the Proposed DSM-5 Alcohol Use Disorder Criteria Using Australian National Data," 947.

321   *"I wanted to avoid a repeat of Axis 5"*: Roger Peele interview, August 2, 2012.

323   *"Conceptual questions are not minor 'side issues'"*: Kendler et al., "Issues for DSM-V," 175.

324   *"Yes," he said, "but I do like a challenge"*: Michael First e-mail, May 12, 2012.

324   *"I felt if I just addressed"*: Swedo, "Making National Headlines," American Psychiatric Association annual meeting, May 6, 2012.

328   *"Newsflash from APA Meeting"*: See http://www.huffingtonpost.com/allen-frances/ dsm-5-reliability-tests_b_1490857.html.

329   *"The controversy stirred by my critique"*: Allen Frances e-mail, June 29, 2012.

Chapter 20

336   *"Melancholia," they wrote*: Parker et al., "Issues for DSM-5: Whither Melancholia?," 745.

336   *"distinct, identifiable, and specifically treatable"*: Ibid., 747.

337   *"I believe the inclusion of a biological measure"*: William Coryell e-mail to Max Fink, October 16, 2008.

337   *"I [am] flabbergasted"*: Max Fink e-mail to William Coryell, April 9, 2010.

338   *"I believe you and your colleagues"*: William Coryell e-mail to Max Fink, April 12, 2010.

338   *"The APA owns all products"*: http://www.dsm5.org/Pages/PermissionsPolicy.aspx.

339   *"arrogance, secretiveness"* . . . *"is no longer capable"*: Allen Frances, "Diagnosing the DSM," *The New York Times*, May 11, 2012.

339   *"Our resources are more likely"*: Thomas Insel e-mail, October 13, 2010.

340   *What Insel heard "over and over again"*: Thomas Insel and Bruce Cuthbert interview, December 12, 2011.

340   *"So many of our disorders"*: Ibid.

343   *"We call this attention deficit/hyperactivity disorder"*: Thomas Insel, "Rethinking Mental Illness," American Psychiatric Association annual meeting, May 14, 2011.

346   *"Why do you hate psychiatrists"*: Allen Frances e-mail, October 20, 2012.

347   *"DSM-IV-TR attempts to describe"*: Sadock and Sadock, *Kaplan & Sadock's Concise Textbook of Clinical Psychiatry*, 33.

348   *"difficulty of distinguishing a manic episode"*: Ibid., 218.

348   *"depressive symptoms are present"*: Ibid.

348   *"every sign or symptom seen in schizophrenia"*: Ibid., 167.

348   *"Once a diagnosis has been established"*: Ibid., 222.

348   *"no one drug is predictably effective"*: Ibid., 224.

348   *"Often," advise Sadock and Sadock, "it is necessary"*: Ibid.

page

348 *"the objective of pharmacologic treatment"*: Ibid.

349 *"Not everyone needs to see"*: Allen Frances e-mail, October 20, 2012.

351 *"Whatever we've been doing for five decades"*: Thomas Insel and Bruce Cuthbert interview, December 12, 2011.

353 *Seventy-two percent*: Mojtabai and Olfson, "Proportion of Antidepressants Prescribed Without a Psychiatric Diagnosis Is Growing," 1436.

353 *"abnormal sensations" and "nonspecific pain"*: Ibid., 1437.

356 *"The future belongs to illness"*: Sedgwick, "Illness—Mental and Otherwise," 37.

Afterword

359 *an occasion to release some details:* "American Psychiatric Association Board of Trustees Approves DSM-5," news release, December 1, 2012.

360 *"We do ask that you focus"*: This e-mail was provided to me by Roger Peele.

360 *one article—in* The Washington Post: Peter Whoriskey, "Antidepressants to Treat Grief? Psychiatry Panelists with Ties to Drug Industry Say Yes," *The Washington Post*, December 26, 2012.

360 *"DSM-5 includes material"*: Statement of David Kupfer, http://www.psychnews .org/files/Response_to_Wash_Post.pdf.

361 *Dilip Jeste, the APA president, told Congress:* Letter from Dilip Jeste to Harry Reid, John Boehner, Mitchell McConnell, and Nancy Pelosi, http://www.psychiatry .org/advocacy—newsroom/advocacy/apa-sends-letter-to-congress-regarding-recent-shooting-in-newtownct.

361 *Not only was LaPierre's language "offensive"*: "American Psychiatric Association Responds to NRA Comments," news release, December 23, 2012, http://www .psychiatry.org/File%20Library/Advocacy%20and%20Newsroom/Press%20Releases/ 2012%20Releases/12-45-APA-Response-to-NRA-Comments.pdf.

361 *"The saddest day"*: Allen Frances, "DSM 5 Is Guide Not Bible—Ignore Its Ten Worst Changes," *DSM-5 in Distress* (blog), http://www.psychologytoday.com/blog/ dsm5-in-distress/201212/dsm-5-is-guide-not-bible-ignore-its-ten-worst-changes.

361 *"one last act"*: Allen Frances, "One Last Chance for the APA to Make the DSM-5 Safer," *The Huffington Post* (blog), http://www.huffingtonpost.com/allen-frances/ one-last-chance-for-the-apa-to-make-the-dsm-5-safer_b_2294868.html.

362 *"Any new boycott must unify the diverse opposition"*: Allen Frances, "DSM 5 Boycotts and Petitions: Too Many, Too Sectarian," *Saving Normal: Mental Health and What Is Normal* (blog), February 8, 2013, http://www.psychologytoday.com/blog/saving-normal/201302/dsm-5-boycotts-and-petitions.

362 *"I can confirm"*: Michael First e-mail, November 27, 2012.

362 *"The good news"*: Michael First e-mail January 7, 2013.

Bibliography

Akinbami, Lara J., Xiang Liu, Patricia M. Pastor, and Cynthia A. Reuben. "Attention Deficit Hyperactivity Disorder Among Children Aged 5–17 Years in the United States 1998–2009." *NCHS Data Brief*, no. 70 (August 2011).

American Psychiatric Association. *Diagnostic and Statistical Manual, Mental Disorders (DSM-I)*. Washington, DC: American Psychiatric Association, 1952.

American Psychiatric Association. *Diagnostic and Statistical Manual of Mental Disorders: DSM-III*. Washington, DC.: American Psychiatric Association, 1980.

American Psychiatric Association. *Diagnostic and Statistical Manual of Mental Disorders: DSM-III-R*. Washington, DC: American Psychiatric Association, 1987.

American Psychiatric Association. *Diagnostic and Statistical Manual of Mental Disorders: DSM-IV-TR*. Washington, DC: American Psychiatric Association, 2000.

American Psychiatric Association. *Statistical Manual for the Use of Hospitals for Mental Diseases*. Albany, NY: State Hospitals Press, 1942.

Anglada, Tracy, Toby Ferguson, and Jennifer Taylor. *Brandon and the Bipolar Bear: A Story for Children with Bipolar Disorder*. Victoria, Canada: Trafford, 2004.

Ash, P. "The Reliability of Psychiatric Diagnosis." *Journal of Abnormal and Social Psychology* 44 (1949): 272–77.

Bayer, Ronald. *Homosexuality and American Psychiatry: The Politics of Diagnosis*. New York: Basic Books, 1981.

Beard, George Miller. *American Nervousness: Its Causes and Consequences; A Supplement to Nervous Exhaustion (Neurasthenia)*. New York: G. P. Putnam's Sons, 1881.

Beck, Aaron T. "Reliability of Psychiatric Diagnoses: 1. A Critique of Systematic Studies." *American Journal of Psychiatry* 119 (1962): 210–16.

Biederman, Joseph. "Pediatric Bipolar Disorder Coming of Age." *Biological Psychiatry* 53, no. 11 (2003): 931–34.

Biederman, Joseph. "Resolved: Mania Is Mistaken for ADHD in Prepubertal Children (Affirmed)." *Journal of the American Academy of Child and Adolescent Psychiatry* 37, no. 10 (October 1998): 1091–93.

Blanchard, Ray. "The Concept of Autogynephilia and the Typology of Male Gender Dysphoria." *The Journal of Nervous and Mental Disease* 177, no. 10 (1989): 616–23.

Blanchard, Ray, Amy D. Lykins, Diane Wherrett, et al. "Pedophilia, Hebephilia, and the DSM-V." *Archives of Sexual Behavior* 38, no. 3 (2009): 335–50.

Blanchard, Ray, Nathan J. Kolla, James M. Cantor, et al. "IQ, Handedness, and Pedophilia in Adult Male Patients Stratified by Referral Source." *Sexual Abuse: A Journal of Research and Treatment* 19, no. 3 (2007): 285–309.

Carley, Michael John. *Asperger's from the Inside Out: A Supportive and Practical Guide for Anyone with Asperger's Syndrome*. New York: Perigee, 2008.

Carpenter, W. T. "Anticipating DSM-V: Should Psychosis Risk Become a Diagnostic Class?" *Schizophrenia Bulletin* 35, no. 5 (2009): 841–43.

Cartwright, Samuel. "Diseases and Peculiarities of the Negro Race," Part 1. In *DeBow's Review*, Vol. 11, Series 4 (New Orleans, 1851): 331–36.

Cartwright, Samuel. "Diseases and Peculiarities of the Negro Race," Part 2. In *DeBow's Review*, Vol. 11, Series 4 (New Orleans, 1851): 504–8.

Charman, Tony. "The Highs and Lows of Counting Autism." *American Journal of Psychiatry* 168, no. 9 (2011): 873–75.

Clayton, Paula J., J. A. Halikes, and W. L. Maurice. "The Bereavement of the Widowed." *Diseases of the Nervous System* 32, no. 9 (1971): 597–604.

Cornblatt, Barbara A., and Christoph U. Correll. "A New Diagnostic Entity in DSM-5?" *Medscape*, September 3, 2010.

Cosgrove, Lisa, Sheldon Krimsky, Manisha Vijayaraghavan, and Lisa Schneider. "Financial Ties Between DSM-IV Panel Members and the Pharmaceutical Industry." *Psychotherapy and Psychosomatics* 75, no. 3 (2006): 154–60.

Feighner, John. P., Eli Robins, Samuel B. Guze, George Winokur, Robert A. Woodruff, Jr., and Rodrigo Muñoz. "Diagnostic Criteria for Use in Psychiatric Research." *Archives of General Psychiatry* 26 (1972): 57–63.

First, Michael B., Carl C. Bell, Bruce Cuthbert, et al. "Personality Disorders and Relational Disorders: A Research Agenda for Addressing Crucial Gaps in DSM." In *A Research Agenda for DSM-V*, ed. David J. Kupfer, Michael B. First, and Darrel A. Regier, 123–200. Washington, DC: American Psychiatric Association, 2002.

Fombonne, Eric. "The Epidemiology of Autism: A Review." *Psychological Medicine* 29 (1999): 769–86.

Foucault, Michel. *Madness and Civilization: A History of Insanity in the Age of Reason*. New York: Pantheon Books, 1965.

Frances, Allen. "Dimensional Diagnosis of Personality—Not Whether but When and Which." *Psychological Inquiry* 4, no. 2 (1993): 110–11.

Frances, Allen. "DSM in Philosophyland: Curiouser and Curiouser." *AAPP Bulletin* 17, no. 2 (2010), 3–7.

Frances, Allen. "The DSM-III Personality Disorders Section: A Commentary." *American Journal of Psychiatry* 137, no. 9 (1980): 1050–54.

Frankfurt, Harry G. *On Bullshit*. Princeton, NJ: Princeton University Press, 2005.

Freud, Sigmund. *The Joke and Its Relation to the Unconscious*. New York: Penguin Books, 2003.

Freud, Sigmund. *The Question of Lay Analysis: Conversations with an Impartial Person*. New York: W. W. Norton, 1989.

Gay, Peter. *Freud: A Life for Our Time*. New York: W. W. Norton, 1988.

Glenmullen, Joseph. *Prozac Backlash: Overcoming the Dangers of Prozac, Zoloft, Paxil, and Other Antidepressants with Safe, Effective Alternatives*. New York: Simon & Schuster, 2000.

Goffman, Erving. *Asylums: Essays on the Social Situation of Mental Patients and Other Inmates*. Garden City, NY: Anchor Books, 1961.

Gould, Stephen Jay. *Wonderful Life: The Burgess Shale and the Nature of History*. New York: W. W. Norton, 1989.

Greenberg, Gary. *Manufacturing Depression: The Secret History of a Modern Disease*. New York: Simon & Schuster, 2010.

Grob, Gerald N. "Origins of DSM-I: A Study in Appearance and Reality." *American Journal of Psychiatry* 148, no. 4 (April 1991): 421–31.

Hales, Robert E., Stuart C. Yudofsky, and Robert H. Chew. *What Your Patients Need to Know About Psychiatric Medications.* Washington, DC: American Psychiatric Publishing, 2005.

Healy, David. *The Creation of Psychopharmacology.* Cambridge, MA: Harvard University Press, 2002.

Horwitz, Allan V., and Jerome C. Wakefield. *The Loss of Sadness: How Psychiatry Transformed Normal Sorrow into Depressive Disorder.* Oxford, England: Oxford University Press, 2007.

Hunt, S. B. "Dr. Cartwright on 'Drapetomania.'" *Buffalo Medical Journal and Monthly Review of Medical and Surgical Science* 10 (1855): 438–43.

Hyman, Steven E. "The Diagnosis of Mental Disorders: The Problem of Reification." *Annual Review of Clinical Psychology* 6, no. 1 (2010): 155–79.

James, Henry. Preface. In *The Tragic Muse*, 3–12. Digireads.com, 2011.

Jarvis, Edward. *Relation of Education to Insanity.* Report. Washington, DC: Government Printing Office, 1872.

Johnson, Steven. *The Ghost Map: The Story of London's Most Terrifying Epidemic—and How It Changed Science, Cities, and the Modern World.* New York: Riverhead Books, 2006.

Kandel, Eric R. "The New Science of Mind." In *Best of the Brain from Scientific American*, ed. Floyd E. Bloom, 68–75. New York: Dana Press, 2007.

Kendell, R. E., J. E. Cooper, A. J. Gourlay, J. R. M. Copeland, L. Sharpe, and B. J. Gurland. "Diagnostic Criteria of American and British Psychiatrists." *Archives of General Psychiatry* 25, no. 2 (1971): 123–30.

Kendler, Kenneth S. "An Historical Framework for Psychiatric Nosology." *Psychological Medicine* 39, no. 12 (December 2009): 1935–41.

Kendler, Kenneth S: "The Nosologic Validity of Paranoia (Simple Delusional Disorder): A Review." *Archives of General Psychiatry* 37 (1980): 699–706.

Kendler, Kenneth S., Paul S. Appelbaum, Carl C. Bell, et al. "Issues for DSM-V: DSM-V Should Include a Conceptual Issues Work Group." *American Journal of Psychiatry* 165, no. 2 (2008): 174–75.

Kendler, Kenneth S., Rodrigo A. Munoz, and George Murphy. "The Development of the Feighner Criteria: A Historical Perspective." *American Journal of Psychiatry* 167, no. 2 (2010): 134–42.

Kessler, Ronald C. "Mild Disorders Should Not Be Eliminated from the DSM-V." *Archives of General Psychiatry* 60, no. 11 (2003): 1117–22.

Kessler, Ronald C., Katherine A. McGonagle, Shanyang Zhao, et al. "Lifetime and 12-Month Prevalence of DSM-III-R Psychiatric Disorders in the United States: Results from the National Comorbidity Survey." *Archives of General Psychiatry,* 51, no. 1 (1994), 8–19.

Kim, Y. S., B. L. Leventhal, Y. J. Koh, et al. "Prevalence of Autism Spectrum Disorders in a Total Population Sample." *American Journal of Psychiatry* 168, no. 9 (2011): 904–12.

Kirk, Stuart A., and Herb Kutchins. *The Selling of DSM: The Rhetoric of Science in Psychiatry.* New York: A. De Gruyter, 1992.

Kirsch, Irving. *The Emperor's New Drugs: Exploding the Antidepressant Myth.* New York: Basic Books, 2010.

Klein, Rachel G., Daniel S. Pine, and Donald F. Klein. "Resolved: Mania Is Mistaken for ADHD in Prepubertal Children (Negative)." *Journal of the American Academy of Child & Adolescent Psychiatry* 37, no. 10 (October 1998): 1093–95.

Kleinman, Arthur. "Culture, Bereavement, and Psychiatry." *The Lancet* 379, no. 9816 (February 18, 2012): 608–9.

Kowatch, Robert A., Mary Fristad, Boris Birmaher, Karen Dineen Wagner, Robert L. Findling, and Martha Hellander. "Treatment Guidelines for Children and Adolescents with Bipolar Disorder." *Journal of the American Academy of Child & Adolescent Psychiatry* 44, no. 3 (2005): 213–35.

Kraemer, Helena C., David J. Kupfer, Diana E. Clarke, William E. Narrow, and Darrel A. Regier. "DSM-5: How Reliable Is Reliable Enough?" *American Journal of Psychiatry* 169, no. 1 (2012): 13–15.

Kraepelin, Emil. *Lectures on Clinical Psychiatry.* New York: Hafner, 1968.

Kraepelin, Emil. "The Manifestations of Insanity." *History of Psychiatry* 3, no. 12 (1992): 504–8.

Kupfer, David J., Michael B. First, and Darrel A. Regier. Introduction. In *A Research Agenda for DSM-V*, xv–xxiii. Washington, DC: American Psychiatric Association, 2002.

Kutchins, Herb, and Stuart A. Kirk. *Making Us Crazy: DSM: The Psychiatric Bible and the Creation of Mental Disorders.* New York: Free Press, 1997.

Lahey, B. B., B. Applegate, K. McBurnett, et al. "DSM-IV Field Trials for Attention Deficit Hyperactivity Disorder." *American Journal of Psychiatry* 151, no. 11 (1994): 1673–85.

Leibenluft, Ellen. "Severe Mood Dysregulation, Irritability, and the Diagnostic Boundaries of Bipolar Disorder in Youths." *American Journal of Psychiatry* 168, no. 2 (February 2011): 129–42.

Leibenluft, Ellen, Donald S. Charney, Kenneth E. Towbin, Robinder K. Banghoo, and Daniel S. Pine. "Defining Clinical Phenotypes of Juvenile Mania." *American Journal of Psychiatry* 160, no. 3 (2003): 430–37.

Lethem, Jonathan. *The Ecstasy of Influence: Nonfictions, Etc.* New York: Doubleday, 2011.

LeVay, Simon. *Queer Science: The Use and Abuse of Research into Homosexuality.* Cambridge, MA: MIT Press, 1996.

Livesley, W. John. "Confusion and Incoherence in the Classification of Personality Disorder." *Psychological Injury and Law* 3, no. 4 (2010): 304–13.

Lord, Catherine, Eva Petkova, Vanessa Hus, Weijin Gan, Feihan Lu, and Donna Martin. "A Multisite Study of the Clinical Diagnosis of Different Autism Spectrum Disorders." *Archives of General Psychiatry* 69, no. 6 (2012): 303–13.

Lyons, Viktoria, and Michael Fitzgerald. "Asperger (1906–1980) and Kanner (1894–1981), the Two Pioneers of Autism." *Journal of Autism and Developmental Disorders* 37, no. 10 (2007): 2022–23. doi:10.1007/s10803-007-0383-3.

McClellan, Jon. "Commentary: Treatment Guidelines for Child and Adolescent Bipolar Disorder." *Journal of the American Academy of Child & Adolescent Psychiatry* 44, no. 3 (March 2005): 236–39.

Melville, Herman. *The Confidence-Man: His Masquerade.* New York: New American Library, 1964.

Menninger, Karl A. *The Vital Balance: The Life Process in Mental Health and Illness.* New York: Viking Press, 1963.

Mewton, Louise, Tim Slade, Orla McBride, Rachel Grove, and Maree Teesson. "An Evaluation of the Proposed DSM-5 Alcohol Use Disorder Criteria Using Australian National Data." *Addiction* 106, no. 5 (2011): 941–50.

Meyer, Adolf. "The Aims and Meaning of Psychiatric Diagnosis." *American Journal of Psychiatry* 74 (1917): 163–68.

Mill, James. *Analysis of the Phenomena of the Human Mind*, vol. 2, ed. John Stuart Mill. London: Longmans Green Reader and Dyer, 1869.

Mojtabai, Ramin, and Mark Olfson. "Proportion of Antidepressants Prescribed Without a Psychiatric Diagnosis Is Growing." *Health Affairs* 30, no. 8 (August 2011): 1434–42.

Montesquieu, Baron de (Charles de Secondat). *The Spirit of Laws.* Great Books in Philosophy. Amherst, NY: Prometheus Books, 2002.

Moreno, C., G. Laje, C. Blanco, H. Jiang, A. B. Schmidt, and M. Olfson. "National Trends in the Outpatient Diagnosis and Treatment of Bipolar Disorder in Youth." *Archives of General Psychiatry* 64, no. 9 (2007): 1032–39.

Narrow, William E., Donald S. Rae, Lee N. Robins, and Darrel A. Regier. "Revised Prevalence Estimates of Mental Disorders in the United States." *Archives of General Psychiatry* 59, no. 2 (2002): 115–23.

Olmsted, Frederick Law. *Journeys and Explorations in the Cotton Kingdom*, vol. 1. London: Sampson Low and Son, 1861.

Pantony, Kaye-Lee, and Paula J. Caplan. "Delusional Dominating Personality Disorder: A Modest Proposal for Identifying Some Consequences of Rigid Masculine Socialization." *Canadian Psychology* 32, no. 2 (1991): 120–35.

Papolos, Demitri F., and Janice Papolos. *The Bipolar Child: The Definitive and Reassuring Guide to Childhood's Most Misunderstood Disorder.* 3rd ed. New York: Broadway Books, 2006.

Parker, Gordon, Max Fink, Edward Shorter, et al. "Issues for DSM-5: Whither Melancholia? The Case for Its Classification as a Distinct Mood Disorder." *American Journal of Psychiatry* 167, no. 7 (2010): 745–47.

Plato. *Phaedrus.* Trans. Benjamin Jowett. Teddington, England: Echo Library, 2006.

Quétel, Claude. *History of Syphilis.* Baltimore: Johns Hopkins University Press, 1990.

Regier, Darrel A. "Diagnostic Threshold Considerations for DSM-5." In *Philosophical Issues in Psychiatry II: Nosology*, ed. Kenneth S. Kendler and Josef Parnas, 285–97. New York: Oxford University Press, 2012.

Regier, Darrel A., Irving D. Goldberg, and Carl M. Taube. "The De Facto U.S. Mental Health Services System." *Archives of General Psychiatry* 35 (June 1978): 685–93.

Regier, Darrel A., William E. Narrow, Emily A. Kuhl, and David J. Kupfer. "The Conceptual Development of DSM-V." *American Journal of Psychiatry* 166 (2009): 645–50.

Robins, Eli, and Samuel B. Guze. "Establishment of Diagnostic Validity in Psychiatric Illness." *American Journal of Psychiatry* 126, no. 7 (1970): 983–87.

Robins, Lee N., and Darrel A. Regier. *Psychiatric Disorders in America: The Epidemiologic Catchment Area Study.* New York: Free Press, 1991. "Appendix B," 399–426.

Sadock, Benjamin J., and Virginia A. Sadock. *Kaplan & Sadock's Concise Textbook of Clinical Psychiatry.* 10th ed. Philadelphia: Wolters Kluwer/Lippincott Williams & Wilkins, 2008.

Salmon, Thomas W., Owen Copp, James V. May, E. Stanley Abbot, and Henry A. Cotton. "Report of the Committee on Statistics of the American Medico-Psychological Association." *American Journal of Insanity* 74 (October 1917): 255–61.

Sandifer, Myron G., Anthony Hordern, Gerald C. Timbury, and Linda M. Green. "Psychiatric Diagnosis: A Comparative Study in North Carolina, London and Glasgow." *The British Journal of Psychiatry* 114, no. 506 (1968): 1–9.

Schatzberg, Alan F. "Presidential Address." *American Journal of Psychiatry* 167 (2010): 1161–65.

Schildkraut, Joseph. "The Catecholamine Hypothesis of Affective Disorders." *American Journal of Psychiatry* 122 (1965): 509–22.

Sedgwick, Peter. "Illness—Mental and Otherwise." *Hastings Center Studies* 1, no. 3 (1973): 19–40.

Shedler, Jonathan, Aaron Beck, Peter Fonagy, et al. "Personality Disorders in DSM-5." *American Journal of Psychiatry* 167, no. 9 (2010): 1026–28.

Shorter, Edward. *A History of Psychiatry: From the Era of the Asylum to the Age of Prozac.* New York: John Wiley & Sons, 1997.

Shorter, Edward, and David Healy. *Shock Therapy: A History of Electroconvulsive Treatment in Mental Illness.* New Brunswick, NJ: Rutgers University Press, 2007.

Siever, Larry J., and Howard Klar. "A Review of DSM-III Criteria for the Personality Disorders." In *Psychiatry Update: American Psychiatric Association Annual Review,* ed. Allen Frances and Robert E. Hales, 279–314. Washington, DC: American Psychiatric Press, 1986.

Skodol, Andrew E., Donna S. Bender, Leslie C. Morey, et al. "Personality Disorder Types Proposed for DSM-5." *Journal of Personality Disorders* 25, no. 2 (2011): 136–69.

Spiegel, Alix. "The Dictionary of Disorder." *The New Yorker,* January 3, 2005.

"Spitzer Reassesses His 2003 Study of Reparative Therapy." Letter from Robert Spitzer. In *Archives of Sexual Behavior.* 4th ed. Vol. 41 (2012).

Spitzer, Robert L. "Can Some Gay Men and Lesbians Change Their Sexual Orientation? 200 Participants Reporting a Change from Homosexual to Heterosexual Orientation." *Archives of Sexual Behavior* 32, no. 5 (October 2003): 403–17.

Spitzer, Robert L., and Jean Endicott. *Critical Issues in Psychiatric Diagnosis.* Ed. Robert L. Spitzer and Donald F. Klein, 15–39. New York: Raven Press, 1978.

Spitzer, Robert L., Jean Endicott, and Eli Robins. "Research Diagnostic Criteria: Rationale and Reliability." *Archives of General Psychiatry* 35, no. 6 (June 1978): 773–82.

Spitzer, Robert L., Janet B. W. Forman, and John Nee. "DSM-III Field Trials: I. Initial Interrater Diagnostic Reliability." *American Journal of Psychiatry* 136, no. 6 (1979): 815–17.

Srole, Leo, Thomas S. Langner, Stanley T. Michael, Marvin K. Opler, and Thomas A. C. Rennie. *Mental Health in the Metropolis: The Midtown Manhattan Study.* New York: McGraw-Hill, 1962.

Stevens, Wallace, and Holly Stevens. *The Palm at the End of the Mind: Selected Poems and a Play.* New York: Alfred A. Knopf, 1971.

Stotland, Nada L. "Presidential Address." *American Journal of Psychiatry* 166 (2009): 1100–04.

Üçok, Alp, and Wolfgang Gaebel. "Side Effects of Atypical Antipsychotics: A Brief Overview." *World Psychiatry* 7, no. 1 (February 2008): 58–62.

Ullmann, A. "Pasteur–Koch: Distinctive Ways of Thinking About Infectious Diseases." *Microbe* 2, no. 8 (2007): 383–87.

Volkmar, Fred R., Ami Klin, Bryna Siegel, et al. "Field Trial for Autistic Disorder in DSM-IV." *American Journal of Psychiatry* 151, no. 9 (1994): 1361–67.

Wakefield, Jerome, and Michael First. "Validity of the Bereavement Exclusion to Major Depression: Does the Empirical Evidence Support the Proposal to Eliminate the Exclusion in DSM-5?" *World Psychiatry* 11 (2012): 3–10.

Wakefield, Jerome C., Mark F. Schmitz, Michael B. First, and Allan V. Horwitz. "Extending the Bereavement Exclusion for Major Depression to Other Losses: Evidence from the National Comorbidity Survey." *Archives of General Psychiatry* 64, no. 4 (2007): 433–40.

Wakefield, Jerome C., and Robert L. Spitzer. "Lowered Estimates—but of What?" *Archives of General Psychiatry* 59, no. 2 (2002): 129–30.

Whitaker, Robert. *Anatomy of an Epidemic: Magic Bullets, Psychiatric Drugs, and the Astonishing Rise of Mental Illness in America.* New York: Crown, 2010.

Widiger, Thomas A., and Erik Simonsen. "Alternative Dimensional Models of Personality Disorder: Finding a Common Ground." *Journal of Personality Disorders* 19, no. 2 (2005): 110–30.

Wilson, Mitchell. "DSM-III and the Transformation of American Psychiatry." *American Journal of Psychiatry* 150, no. 3 (1993): 399–410.

Wing, Lorna. "Asperger's Syndrome: A Clinical Account." *Psychological Medicine* 11, no. 1 (1981): 115–29.

Wing, Lorna. "Reflections on Opening Pandora's Box." *Journal of Autism and Developmental Disorders* 35, no. 2 (April 2005): 197–203.

Woods, Scott W., Jean Addington, and Kristin S. Cadenhead. "Validity of the Prodromal Risk Syndrome for First Psychosis: Findings from the North American Prodrome Longitudinal Study." *Schizophrenia Bulletin* 35, no. 5 (2009): 894–908.

Wozniak, Janet, Joseph Biederman, Kathleen Kiely, J. Stuart Ablon, Stephen V. Faraone, Elizabeth Mundy, and Douglas Mennin. "Mania-Like Symptoms Suggestive of Childhood-Onset Bipolar Disorder in Clinically Referred Children." *Journal of the American Academy of Child & Adolescent Psychiatry* 34, no. 7 (July 1995): 867–76.

Yeargin-Alsopp, Marshalyn, Catherine Rice, Tanya Karapurkar, Nancy Doernberg, Colleen Boyle, and Catherine Murphy. "Prevalence of Autism in a U.S. Metropolitan Area." *JAMA: The Journal of the American Medical Association* 289, no. 1 (2003): 49–55.

Zaretsky, Eli. *Secrets of the Soul: A Social and Cultural History of Psychoanalysis.* New York: Alfred A. Knopf, 2004.

Zisook, Sidney, and Kenneth S. Kendler. "Is Bereavement-Related Depression Different Than Non-Bereavement-Related Depression?" *Psychological Medicine* 37, no. 6 (June 2007): 779–94.

Zisook, Sidney, Steven R. Schuchter, Paola Pedrelli, Jeremy Sable, and Simona C. Deaciuc. "Bupropion Sustained Release for Bereavement: Results of an Open Trial." *The Journal of Clinical Psychiatry* 62, no. 4 (2001), 227–30.

Zisook, Sidney, Katherine Shear, and Kenneth S. Kendler. "Validity of the Bereavement Exclusion Criterion for the Diagnosis of Major Depressive Episode." *World Psychiatry* 6, no. 2 (2007): 102–7.

Zucker, Kenneth J., and Susan J. Bradley. *Gender Identity Disorder and Psychosexual Problems in Children and Adolescents.* New York: Guilford Press, 1995.

Index